Herbal Secrets
of the Rainforest

LESLIE TAYLOR

Herbal Secrets
of the Rainforest

The Healing Power of
Over 50 Medicinal Plants
You Should Know About

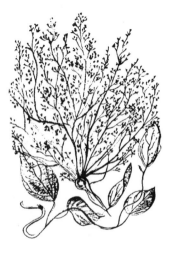

PRIMA HEALTH
A Division of Prima Publishing

Warning—Disclaimer

This book is not intended to provide medical advice and is sold with the understanding that the publisher and the author are not liable for the misconception or misuse of information provided. The author and Prima Publishing shall have neither liability nor responsibility to any person or entity with respect to any loss, damage, or injury caused or alleged to be caused directly or indirectly by the information contained in this bok or the use of any products mentioned. Readers should not use any of the products discussed in this book without the advice of a medical professional.

Library of Congress Cataloging-in-Publication Data

Taylor, Leslie.
 Herbal secrets of the rainforest: the healing power of over 50 medicinal plants you should know about / Leslie Taylor.
  p.   cm.
 Includes index.
 ISBN 0-7615-1734-0
 1. Rain forest plants—Amazon River Valley—Therapeutic use. 2. Herbs—Amazon River Valley—Therapeutic use. I. Title.
RM666.H33T39 1998
615'.321—dc21   98-28208
                                                                CIP

    03 04 05 MP 10 9 8 7 6 5 4 3
Printed in the United States of America

This book is dedicated to the Indigenous Peoples of the Amazon Rainforest.

~~~~~~

WE, THE INDIGENOUS PEOPLES, have been an integral part of the Amazon Biosphere for millennia. We used and cared for the resources of that biosphere with respect, because it is our home, and because we know that our survival and that of our future generations depend on it. Our accumulated knowledge about the ecology of our home, our models for living within the Amazonian Biosphere, our reverence and respect for the tropical forest and its other inhabitants, both plant and animal, are the keys to guaranteeing the future of the Amazon Basin, not only for our peoples, but also for all humanity.

Our experience, especially during the past 100 years, has taught us that when politicians and developers take charge of our home, they are capable of destroying it because of their short-sightedness, their ignorance, and their greed.

We are concerned that the Amazon peoples, and in particular the Indigenous Peoples, have been left out of the environmentalists' vision of the Amazonian Biosphere. The focus of concern of the environmental community has typically been the preservation of the tropical forests and its plant and animal inhabitants. Little concern has been shown for its human inhabitants who are also part of that biosphere.

We are concerned that the Indigenous Peoples and their representative organizations have been left out of the political process which is determining the future of our homeland. The environmentalist community has at times lobbied on our behalf; it has spoken out and written in the name of the Amazonian Indians. While we appreciate these efforts, it should be made clear that we never delegated this power to the environmentalist community nor to any individual or organization within that community.

The most effective defense of the Amazonian Biosphere is the recognition and defense of the territories of the region's Indigenous Peoples and the promotion of their models for living within that Biosphere and for managing its resources in a sustainable way.

Coordinating Body for the Indigenous Organizations of the Amazon Basin (COICA), adapted from COICA's "To the Community of Concerned Environmentalists" (1989)

Contents

Introduction

~~~~~~

A TALL, FAIR-SKINNED BLONDE woman traveling down the Amazon River and into the remote areas of the Amazon rainforest is an oddity of sorts. However, for most of my life I've been told that I'm odd. Admittedly, trekking through jungles, studying the plant knowledge of indigenous Indian shamans and South American herbal healers, getting harassed in airport customs with a suitcase full of strange-looking murky liquids, bark, leaves, and roots, and running a large corporation in the process, is not your everyday career. The question that I am always asked, whether I'm in the jungle or in the States, is, "How did you ever get into a profession like this?" Looking back, a series of journeys seems to have redirected the course of my life and shaped it into what it is today. I have to go back about fifteen years to my most memorable journey, which started me onto this odd path where I find myself today.

I first became interested in herbal medicine and alternative health when, in my mid-twenties, I was diagnosed with acute myceoblastic leukemia. Conventional medicine gave up on me after two years of traditional chemotherapy and cancer treatments and sent me home to die. But being the odd, determined, stubborn, rebellious individual that most people described me as, I didn't give up.

Fifteen years ago it was even harder than it is now to access accurate information on herbs and alternative therapies. But you might say that I had a "dying need to know," and I began studying alternative health with a vengeance. With a combination of herbal medicine, diet, nutrition, and other natural healing modalities, I was diagnosed as cancer-free eighteen months later. Not only was my cancer gone, but the extensive damage that was done to my body and internal organs from the conventional cancer treatments was healed or on the mend. Another real oddity, I was told. My oncologist, who scoffed at anything herbal or unconventional, believes that I was simply too stubborn to die. I know there is some truth in that statement, but I also believe that herbal medicine went a long way in healing my body.

What I didn't understand then (or now, really) is why they call "that" conventional medicine and refer to herbal medicine as "alternative." My personal journey showed me that herbal medicine was much more conventional. It dates back literally centuries in time, with the less-than-100-year-old pharmaceutical industry offering the "alternatives" to the plant medicines we've used since before human beings even learned how to chronicle their uses. At least for me, herbal medicine was much more effective than the "alternatives" conventional medicine offered me in my battle with cancer.

After winning this battle, I continued on in my business career in Texas—starting companies in several different industries and selling them when I became bored with their day-to-day management. In business I was considered "successful," and that success resulted in a ballistic, workaholic lifestyle. I continued studying herbal medicine and alternative health as a hobby, choosing to use herbs and natural health rather than drugs for my and my family's health. They thought I was pretty odd too but accepted the strange herbal potions and nutritional remedies I gave them when they were sick.

Then, in 1989, I took a much-needed vacation that changed the course of my life yet again. Maybe it was just the first time I had taken a breath or a break in many years, but a journey to the wilds of Africa somehow reconnected me to the land, nature, and wildlife. It showed me that I needed to make a change in the hectic, harried life I had created, which was involved in the ego of success and the power of money and which wasn't really personally fulfilling. So, when I returned from Africa, I sold my companies, bought a ranch in the hill country of Texas, and "retired."

There—in a conventional, sort of backwards, rural Texas community north of Austin—I quickly became "the odd woman at Clear Creek Ranch" to the local farmers and ranchers. I grew weird plants, herbs, and vegetables, raised a motley menagerie of teenage boys and exotic animals (which hardly ever acted like they were supposed to), had too much land that was "unproductive," and was obviously in dire need of a husband to make her do things right. Leastwise, that's what the locals would tell you. That didn't keep them from dropping by to tell me about their aches and pains to see what kind of odd concoction of plants I might pick out of the gardens and give them, and which somehow mysteriously worked. Often, they'd just drop by to see what odd thing I was up to that day.

Wanting to give something back (and a bit bored with farm life), I started a small consulting company there on the ranch. The company (me) researched and disseminated information on cancer and AIDS therapies that were being used in other places in the world and taught cancer patients how they could access them. Burying eight miles of phone cables to the ranch—to get a non-party fax and modem line to connect to the Internet to research university and government databases worldwide—was another odd thing to do, I guess, at least to the locals. But they just shook their heads, as they normally did when talking about "that odd woman," and drove around the construction crews on the county road. My personal mission was to compile all the research on alternative therapies and to make the information available to those faced with the same struggle that I had once confronted. It had been a great source of frustration and a committed struggle for me to try to access this type of information when I had cancer, especially at a time when I had little enough energy to just get through a day.

It was during this research that I came across an herbal extract that was being used in Europe for cancer and AIDS patients, with some interesting results. When I determined that it was a simple extract of a natural plant that could be sold here as an herbal supplement (for a lot less money than the European company was charging), I decided to go to the source where the plant grew. My mission then was to try to import the plant into the United States. The plant was called cat's claw *(Uncaria tomentosa)*, and the source was the Amazon rainforest in Peru. This new journey into the Amazon rainforest changed the course of my life yet again.

It is extraordinarily hard to try to describe a rainforest to someone who has never experienced it. The first thing that hits you when you step into the rainforest is the air. It's so heavy with oxygen and humidity that it is almost a tangible thing that envelops you. There is a heavy, rich stillness to it . . . because in the heart of a primary rainforest, very little wind makes it down below the unbroken green canopy of trees. The clean, oxygen-filled air and the sheer magnitude of living things all around you overwhelm and energize you all at once. The vibrancy of life you feel flowing around you and through you almost resonates. It's as if all of Earth's core elements surround you in an abundance that you've never experienced before.

The next thing that hits you is the sheer immensity of the trees and the incredible number of different types of vegetation that surround you. It's an amazing display of Nature in her most flamboyant expression of life. Literally everything around you is in a state of flux—living, breathing, growing, decaying, or dying. You can actually see some of the plants growing with the naked eye. Huge fallen trees that would take years to return to the earth in a temperate forest are reduced to compost in a month or two.

Trees the size of skyscrapers, leaves the size of umbrellas, and enormous vines of incredible shapes and sizes seemingly knitting everything together are everywhere you look. It's hard to take it all in at once. The "everything is bigger in Texas" brag I grew up with certainly seemed to pale in comparison to the Amazon rainforest. Maybe that is why so many people (and even Texans) describe their first trip into a rainforest as a "humbling experience." For me, there was a feeling of coming home.

On that first journey into the rainforest, I fell in love. I fell in love with the jungle, the people, the culture, the lifestyle and attitude, the plants and trees, the incredible rivers . . . all of which make up the Amazon rainforest. I also saw, on that first trip, the incredible amount of destruction that was happening in the Amazon. I saw that it was possible that the whole thing could go up in smoke and be wiped off the face of the Earth, conceivably in my lifetime. Waiting for my flight home in the Lima airport in Peru, I sat there sunburned, bug-bit, tired, and excited and decided that not only did I want to start a new company in the States to begin importing this wonderful plant called cat's claw; I also had to try to make a difference to help stop the destruction of the Amazon rainforest. I didn't quite know how then, but I knew that an odd, determined, stubborn, rebellious sort of person such as myself had as good a chance as anyone else did.

That was the beginning of a group of companies that I founded in my thoughts sitting in the Lima airport, and officially two days later in Austin, Texas. I came out of "retirement" and began importing cat's claw into the United States shortly thereafter. Through my ongoing work with the company and the many subsequent trips to the Amazon, I learned more and more about the other medicinal plants that were used as natural medicines by the indigenous peoples in the rainforest and began importing those as well. Oddly enough, of all the businesses I have founded and managed in my career, this is the only one that I've never had to determinedly push, market, make work, or direct. Since they were created, I have literally been running behind them trying to keep up. They seem to have a life of their own; and I have never worked so hard, had so much fun and adventure, and been as personally fulfilled as I am today. However odd it is, I feel I am truly blessed to be on the path I find myself on today. And believe it or not, I haven't been bored—not once—in the last four years!

In my work with the Raintree Group of companies, I have been setting up botanical harvesting programs with rural Amazon communities and tribes that are today sustainably harvesting over eighty medicinal plants. I am fortunate enough to work with indigenous shamans and healers to document and learn their amazing empirical plant knowledge and natural plant remedies. Another part of my job is to scientifically research and document these important medicinal plants so that I can teach consumers and practitioners how to positively affect their health with them. Sadly, wherever I go in the Amazon, I find that I am teaching this same plant knowledge to the people living there. Despite the fact that these plants grow in their yards and gardens and in the forests surrounding them, the people living in the Amazon (who have little or no access to any type of health care or prescription drugs) today know very little about natural medicine and how to use their plants effectively.

Being the businessperson I am, I approached the rainforest and rainforest conservation in a business-like manner and began to look for business solutions to rainforest destruction. This was odd to the activists and conservationists I came across, but again, I was used to being called odd. I believed then and now that, wherever you are in the world, basic business strategies still apply. Greed is greed and profits are profits, even in the remote jungles. If you want someone to do something, make it profitable for them to do and it's not so hard to convince them. So I set about showing people in the rainforest how they could make more money sustainably harvesting medicinal plants like cat's claw than they could make at timber harvesting, grazing livestock, agriculture, or subsistence cropping, practices that destroy the forest. It sounds almost too simple, but it's effective and it works.

The only component left to make this business strategy work is to create the market demand for these sustainable forest resources so that it *can* result in profits for those participating. That's not as hard as it sounds either. The alternative health and natural/herbal products industry in the United States is growing at an unprecedented rate. Recent statistics show that consumers have spent more out-of-pocket funds on alternative health and alternative health products and supplements than they have for conventional medicine over the past few years. And the rainforest *does* provide a wealth of beneficial natural products and highly effective medicinal plants for that industry.

This book represents four years of my personal research and documentation on these important medicinal plants in the Amazon rainforest during my journeys into the South American jungles and in my journey with Raintree. I firmly believe that medicinal plants, such as those found in this book, are the true wealth of the rainforest and the means by which it can be saved from destruction. They have for centuries positively affected the health and well-being of the inhabitants of the forest. Through their sustainable harvesting, they can and will positively affect the health, well-being, and continuance of the rainforest itself.

It is my sincere hope that you, the reader of this book, will learn an appreciation of the rainforest and why it is so important to be saved; learn more about the wealth of beneficial medicinal plants it provides us; and learn how you can take part in positively affecting your health and the health of the rainforest with these wonderful plants.

Yours in health,
Leslie Taylor

How to Use This Book

~~~~~~

THIS BOOK IS divided into three main sections. Part 1, Rainforest Destruction and Survival, discusses the rainforest, the Amazon rainforest in particular, and the issues involved in its destruction and preservation. Part 2, Medicinal Plants of the Rainforest, provides detailed documentation on fifty-four different medicinal plants of the rainforest. Part 3, Rainforest Resources, includes recipes for herbal remedies, tables that summarize the documented medicinal properties and ethnic uses of rainforest plants, a listing of nonprofit rainforest organizations, and a listing of sustainable rainforest products.

A helpful element of this book is the Quick Guide to Herbal Terms, Uses, and Disorders. In this section you will find definitions of medical and herbal terms, and it also serves as a quick reference for matching a condition to the plants that are used to treat it.

READING THE PLANT INFORMATION IN PART 2

PART 2, MEDICINAL Plants of the Rainforest, describes fifty-four rainforest plants, trees, and herbs. You will find the following information on each plant: family, genus, and species; common names; parts used; medicinal properties; main text on the plant; worldwide uses of the plant; and phytochemical information.

Medicinal Properties

Scientists, herbalists, and practitioners refer to the biological or pharmacological properties or actions of medicinal plants using specifically defined words like *anti-inflammatory, diuretic, spasmolytic,* and so on. These terms describe the documented actions or properties of the plant. Some, such as *anti-inflammatory* and *antibacterial,* are pretty self-explanatory. Others, like *febrifuge* or *vulnerary,* may be less familiar. If you are unfamiliar with the meaning of any of these specific property and action terms, you can find their definitions in the Quick Guide to Herbal Terms, Uses, and Disorders. The listing of medicinal properties of each plant summarizes the documented actions and properties that have been attributed to the plant *either* through clinical laboratory research or practitioner uses and observations (and it's for all parts of the plant as well). These properties and actions are then discussed in more detail in the text section on the plant.

Main Text on the Plants

The main text provides well-referenced information about each plant. This information includes

+ what the plant looks like

+ where and how it grows

+ the history of its uses by rainforest inhabitants and Indian tribes

+ current uses in different countries and in herbal medicine

+ methods of preparation

+ how various parts of the plants are used

+ a summary of the results of scientific research conducted on the plant

An overview of scientific research and clinical data about each plant is provided in the text. Complete citations of the studies that are footnoted in the text are found in the Notes section in the back of the book. You also will see the distinction as to whether the research was performed *in vivo* or *in vitro*. *In vivo* studies refer to research that has been performed on animals or humans to determine a drug's effects on mammals. *In vitro* studies refer to research that is conducted "in the test tube." A good example is studies performed on parasites. An *in vitro* study would place the parasite in a test tube or a petrie dish and place the plant or some form of liquid extract of the plant in with the parasite to determine whether or not it kills the parasite. An *in vivo* study would inoculate an animal with a parasite, and then administer the plant or extract to the animal to determine the effectiveness of the dosage administered in treating the parasitic infection in the animal. Clearly, *in vivo* studies are much more effective in verifying a plant's uses and how it might affect a tested mechanism or affect you. Yet this is just a point of reference as well. How a plant might affect a rat or mouse does not always relate to how it will affect humans. Readers should also understand that scientific research is in no manner standardized, and different results will be demonstrated based on the methods employed by the researcher. As stated earlier, wherever possible the summary of research provided herein will differentiate whether the study was performed *in vitro* or *in vivo* and will give information on the types of methods or types of extracts that were used.

Worldwide Uses Table

Ethnic uses of plants can be very important. If a plant has been used in a specific way for a specific purpose for many years and in many different geographical areas, there certainly is a reason for it: It's effective. It is this ethnobotany that helps scientists target which plants to research first and what to study them for. In fact, the majority of our plant-based drugs or pharmaceuticals were discovered through this ethnobotanical research and documentation process.

The Worldwide Uses table summarizes the documented ethnobotany or ethnic uses of the plant. This information includes the plant's properties and actions as well as specific conditions and illnesses for which the plant has been utilized by people around the world. It includes tribal or indigenous uses, as well as current uses in herbal medicine. This information summarizes how all parts of the plants are employed, *without distinction*. The information shown in the table should only be used as a reference, and the main body of the text will review it in more detail.

You must be observant when reviewing the ethnobotany documentation provided. Although a plant may be documented to be anti-inflammatory, the ethnic use may well be as a *topical* inflammatory aid for something such as skin rashes rather than taken *internally* for arthritis or stomach inflammation. Or, many tribal remedies documented and employed by indigenous people call for a specific plant to be placed in bath water for a "bathing remedy" rather than taken internally. Other times, a disease or condition like herpes or malaria may be documented and listed in the Worldwide Uses table; the text, however, may reveal that the specific plant has been employed as an aid to treat such *symptoms* as fever or lesions rather than being used as an antiviral or antimalarial aid to directly affect the illness. For these reasons, it is important to read the main text on the plant and use the ethnobotany tables only as a general reference.

The information on the ethnic uses of the plants, as well as their current uses in herbal medicine, has been compiled from many publications, journals, and books by various authors, herbalists, botanists, and ethnobotanists. These documents are listed in the References section in the back of the book.

Phytochemical Information

The last table in each plant entry shows phytochemical data. *Phyto* means plant, so *phytochemicals* simply refers to the chemicals that are found in the plant. Many readers will never need or use this type of information. Phytochemical data, however, is sometimes very difficult to access, and many medical professionals, pharmacists, botanists, ethnobotanists, researchers, scientists, and alternative health professionals will value this compiled information. Often, the plant's effective uses or actions will be closely tied to specific chemicals found in the plant that have been tested and documented to have specific pharmacological and biological activities. In other words, it helps explain why the plant works for certain things.

Again, the phytochemical data provided is a *summary* of chemicals that have been documented to exist in the plant. It does not include every known chemical in the plant, and no distinction has been made as to which chemicals are found in the different parts of the plant (leaves, fruit, bark, and so on). Therefore, the phytochemical data may or may not be all-inclusive or complete. It is provided for a general reference for the more experienced reader.

READING THE INFORMATION IN PART 3

THE INFORMATION SUMMARIZED in Table 1, Documented Properties and Actions of Rainforest Plants, and Table 2, Documented Worldwide Ethnic Uses of Rainforest Plants, is just that: *summaries* of all the documentation on *all* of the plant parts. This is why it is important to read *all* of the information in Part 2 on each plant before using it. The information provided in the text on each plant reviews how different parts of the plant are prepared for different purposes.

The information contained in this book is for informational and educational purposes and is not intended to be used to diagnose, prescribe, or treat any illness, nor to replace proper medical care.

Quick Guide to Herbal Terms, Uses, and Disorders

~~~~~~

HERBAL MEDICINE PRACTITIONERS use specific terms to help identify the properties and actions of plants. In this section you will find definitions for many of these medical and herbal terms. The section also serves as a quick reference for matching a disorder or condition to the plants that are used to treat it. For full descriptions of the plants listed, turn to the appropriate entries in Part 2.

The following information was compiled from more than 500 published sources of documentation referenced in the Notes section of this book.

This information is for informational purposes and is not intended to be used to diagnose, prescribe, or treat any illness nor to replace proper medical care.

Abortifacient . . . . *A substance that induces abortion.*
Erva tostão, fedegoso, gervão, manacá, vassourinha

Abscess . . . . *A localized collection of pus surrounded by inflamed tissue.*
Balsam, cat's claw, erva tostão, fedegoso, jurubeba (internal), picao preto, samambaia

Acne . . . . Abuta, cat's claw, espinheira santa, fedegoso, sarsaparilla, tayuya

Adaptogen . . . . *See Alterative.*

Adrenal Disorders . . . . . Chuchuhuasi, espinheira santa, suma, tayuya

AIDS/HIV . . . . Cat's claw, catuaba, chanca piedra, macela, pau d'arco

Allergies . . . . Amor seco, carqueja, cat's claw, gervão, jatoba, nettle, pau d'arco, picao preto, yerba mate

Alopecia . . . . *Hair loss.*
Catuaba, gervão, jaborandi, muira puama, mutamba, nettle, sarsaparilla

Alterative . . . . *A substance that stimulates changes of a defensive or healing nature in metabolism or tissue function when there is chronic or acute disease or that restores in some unknown way the normal functions of an organ or system; sometimes referred to as an adaptogen.*
Cat's claw, maca, manacá, sarsaparilla, suma, yerba mate

Amebicide . . . . *A substance used to kill amebas.*
Erva tostão, simaruba

Amenorrhea . . . . *Abnormal absence of menses.*
Balsam, Brazilian peppertree, cat's claw, chuchuhuasi, gervão, macela

Analgesic . . . . *A substance that relieves pain.*
Abuta, andiroba, boldo, Brazilian peppertree, carqueja, chanca piedra, chuchuhuasi, espinheira santa, fedegoso, gervão, graviola, guarana, iporuru, macela, manacá, maracuja, mullaca, mulungu, nettle, pau d'arco, simaruba, suma, tayuya, vassourinha

Anaphylactic . . . . *A substance that blocks an allergic reaction.*
Amor seco, gervão, picao preto, yerba mate

Anemia . . . . *A condition in which the blood is deficient in red blood cells, in hemoglobin, or in total volume.*
Alcachofra, carqueja, erva tostão, fedegoso, espinheira santa, jurubeba, maca, pau d'arco, simaruba, suma, vassourinha

Anesthetic . . . . *A substance that decreases nerve sensitivity to pain.*
Iporuru, manacá, tayuya

Angina . . . . *Short for angina pectoris; a sharp, suffocating pain in the chest normally caused when the demand of blood by the heart exceeds the supply of the coronary artery.*
Carqueja, picao preto

Anodyne . . . . *See Analgesic.*

Antacid . . . . *A substance that reduces and/or neutralizes stomach acid.*
Carqueja, espinheira santa, gervão, jurubeba, vassourinha

Anthelmintic . . . . *See Vermifuge.*

Antibacterial . . . . *A substance that kills or inhibits bacteria.*
Andiroba, annatto, balsam, Brazilian peppertree, catuaba, chanca piedra, copaiba, erva tostão, fedegoso, graviola, guava, iporuru, jatoba, macela, mutamba, nettle, pau d'arco, picao preto, simaruba, tayuya

Antibiotic . . . . *A substance that kills or inhibits the growth of microorganisms and treats infections caused by bacteria and other microorganisms.*
Brazilian peppertree, espinheira santa, mutamba, sangre de grado, sarsaparilla

Anticarcinomic . . . . *A substance that kills or inhibits carcinomas (any cancer that arises in epithelium cells).*
Abuta, pau d'arco

Antidepressant . . . . *A substance meant to oppose depression or sadness.*
Brazilian peppertree, cat's claw, damiana, graviola, maracuja, muira puama, mulungu, tayuya

Antifungal . . . . *An agent that kills or inhibits fungi.*
Balsam, Brazilian peppertree, fedegoso, jatoba, mulateiro, pau d'arco, picao preto, sangre de grado, stevia, tayuya

Antihemorrhagic . . . . . . *See Hemostatic.*

Antihepatotoxic . . . . *A substance used to protect the liver from toxins.*
Carqueja, chanca piedra, manacá, mullaca, mutamba

Antihistamine . . . . *See Anaphylactic.*

Anti-inflammatory . . . . . *A substance used to reduce inflammation.*
Abuta, alcachofra, amor seco, andiroba, annatto, balsam, cajueiro, camu-camu, carqueja, cat's claw, chanca piedra, chuchuhuasi, copaiba, erva tostão, fedegoso, gervão, iporuru, jaborandi, jatoba, jurubeba, macela, manacá, maracuja, mullaca, mulungu, pau d'arco, picao preto, sangre de grado, sarsaparilla, tayuya, vassourinha

Antileukemic . . . . *A substance that kills or inhibits leukemia.*
Abuta, espinheira santa, mullaca, pau d'arco, simaruba

Antimicrobial . . . . *A substance that destroys or inhibits growth of disease-causing bacteria and other microorganisms.*
Brazilian peppertree, copaiba, guava, iporuru, jatoba, macela, mutamba, pau d'arco, picao preto, samambaia, simaruba, tayuya

Antimutagenic .... *A substance that can reduce, prevent, or reverse the action of a mutagen.*

Cat's claw, graviola, macela, mullaca, pau d'arco, suma

Antioxidant .... *A substance that protects against free radical activity and lipid peroxidation by preventing oxidation.*

Acerola, annatto, Brazil nut, camu-camu, cat's claw, jatoba, tayuya, yerba mate

Antiparasitic .... *A substance that kills parasites.*

Amor seco, andiroba, annatto, balsam, boldo, carqueja, cat's claw, fedegoso, gervão, graviola, jatoba, macela, maracuja, mulateiro, mullaca, pau d'arco, picao preto, simaruba

Antipyretic .... *An agent that reduces fever. See Febrifuge.*

Antiseptic .... *A substance that destroys or inhibits germs, disease-causing bacteria, and other microorganisms, and is sufficiently nontoxic to cleanse wounds and prevent infections.*

Abuta, andiroba, balsam, boldo, Brazilian peppertree, espinheira santa, fedegoso, macela, mullaca, nettle, sangre de grado, sarsaparilla, vassourinha

Antispasmodic .... *A substance that relieves spasm of smooth muscle.*

Abuta, amor seco, Brazilian peppertree, chanca piedra, chuchuhuasi, erva tostão, fedegoso, gervão, graviola, guava, jatoba, macela, maracuja, mulungu

Antitussive .... *A substance that depresses coughing.*

Amor seco, annatto, balsam, cajueiro, copaiba, jatoba, mullaca, vassourinha

Antiulcerogenic .... *A substance that protects against the formation of ulcers or is used for the treatment of ulcers. See Ulcer for specific type.*

Antiviral .... *A substance that destroys or inhibits the proliferation and viability of infectious viruses.*

Brazilian peppertree, cat's claw, catuaba, chanca piedra, erva tostão, macela, pau d'arco, sangre de grado, vassourinha

Aperient .... *A substance that acts as a mild laxative.*

Abuta, carqueja, chanca piedra, jatoba, muira puama, yerba mate

Aperitif .... *An alcoholic beverage taken before a meal as an appetizer.*

Chanca piedra, espinheira santa, muira puama, sarsaparilla

Aphrodisiac .... *A substance that stimulates sexual activity and libido.*

Amor seco, cajueiro, catuaba, chuchuhuasi, damiana, erva tostão, guarana, iporuru, maca, muira puama, sarsaparilla, suma, vassourinha

Arrhythmia . . . . *Erratic heartbeat.*
Brazilian peppertree

Arteriosclerosis . . . . *A chronic disease characterized by abnormal thickening and hardening of the arterial walls with resulting loss of elasticity.*
Alcachofra, cat's claw, guarana, suma, yerba mate

Arthritis . . . . Abuta, amor seco, andiroba, cat's claw, chuchuhuasi, espinheira santa, graviola, iporuru, jatoba, manacá, mullaca, mulungu, nettle, pau d'arco, sarsaparilla, suma, tayuya, yerba mate

Ascaricide . . . . *A substance used to destroy or inhibit Ascaris lumbricoides, an intestinal parasitic worm.*
Boldo

Asthma . . . . Abuta, amor seco, balsam, Brazilian peppertree, cajueiro, cat's claw, chanca piedra, chuchuhuasi, erva tostão, espinheira santa, fedegoso, gervão, graviola, jatoba, macela, maracuja, muira puama, mullaca, mulungu, mutamba, nettle, sarsaparilla, suma

Astringent . . . . *A substance that contracts blood vessels and certain body tissues (such as mucous membranes) with the effect of reducing secretion and excretion of blood and/or fluids.*
Acerola, annatto, Brazilian peppertree, cajueiro, camu-camu, damiana, fedegoso, graviola, guarana, guava, jatoba, mutamba, nettle, pedra hume caa, picao preto, sangre de grado, vassourinha, yerba mate

Balsamic . . . . *A soothing, healing, oily substance.*
Andiroba, balsam, Brazilian peppertree, copaiba

Bladder Disorders . . . . . Abuta, alcachofra, chanca piedra, jatoba, jurubeba, sarsaparilla

Blennorrhagia . . . . *A discharge of mucus in the urethra and/or urinary tract. Normally a symptom/side effect of urethritis, some kidney infections, and/or severe prostatitis.*
Abuta, amor seco, Brazilian peppertree, chanca piedra, erva tostão, jatoba, picao preto, tayuya, vassourinha

Blood Disorders . . . . Alcachofra (uremia), amor seco, cat's claw, erva tostão, nettle, sarsaparilla

Boils . . . . Abuta, erva tostão, cat's claw, gervão, graviola, jurubeba, mullaca, pau d'arco, picao preto, samambaia

Bowel/Intestinal Disorders . . . . Boldo, cat's claw, catuaba, chanca piedra, copaiba, damiana, espinheira santa, guava, jatoba, jurubeba, macela, muira puama, mullaca, mutamba, picao preto, tayuya

Bronchitis . . . . Abuta, amor seco, balsam, Brazilian peppertree, cajueiro, chanca piedra, chuchuhuasi, copaiba, fedegoso, gervão, jaborandi, jatoba, manacá, maracuja, mulungu, mutamba, nettle, picao preto, samambaia, suma, vassourinha

Burns .... Annatto, fedegoso, mutamba, nettle, sarsaparilla

Bursitis .... *Inflammation of a bursa (sac) that contains fluid that lubricates joints.*
Cat's claw, jatoba

Calculus .... *A concentration of mineral salts; tartar.*
Abuta, alcachofra, carqueja, chanca piedra, erva tostão

Cancer .... Alcachofra, andiroba, annatto, balsam, cat's claw, catuaba (skin), chanca
piedra, chuchuhuasi (skin), erva tostão (abdominal), espinheira santa (skin),
jurubeba (tumors), macela, mullaca, mulungu (stomach), nettle, pau d'arco,
picao preto, samambaia, sarsaparilla, suma

Candida .... *Any of a genus (Candida) of parasitic fungi that resemble yeasts and occur in
the mouth, vagina, and intestinal tract and that are usually benign but can be-
come pathogenic, especially C. albicans, which causes thrush.*
Brazilian peppertree, cat's claw, fedegoso, jatoba, mulateiro, pau d'arco, sangre
de grado, stevia, suma

Cardiotonic .... *A substance that strengthens, tones, or regulates heart functions without overt
stimulation or depression.*
Cat's claw, erva tostão, fedegoso, gervão, graviola, guarana, jatoba, muira
puama, mulungu, stevia, yerba mate

Carminative .... *A substance used to expel gas from the stomach and intestines.*
Chanca piedra, fedegoso, jurubeba, macela, picao preto, sarsaparilla

Catarrh .... *Inflamed mucous membranes and/or an increase in mucous discharge. It is an
older medical/herbal term that usually implies excess secretions in the upper
respiratory tract, particularly with congestion.*
Balsam, copaiba, damiana, guava, jatoba, jurubeba, nettle, picao preto

Cathartic .... *See Laxative.*

**Central Nervous
System** .... *See CNS Disorders, CNS Stimulant.*

Cholagogue .... *A substance that increases the production and flow of bile in the liver.*
Alcachofra, boldo, erva tostão, fedegoso, jurubeba

Cholera .... Abuta, erva tostão, guava, tayuya

Choleretic .... *A substance that increases the flow of bile from the gallbladder.*
Alcachofra, boldo, chanca piedra, erva tostão, tayuya

Cholesterol Problems . *See Hypocholesterolemic.*

Choliokinetic .... *A substance that increases the contractive power of the bile duct.*
Alcachofra

**Chronic Fatigue
Syndrome (CFS)** ...... Cat's claw, chuchuhuasi, guarana, jatoba, maca, suma, yerba mate

Cicatrizant .... *A substance that promotes wound healing and the formation of new tissue.*
Andiroba, annatto, balsam, Brazilian peppertree, espinheira santa, graviola, guava, sangre de grado, vassourinha

Circulation Problems .. Alcachofra, carqueja, cat's claw, guarana, pau d'arco, suma

CNS Disorders .... Catuaba, guarana, muira puama, mulungu

CNS Stimulant .... *A substance that stimulates the central nervous system.*
Catuaba, muira puama

Colds/Flu .... Abuta, amor seco, andiroba, annatto, balsam, boldo, Brazilian peppertree, cajueiro, camu-camu, cat's claw, chanca piedra, damiana, fedegoso, gervão, graviola, jaborandi, macela, manacá, mullaca, mutamba, pau d'arco, picao preto, samambaia, sangre de grado, sarsaparilla, simaruba

Colic .... *Acute, spasmodic abdominal pain.*
Amor seco, balsam, Brazilian peppertree, cajueiro, cat's claw, chanca piedra, espinheira santa, fedegoso, guava, macela, mullaca, picao preto, simaruba, vassourinha

Colon Disorders ...... Boldo, carqueja, cat's claw, gervão, jaborandi, jurubeba, macela, pau d'arco

Conjunctivitis .... Abuta, annatto, Brazilian peppertree, picao preto, sarsaparilla, vassourinha

Constipation .... Abuta, amor seco, boldo, cajueiro, carqueja, chanca piedra, damiana, espinheira santa, fedegoso, jatoba, manacá, mutamba, nettle, pau d'arco, tayuya, yerba mate

Convulsion .... Abuta, amor seco, erva tostão, guava, macela, maracuja

Cough .... Abuta, amor seco, andiroba, balsam, Brazilian peppertree, cajueiro, chanca piedra, damiana, erva tostão, gervão, graviola, guava, iporuru, jatoba, maracuja, mullaca, mulungu, mutamba, pau d'arco, picao preto, samambaia, sarsaparilla, vassourinha

Crohn's Disease ...... Boldo, Brazilian peppertree, carqueja, cat's claw, jurubeba, macela

Cystitis .... *Inflammation of the urinary bladder.*
Abuta, alcachofra, annatto, Brazilian peppertree, chanca piedra, copaiba, erva tostão, jatoba

Cytotoxic . . . . *A substance used to damage or destroy cancerous cells.*

Brazilian peppertree, cat's claw, graviola, macela, mutamba, pau d'arco, simaruba

Decoction . . . . *See page 237.*

Decongestant . . . . *A substance that relieves or reduces nasal congestion.*

Jatoba, jurubeba

Demulcent . . . . *An agent that soothes internal membranes; traditionally separated from external soothing agents, emollients.*

Boldo, samambaia

Depression . . . . *See Antidepressant.*

Depurative . . . . *A substance used to cleanse or purify the blood.*

Alcachofra, amor seco, annatto, boldo, carqueja, gervão, graviola, mullaca, mutamba, nettle, samambaia, sarsaparilla, tayuya, vassourinha, yerba mate

**Dermatosis/
Dermatitis** . . . . *Disease/inflammation of the skin.*

Cajueiro, cat's claw, chanca piedra, copaiba, fedegoso, graviola, guava, mullaca, mutamba, sarsaparilla

Detoxifier . . . . *A substance that promotes the removal of toxins from a system and/or organ.*

Alcachofra, amor seco, boldo, Brazilian peppertree, carqueja, cat's claw, chanca piedra, espinheira santa, fedegoso, gervão, graviola, guarana, jurubeba, muira puama, mutamba, nettle, pata de vaca, pau d'arco, picao preto, samambaia, sarsaparilla, tayuya, vassourinha, yerba mate

Diabetes . . . . *Abuta, alcachofra, annatto, cajueiro, carqueja, cat's claw, chanca piedra, damiana, fedegoso, guava, iporuru, macela, mulateiro, mullaca, pata de vaca, pau d'arco, pedra hume caa, picao preto, sarsaparilla, stevia, suma, vassourinha*

Diaphoretic . . . . *A substance that induces increased perspiration.*

Fedegoso, gervão, jaborandi, macela, manacá, mutamba, samambaia, sarsaparilla, simaruba, yerba mate

Diarrhea . . . . *Abuta, acerola, amor seco, boldo, Brazilian peppertree, cajueiro, carqueja, chanca piedra, chuchuhuasi, copaiba, fedegoso, gervão, graviola, guarana, guava, iporuru, jatoba, macela, maracuja, mullaca, mutamba, pedra hume caa, picao preto, simaruba, tayuya, vassourinha*

Digestive . . . . *A substance that stimulates, promotes, or assists digestion.*

Alcachofra, amor seco, boldo, carqueja, chanca piedra, guava, jurubeba, macela, tayuya

Digestive Disorders ... Abuta, alcachofra, boldo, Brazilian peppertree, carqueja, cat's claw, chanca piedra, espinheira santa, fedegoso, gervão, graviola, jatoba, jurubeba, macela, manacá, mutamba, pau d'arco, sarsaparilla, suma, tayuya, yerba mate

Disinfectant .... *A substance that prevents the spread of infection, bacteria, or communicable disease.*

Brazilian peppertree, copaiba, espinheira santa, maracuja, mullaca, mulungu

Diuretic .... *A substance that increases urination.*

Abuta, alcachofra, amor seco, annatto, boldo, Brazilian peppertree, cajueiro, carqueja, cat's claw, chanca piedra, copaiba, damiana, erva tostão, espinheira santa, fedegoso, graviola, guarana, jaborandi, jatoba, jurubeba, manacá, maracuja, mullacá, mutamba, nettle, pata de vaca, picao preto, samambaia, sarsaparilla, tayuya, vassourinha, yerba mate

Dropsy (Edema)....... *Accumulation of fluid in tissues (swelling).*

Abuta, alcachofra, Brazilian peppertree, chanca piedra, erva tostão, fedegoso, gervão, jaborandi, nettle, picao preto, tayuya

Dysentery .... Abuta, acerola, amor seco, annatto, cajueiro, cat's claw, chanca piedra, chuchuhuasi, damiana, fedegoso, gervão, graviola, guava, jatoba, macela, muira puama, mutamba, pau d'arco, pedra hume caa, picao preto, simaruba, vassourinha

Dysmenorrhea/
Dysmenorrhagia ...... *Painful menstruation.*

Balsam, Brazilian peppertree, cat's claw, chuchuhuasi, damiana, erva tostão, fedegoso, gervão, maca, macela, maracuja, picao preto, vassourinha

Dyspepsia .... *Indigestion.*

Abuta, alcachofra, boldo, cajueiro, carqueja, chanca piedra, damiana, erva tostão, espinheira santa, fedegoso, gervão, graviola, guava, jatoba, jurubeba, simaruba, tayuya

Earache .... Boldo, fedegoso, mullaca, picao preto, vassourinha

Eczema.............. Cajueiro, fedegoso, gervão, graviola, pau d'arco, samambaia, sangre de grado, sarsaparilla, tayuya, vassourinha

Edema............... *See Dropsy.*

Emetic .... *An agent that induces vomiting.*

Erva tostão, gervão, graviola, jaborandi, sarsaparilla, simaruba, vassourinha

Emmenagogue . . . . *A substance that stimulates, initiates, and/or promotes menstrual flow. Emmenagogues are used to balance and restore the normal function of the female reproductive system.*

Abuta, Brazilian peppertree, chanca piedra, damiana, fedegoso, gervão, guava, jurubeba, macela, manacá, nettle, picao preto, simaruba, vassourinha

Emollient . . . . *An agent that has a protective and soothing action on the surfaces of the skin and membranes.*

Andiroba, annatto, Brazil nut, camu-camu, copaiba, mulateiro, mutamba, picao preto, vassourinha

Emphysema . . . . Jatoba, macela, manacá

Enteritis . . . . *Inflammation of the intestines*
Carqueja, pedra hume caa

Epilepsy . . . . Abuta, annatto, erva tostão, guava, macela, mulungu, tayuya

Epstein-Barr Virus . . . . . Cat's claw, suma, tayuya

Erysipelas . . . . *An infection of the skin and underlying tissues with the bacterium Streptococcus pyogenes; most commonly occurs on the face and head.*

Abuta, annatto, erva tostão, fedegoso, gervão, jurubeba, mutamba, tayuya, vassourinha

Expectorant . . . . *An agent that increases bronchial mucous secretion by promoting liquefaction of the sticky mucus and its expulsion from the body.*

Abuta, annatto, balsam, Brazilian peppertree, copaiba, erva tostão, jatoba, mullaca, vassourinha

Fatigue . . . . Cat's claw, catuaba, chuchuhuasi, erva tostão, fedegoso, guarana, jatoba, maca, muira puama, simaruba, suma, tayuya, yerba mate

Febrifuge . . . . *A substance that reduces high body temperatures, as in fevers, or that is used to treat feverish conditions.*

Abuta, acerola, andiroba, annatto, Brazilian peppertree, cajueiro, carqueja, chanca piedra, chuchuhuasi, erva tostão, fedegoso, gervão, graviola, guarana, jaborandi, jurubeba, manaca, mullaca, mulungu, mutamba, pau d'arco, picao preto, samambaia, sarsaparilla, simaruba, tayuya, vassourinha

Fever . . . . *See Febrifuge.*

Fibromyalgia . . . . *A group of common nonarticular rheumatic disorders characterized by achy pain, tenderness, and stiffness of fibrous tissues like muscles, tendons, ligaments, and other "white" connective tissues.*

Cat's claw, catuaba, erva tostão, iporuru, tayuya

Fractures . . . . Amor seco, Brazilian peppertree, mutamba

Fungal Infection . . . . . . *See Antifungal.*

Galactagogue . . . . *A substance that increases or stimulates milk flow or production.*
Amor seco, erva tostão, gervão, graviola, jaborandi, mulungu, picao preto

Gallbladder Disorders,
Gallstones . . . . Abuta, alcachofra, boldo, carqueja, chanca piedra, erva tostão, graviola,
mullaca

Gastritis . . . . *Inflammation of the mucous membrane of the stomach.*
Boldo, carqueja, cat's claw, chanca piedra, espinheira santa, jurubeba, macela,
muira puama, mutamba, pau d'arco, vassourinha

Gastrotonic . . . . *A substance that is tonic to the gastrointestinal system.*
Carqueja, gervão, jurubeba, macela

Gingivitis . . . . *Inflammation of the gums.*
Brazilian peppertree, guava

Gonorrhea . . . . Abuta, annatto, boldo, Brazilian peppertree, cat's claw, chanca piedra, copaiba,
erva tostão, fedegoso, gervão, mullaca, mutamba, sarsaparilla, simaruba,
vassourinha

Gout . . . . *Painful inflammation of the joints.*
Alcachofra, balsam, boldo, Brazilian peppertree, carqueja, nettle, samambaia,
sarsaparilla, tayuya

Gravel . . . . *A deposit of small calculous concentrations (stones) in the kidneys and
bladder.*
Abuta, vassourinha

Grippe . . . . *An older term that has mostly been replaced/redefined in the United States as
"influenza." The term is still used in developing countries to describe general
flu-like symptoms and conditions typically not tested/identified through bacte-
rial/viral culture tests. See Colds/Flu.*

Headaches and
Migraine . . . . Annatto, balsam, damiana, fedegoso, gervão, guarana, iporuru, jatoba,
maracuja, picao preto, tayuya, vassourinha, yerba mate

Heartburn . . . . Annatto, espinheira santa

Heart Palpitations/
Disorders . . . . Abuta, cat's claw, erva tostão, fedegoso, gervão, graviola, guarana,
vassourinha, yerba mate

Hemorrhage . . . . *See Hemostatic.*

Hemorrhoids . . . . Cat's claw, chuchuhuasi, copaiba, erva tostão, jatoba, maracuja, mutamba, vassourinha

Hemostatic . . . . *An agent that stops or prevents bleeding or hemorrhages. Other words used for* hemostatic *include* antihemmorrhagic *and* styptic.

Abuta, amor seco, cat's claw, erva tostão, fedegoso, guava, jatoba, mullaca, mutamba, nettle, pedra hume caa, sangre de grado, yerba mate

Hepatic . . . . *Pertaining to the liver.*

Abuta, alcachofra, annatto, boldo, carqueja, erva tostão, gervão, jurubeba, mutamba, picao preto, sarsaparilla, vassourinha

Hepatitis . . . . Acerola, annatto, boldo, chanca piedra, erva tostão, jurubeba, mullaca, mulungu, mutamba, picao preto

Hepatoprotective . . . . . *A substance that helps protect the liver.*

Abuta, alcachofra, annatto, boldo, carqueja, erva tostão, fedegoso, gervão, jatoba, jurubeba, mutamba, picao preto, sarsaparilla, vassourinha

Hepatotonic . . . . *A substance that is tonic to the liver.*

Boldo, carqueja, chanca piedra, erva tostão, fedegoso, jurubeba

Herpes . . . . Andiroba, cat's claw, copaiba, fedegoso, sangre de grado, tayuya, vassourinha

**High Blood
Pressure** . . . . Abuta, alcachofra, annatto, Brazilian peppertree, cajueiro, cat's claw, chanca piedra, fedegoso, gervão, graviola, jurubeba, manacá, maracuja, mullaca, mulungu, nettle, pedra hume caa, samambaia, sarsaparilla, stevia, suma, vassourinha

High Cholesterol . . . . . . *See Hypocholesterolemic.*

Hodgkin's Disease . . . . Pau d'arco

Hormonal (Female) . . . *A substance that has a hormone-like effect similar to that of estrogen.*

Abuta, Brazilian peppertree, cat's claw, chuchuhuasi, damiana, fedegoso, gervão, maca, macela, picao preto, sarsaparilla, suma

Hormonal (Male) . . . . . . *A substance that has a hormone-like effect simlar to that of testosterone.*

Catuaba, chuchuhuasi, damiana, muira puama, nettle, sarsaparilla, suma

Hydropsy . . . . *See Dropsy.*

Hyperglycemia........ *Excess of sugar in the blood.*
Annatto, chanca piedra, macela, stevia, suma, vassourinha

Hypertension .... *See High Blood Pressure.*

Hypocholesterolemic.. *A substance that lowers blood cholesterol levels.*
Alcachofra, annatto, cat's claw, sarsaparilla, suma, vassourinha, yerba mate

Hypoglycemic......... *A substance that helps lower the amount of sugar in or remove sugar from the urine.*
Annatto, cajueiro, carqueja, chanca piedra, guava, macela, nettle, pata de vaca, pedra hume caa, stevia

Hypotensive .... *A substance that lowers blood pressure. See High Blood Pressure.*

Hypothermal......... *A substance that lowers body temperature. See Refrigerant.*

Immune Disorders .... Cat's claw, chanca piedra, chuchuhuasi, espinheira santa, jatoba, maca, macela, mullaca, pau d'arco, samambaia, sarsaparilla, simaruba, suma

Immunostimulant ..... *A substance that stimulates immune system functions.*
Cat's claw, chanca piedra, chuchuhuasi, maca, macela, mullaca, pau d'arco, simaruba, suma, yerba mate

Impotence........... Cajueiro, catuaba, chuchuhuasi, damiana, maca, macela, muira puama, sarsaparilla, suma

Infusion.............. *See page 237.*

Insect Bites .... Amor seco, andiroba, annatto, cat's claw, copaiba, vassourinha

Insecticide, Insect Repellent............. *A substance that kills or repels insects.*
Andiroba, Brazil nut, fedegoso, graviola, macela, vassourinha

Insomnia .... Catuaba, graviola, maracuja, mulungu

Itch................. Abuta, andiroba, balsam, chanca piedra, copaiba, fedegoso, gervão, guava, picao preto, vassourinha

Jaundice............. Abuta, alcachofra, annatto, boldo, chanca piedra, erva tostão, fedegoso, guava, mullaca, picao preto, vassourinha

Kidney Disorders...... Abuta, alcachofra, amor seco, annatto, boldo, carqueja, cat's claw, chanca piedra, erva tostão, espinheira santa, fedegoso, graviola, jatoba, manacá, mullaca, mutamba, sarsaparilla, vassourinha

Kidney Stones .... Abuta, boldo, chanca piedra

Lactagogue . . . . *See Galactagogue.*

Laryngitis . . . . Jaborandi, jatoba, picao preto

Laxative . . . . *A substance that increases or stimulates the evacuation of the bowels.*
Abuta, amor seco, Brazilian peppertree, carqueja, chanca piedra, copaiba, damiana, erva tostão, espinheira santa, fedegoso, gervão, guava, iporuru, jatoba, manaca, pau d'arco, tayuya

Leprosy . . . . Andiroba, cajueiro, carqueja, fedegoso, mutamba, sarsaparilla, vassourinha

Leucorrhoea . . . . *A whitish vaginal discharge.*
Abuta, amor seco, picao preto, sangre de grado, sarsaparilla

Leukemia . . . . Abuta, cat's claw, mullaca, pau d'arco, simaruba

Lice . . . . *See Pediculicide.*

Liver Disorders . . . . Abuta, alcachofra, annatto, boldo, carqueja, cat's claw, catuaba, chanca piedra, erva tostão, espinheira santa, fedegoso, gervão, jurubeba, mullaca, mulungu, mutamba, pau d'arco, picao preto, sarsaparilla, tayuya, vassourinha

Lung Disorders . . . . Manacá, mutamba

Lupus . . . . *A musculoskeletal and/or connective tissue disorder that produces chronic inflammation of connective tissue, including the skin and various internal organs.*
Cat's claw, pau d'arco

Lymph Disorders . . . . . . Manacá

Maceration . . . . *See page 237.*

Malaria . . . . Abuta, amor seco, andiroba, annatto, carqueja, chanca piedra, damiana, fedegoso, gervão, graviola, mullaca, mutamba, pau d'arco, simaruba, vassourinha

Menopause . . . . Abuta, cat's claw, chuchuhuasi, damiana, maca, macela, maracuja, muira puama, sarsaparilla, simaruba, suma

Menorrhagia . . . . *Excess bleeding at menstruation, either in duration or amount of blood flow.*
Abuta, cat's claw, macela, vassourinha

Menstrual Cramps . . . . Abuta, amor seco, chuchuhuasi, erva tostão, fedegoso, gervão, guava, iporuru, macela, manacá, maracuja, muira puama, mulungu, tayuya

**Menstrual
Disorders** . . . . Abuta, balsam, Brazilian peppertree, cat's claw, chuchuhuasi, erva tostão, fedegoso, guava, maca, macela, sarsaparilla, suma, vassourinha

Migraine. . . . . *See Headaches and Migraine.*

Mononucleosis . . . . Cat's claw, suma

Muscle Aches . . . . Abuta, amor seco, andiroba, cat's claw, chuchuhuasi, erva tostão, iporuru, macela, maracuja, nettle, simaruba, suma, tayuya

Muscle Spasms. . . . . . . Abuta, amor seco, andiroba, balsam, cat's claw, erva tostão, fedegoso, graviola, iporuru, jatoba, macela, maracuja, mulungu, sarsaparilla, vassourinha

Nausea . . . . Cajueiro, fedegoso, gervão, guava, mullaca

Nephritis . . . . *Acute or chronic inflammation of the kidney.*
Abuta, erva tostão, guava, mullaca

Nervine. . . . . *A substance that is tonic to or has an effect on the nerves and/or central nervous system.*
Catuaba, damiana, gervão, graviola, guarana, maracuja, muira puama, mulungu

Nervous Disorders . . . . Amor seco, catuaba, damiana, espinheira santa, gervão, graviola, guarana, maracuja, muira puama, mulungu, sarsaparilla, suma, tayuya, vassourinha, yerba mate

Nervousness. . . . . *See Stress.*

Neuralgia . . . . *Acute pain radiating along the course of one or more nerves.*
Abuta, catuaba, gervão, guarana, manacá, maracuja, muira puama, suma, tayuya, yerba mate

Neurasthenic . . . . *A substance used to treat neuralgia, neurasthenia, and nerve pain.*
Muira puama

Obesity. . . . . Annatto, guarana, mutamba, picao preto, yerba mate

Paralysis . . . . Damiana, maracuja, muira puama, nettle

**Parasites,
Parasiticide**. . . . . *See Antiparasitic.*

**Parkinson's
Disease** . . . . Maracuja, pau d'arco

Pectoral. . . . . *Relating to or used for the chest.*
Graviola, mutamba, samambaia, vassourinha

Pediculicide . . . . *A substance used to kill lice.*
Andiroba, balsam, fedegoso, graviola, macela

Pellagra .... *A disease associated with a diet deficient in niacin.*
Graviola

Piles .... *Hemorrhoids.*
Guava, maracuja, mulungu, sangre de grado, vassourinha

Piscicide .... *An agent that kills fish, which is a common indicator that the substance has other properties that make it toxic to parasites or bacteria.*
Abuta, Brazilian peppertree, cajueiro, chanca piedra, graviola, mulungu

Pityriasis .... *A condition marked by dry scaly or scurfy patches of skin.*
Andiroba, cat's claw, fedegoso, samambaia, sarsaparilla

Prostate Disorders .... Annatto, Brazilian peppertree, cat's claw, copaiba, jatoba, mutamba, nettle, pau d'arco, sarsaparilla

Psoriasis .... Andiroba, boldo, cajueiro, cat's claw, chanca piedra, copaiba, fedegoso, gervão, graviola, jaborandi, pau d'arco, samambaia, sarsaparilla, suma

Purgative .... *See Laxative.*

Rash (Skin) .... Andiroba, copaiba, fedegoso, gervão, graviola, mutamba, picao preto, sarsaparilla, vassourinha

Refrigerant .... *A substance to lower the temperature of a part of the body, to reduce the metabolic activity of its tissues, or to provide a local anesthetic effect.*
Cajueiro, carqueja, manacá, mutamba, vassourinha

Renal Disorders .... Annatto, chanca piedra, damiana, erva tostão, jaborandi, pata de vaca, samambaia, vassourinha

Respiratory Disorders .... Amor seco, Brazilian peppertree, espinheira santa, fedegoso, guava, jatoba, macela, manacá, mullaca, mutamba, pau d'arco, samambaia, sangre de grado, vassourinha

Rheumatism .... Abuta, alcachofra, amor seco, andiroba, boldo, Brazilian peppertree, carqueja, cat's claw, chuchuhuasi, erva tostão, espinheira santa, fedegoso, gervão, graviola, iporuru, jaborandi, jatoba, manacá, muira puama, mullaca, nettle, pau d'arco, picao preto, samambaia, sarsaparilla, simaruba, suma, tayuya, yerba mate

Rheumatoid Arthritis .... Alcachofra, andiroba, cat's claw, iporuru

Ringworms, Roundworms .... Amor seco, boldo, fedegoso, graviola, macela, mullaca, picao preto

Scabies............... Balsam, fedegoso, guava

Scleroderma.......... *A disease marked by the deposition of fibrous connective tissue in the skin or internal organs.*
Fedegoso, mulateiro

Sclerosis............. *Hardening of tissue from overgrowth of fibrous tissue.*
Cat's claw (liver), erva tostão (liver), picao preto (glands)

Scrofula.............. *Tuberculosis of lymph nodes, most commonly in the neck.*
Cajueiro, manacá, sarsaparilla

Sedative.............. *A substance that has a calming effect.*
Boldo, gervão, graviola, macela, manacá, maracuja, mullaca, mulungu, suma

Shingles.............. *Common name for herpes zoster.*
Cat's claw, maracuja, nettle

Sialogogue........... *A substance that increases or promotes the excretion of saliva.*
Brazilian peppertree, jaborandi, picao preto

Skin Disorders........ Andiroba, annatto, cajueiro, cat's claw, catuaba, copaiba, fedegoso, gervão, graviola, guava, jurubeba, maracuja, mulateiro, mullaca, mutamba, samambaia, sangre de grado, sarsaparilla, tayuya, vassourinha

Sore Throat.......... Annatto, cajueiro, carqueja, fedegoso, guava, jaborandi, mullaca, picao preto, sangre de grado, vassourinha

Spasmogenic......... *A substance that reduces spasms. See Antispasmodic.*

Spasmolytic.......... *See Antispasmodic.*

Spleen Disorders...... Erva tostão, jurubeba, mulungu, tayuya

Sprains.............. Andiroba, balsam, chuchuhuasi, gervão, nettle

Stimulant............ *A substance that promotes the activity of a body system or function.*
Abuta, alcachofra, boldo, Brazilian peppertree, chuchuhuasi, damiana, guarana, jatoba, maca, sarsaparilla, yerba mate

Stomach Ache........ Abuta, annatto, balsam, boldo, Brazilian peppertree, cajueiro, carqueja, chanca piedra, chuchuhuasi, damiana, espinheira santa, fedegoso, gervão, graviola, guava, jurubeba, mullaca, mulungu, mutamba, picao preto, vassourinha

Stomach Disorders.... Annatto, boldo, cat's claw, catuaba, chanca piedra, espinheira santa, fedegoso, gervão, graviola, jatoba, jurubeba, macela, mullaca, mutamba, pau d'arco, picao preto, simaruba, vassourinha

Stomachic . . . . *A substance that stimulates the secretory activity of the stomach; used as a tonic to improve the appetite and/or digestive processes.*
Abuta, annatto, boldo, Brazilian peppertree, cajueiro, carqueja, chanca piedra, chuchuhuasi, damiana, erva tostão, espinheira santa, fedegoso, gervão, graviola, jatoba, jurubeba, mutamba, nettle, picao preto, sarsaparilla, simaruba, tayuya, yerba mate

Stress, Nervousness . . Amor seco, catuaba, damiana, gervão, graviola, guava, manacá, maracuja, muira puama, mulungu, sarsaparilla, suma, tayuya, vassourinha

Styptic . . . . *See Hemostatic.*

Sudorific . . . . *See Diaphoretic.*

Syphilis . . . . Amor seco, boldo, cajueiro, cat's claw, chanca piedra, copaiba, damiana, gervão, manaca, mutamba, pau d'arco, sarsaparilla, tayuya, vassourinha

**Testicular
Inflammation** . . . . Abuta, jatoba

Tetanus . . . . Andiroba, fedegoso, maracuja

Thrush . . . . *A disease caused by a fungus (Candida albicans) that is marked by white patches in the mouth; also vaginal candidiasis.*
Brazilian peppertree, cajueiro, jatoba, pau d'arco

Tincture . . . . *See page 238.*

Tonic . . . . *A substance that acts to restore, balance, tone, strengthen, or invigorate a body system.*
Abuta, alcachofra, boldo, Brazilian peppertree, cajueiro, carqueja, cat's claw, catuaba, chanca piedra, chuchuhuasi, damiana, erva tostão, espinheira santa, fedegoso, gervão, guarana, jatoba, jurubeba, maca, muira puama, pata de vaca, pedra hume caa, sarsaparilla, simaruba, suma, tayuya, yerba mate

Tuberculosis . . . . Balsam, Brazilian peppertree, fedegoso, maca, manacá

Tumors . . . . Annatto, balsam, Brazilian peppertree, cajueiro, cat's claw, chanca piedra (abdomen), chuchuhuasi, copaiba (prostate), fedegoso, gervão, jurubeba (uterine), macela, mullaca (testicle), nettle, samambaia, sangre de grado, suma, tayuya (joint), vassourinha

Typhoid . . . . Chanca piedra, fedegoso

Ulcer (Mouth) . . . . Brazilian peppertree, cajueiro, pedra hume caa, picao preto, sangre de grado

Ulcer (Skin) . . . . Andiroba, balsam, espinheira santa, fedegoso, gervão, graviola, manacá, mutamba, pau d'arco, sangre de grado

Ulcer (Stomach/ Gastric) . . . . Alcachofra, andiroba, cajueiro, carqueja, cat's claw, copaiba, espinheira santa, fedegoso, gervão, graviola, guava, jatoba, jurubeba, manacá, mutamba, pau d'arco, sangre de grado, suma, tayuya

Uremia . . . . *Accumulation in the blood of substances normally eliminated in the urine, producing a toxic condition. See Blood Disorders.*

Urinary Infections . . . . . Abuta, amor seco, boldo, Brazilian peppertree, cat's claw, chanca piedra, fedegoso, jatoba, picao preto, samambaia

Urinary Tract Disorders . . . . Abuta, alcachofra, amor seco, annatto, boldo, Brazilian peppertree, cat's claw, chanca piedra, damiana, erva tostão, espinheira santa, fedegoso, jatoba, jurubeba, nettle, pata de vaca, pau d'arco, picao preto, sarsaparilla, yerba mate

Uterine Disorders . . . . . Abuta, amor seco, chanca piedra, erva tostão, fedegoso, jurubeba (tumors), manacá, mutamba

Vaginitis . . . . *An inflammation of the vagina, either from simple tissue irritation or from an infection.*
Amor seco, annatto, chanca piedra, picao preto, sangre de grado

Vasodilator . . . . *A substance that causes a widening and/or relaxation of the blood vessels and therefore an increase in blood flow.*
Guarana, nettle, simaruba

Venereal Disease . . . . . Abuta, amor seco, annatto, balsam, Brazilian peppertree, cajueiro, damiana, fedegoso, gervão, jatoba, manacá, samambaia, sarsaparilla, vassourinha

Vermifuge . . . . *A substance used to expel worms from the intestine.*
Amor seco, boldo, carqueja, cat's claw, chanca piedra, erva tostão, fedegoso, gervão, graviola, guava, macela, maracuja, mulateiro, mullacá, nettle, simaruba, vassourinha

Vertigo . . . . Chanca piedra, guava, iporuru

Vulnerary . . . . *A substance used to heal wounds.*
Amor seco, andiroba, balsam, Brazilian peppertree, copaiba, espinheira santa, gervão, guava, mulateiro, picao preto, sangre de grado

Warts . . . . Brazilian peppertree, cajueiro, cat's claw, pau d'arco

Wounds . . . . Amor seco, andiroba, balsam, Brazilian peppertree, cajueiro, cat's claw, copaiba, fedegoso, guava, iporuru, mulateiro, mutamba, nettle, pau d'arco, picao preto, sangre de grado, sarsaparilla, tayuya, vassourinha

Yellow Fever . . . . Fedegoso, gervão, manacá

Herbal Secrets
of the Rainforest

Part One

Rainforest Destruction and Survival

~~~~~~

THE BEAUTY, MAJESTY, and timelessness of a primary rainforest is indescribable. It is impossible to capture on film, to
describe in words, or to explain to those who have never had
the awe-inspiring experience of standing in the heart of a primary
rainforest.

Rainforests have evolved over millions of years to turn into the
incredibly complex environments they are today. A rainforest
represents a store of living and breathing renewable natural resources that for eons, by virtue of their richness in both animal
and plant species, have contributed a wealth of resources for the
survival and well-being of humankind. These have included basic
food supplies, clothing, shelter, fuel, spices, industrial raw materials,
and medicine for all those who have lived sustainably in the
majesty of the forest. However, the inner dynamics of a tropical
rainforest are an intricate and fragile system. Everything is so
interdependent that upsetting one part can lead to unknown
damage or even destruction of the whole. Sadly, it has taken only
a century of human intervention to destroy what nature has
designed to last forever.

In 1950, 15 percent of the Earth's land surface was covered by
rainforest. Today more than half has already gone up in smoke.

More than 20 percent of the Amazon rainforest is already gone, and much more is severely threatened as destruction continues to escalate. Statistics reported in 1996 revealed the Amazon showed a 34 percent increase in deforestation since 1992.[1]

Over 200,000 acres of rainforest are burned every day. That is more than 150 acres lost every minute of every day, and 78 million acres are lost every year!

A new report by a congressional committee says the Amazon is vanishing at a rate of 20,000 square miles a year.[2] That's more than three times the rate of 1994, the last year for which official figures are available. "If nothing is done, the entire Amazon will be gone within fifty years," said the 110-page report's author, Rep. Gilney Vianna of the leftist Worker's Party in the Amazon state of Mato Grosso. Yet another recent report said new figures showed that in the Brazilian Amazon, forest fires increased by more than 50 percent over the 1996 rate.[3]

In less than fifty years, more than half of the world's tropical rainforests have fallen victim to fire and the chain saw, and the rate of destruction is still accelerating. Unbelievably, over 200,000 acres of rainforest are burned every day. That is more than 150 acres lost every minute of every day, and 78 million acres are lost every year![4] The World Wide Fund for Nature reported that more tropical forest burned around the world in 1997 than at any other time in recorded history. "1997 will be remembered as the year the world caught fire," said Jean-Paul Jeanrenaud, head of its forest program.

Massive deforestation brings with it many ugly consequences—air and water pollution, soil erosion, malaria epidemics, the release of carbon dioxide into the atmosphere, the eviction and decimation of indigenous Indian tribes, and the loss of biodiversity through extinction of plants and animals. Fewer rainforests means less rain, less oxygen for us to breathe, and an even greater threat from global warming.

But who is really to blame? Consider what we industrialized Americans have done to our own homeland . . . We converted 90 percent of North America's virgin forests into firewood, shingles, furniture, railroad ties, and paper. Other industrialized countries have done no better. Malaysia, Indonesia, and Brazil, among other tropical countries with rainforests, are often branded as "environmental villains" of the world, mainly due to their reported levels of destruction of their rainforests. But despite the levels of deforestation, up to 60 percent of their territory is still covered by natural tropical forests. In fact, much of the pressure today on their remaining rainforests comes from servicing the needs and markets for wood products in industrialized countries that have already depleted their own natural resources. Industrial countries would not be buying rainforest hardwoods and timber had we not cut down our own trees long ago, nor would poachers in the Amazon jungle be slaughtering jaguar, ocelot, caiman, and otter if we did not provide lucrative markets for their skins in Berlin, Paris, and Tokyo.

THE BIODIVERSITY OF THE RAINFOREST

WHY SHOULD THE loss of tropical forests be of any more concern to us in light of our own poor management of natural resources? The loss of tropical rainforests has a profound and devastating world impact because rainforests are so much more biologically diverse.

> Regardless of which eyes view this forest, there is a wealth of raw materials therein, which can be rationally exploited so that they yield employment and income to tropical forest residents while preserving the forest as an aesthetic, conservational, and economic entity. . . . If Brazil nuts and rubber alone make the standing irreplaceable forest worth more than the cattle farm or soybean farm (Schwartzman and Allegretti, 1987) that might replace it, how much more valuable can green consumerism make that forest?
>
> —James A. Duke,
> *Tropical Botanical Extractives*

Consider these facts:

+ A single pond in Brazil can sustain a greater variety of fish than are found in all of Europe's rivers.

+ A twenty-five-acre plot of rainforest in Borneo may contain over 700 species of trees—a number equal to the total tree diversity of North America.

+ A single rainforest reserve in Peru is home to more species of birds than are found in the entire United States.

+ One single tree in Peru was found to harbor forty-three different species of ants—a total that approximates the entire ant species in the British Isles.

The biodiversity of the tropical rainforest is so immense that less than 1 percent of its millions of species have been studied by scientists for active constituents and their possible uses. When an acre of topical rainforest is lost, the impact to the number of plant, animal, and insect species lost and their possible uses is staggering. Scientific experts estimate that we are losing over 137 species of plants, animals, and insects every single day because of rainforest deforestation.

Scientific experts estimate that we are losing over 137 species of plants, animals, and insects every single day because of rainforest deforestation.

Surprisingly, scientists have a better understanding of how many stars there are in the galaxy than how many species there are on Earth. Estimates of global species diversity have varied from 2 million to 100 million species, with a best estimate of somewhere near 10 million, and only 1.4 million have actually been named. Today rainforests occupy only 2 percent of the entire Earth's surface and 6 percent of the world's land surface, yet these remaining lush rainforests support over half of our planet's wild plants and trees and one-half of the world's wildlife. Hundreds and thousands of these rainforest species are being extinguished before they have even been identified, much less catalogued and studied. The magnitude of this loss to the world was most poignantly described by Harvard's Pulitzer Prize–winning biologist Edward O. Wilson over a decade ago:

> The worst thing that can happen during the 1980s is not energy depletion, economic collapses, limited nuclear war, or conquest by a totalitarian government. As terrible as these catastrophes would be for us, they can be repaired within a few generations. The one process ongoing in the 1980s that will take millions of years to correct is the loss of genetic and species diversity by the destruction of natural habitats. This is the folly that our descendants are least likely to forgive us for.

Yet still the destruction continues. If deforestation continues at current rates, scientists estimate nearly 80 to 90 percent of tropical rainforest ecosystems will be destroyed by the year 2020. This destruction is the main force driving a species extinction rate unmatched in 65 million years.

THE AMAZON RAINFOREST . . . THE LAST FRONTIER ON EARTH

IF AMAZONIA WERE a country, it would be the ninth largest in the world. The Amazon rainforest, the world's greatest remaining natural resource, is the most powerful and bio-actively diverse natural phenomenon on the planet. It has been described as the "lungs of our planet" because it provides the essential environmental world service of continuously recycling carbon dioxide into oxygen. It is estimated that over 20 percent of Earth's oxygen is produced in this area.

It is estimated that over 20% of Earth's oxygen is produced in the Amazon rainforest.

The Amazon rainforest covers over 1.2 billion acres, representing two-fifths of the enormous South American continent, and is found in nine South American countries: Brazil, Colombia, Peru, Venezuela, Ecuador, Bolivia, and the three Guyanas. With 2.5 million square miles of rainforest, the Amazon rainforest represents 54 percent of the total rainforests left on the planet.

The life force of the Amazon rainforest is the mighty Amazon River. It starts as a trickle high in the snow-capped Andes Mountains and flows over 4,000 miles across the South American continent until it enters the Atlantic Ocean at Belem, Brazil, where it is 200 to 300 miles across, depending on the season. Even 1,000 miles inland it is still 7 miles in width. The river is so deep that ocean liners can travel 2,300 miles inland, up its length. The Amazon River flows through the center of the rainforest and is fed by 1,100 tributaries, 17 of which are over 1,000 miles long. The Amazon is by far the largest river system in the world, and over two-thirds of all the fresh water found on Earth is in the Amazon Basin's rivers, streams, and tributaries.

With so much water it's not unusual that the main mode of transportation throughout the area is by boat. The smallest and most common boats used today are still made out of hollowed tree trunks, whether they are powered by outboard motors or more often by human-powered paddles. Almost 14,000 miles of Amazon waterway are navigable, and several million miles through swamps and forests are penetrable by canoe. The enormous Amazon River carries massive amounts of silt from runoff from the rainforest floor. Massive amounts of silt deposited at the mouth of the Amazon River has created the largest river island in the world, Marajo Island, which is roughly the size of Switzerland. With this massive fresh water system, it not unusual that the life beneath the water is as abundant and diverse as the surrounding rainforest's plant and animal species. Over 2,000 species of fish have been identified in the Amazon Basin—more species than in the entire Atlantic Ocean.

The Amazon Basin was formed in the Paleozoic period, somewhere between 500 million and 200 million years ago. The extreme age of the region in geologic terms has much to do with the

Over two-thirds of all the fresh water found on Earth is in the Amazon Basin's rivers, streams, and tributaries.

relative infertility of the rainforest soil and the richness and unique diversity of the plant and animal life. There are more fertile areas in the Amazon River's flood plain, where the river deposits richer soil brought from the Andes, which only formed 20 million years ago. The rich diversity of plant species in the Amazon rainforest is the highest on Earth. Experts show that one hectare (2.47 acres) may contain over 750 types of trees and 1,500 species of higher plants. It is estimated that a single hectare of Amazon rainforest contains about 900 tons of living plants. Altogether it contains the largest collection of living plants and animal species in the world. The Andean mountain range and the Amazon jungle are home to more than half of the world's species of flora and fauna, and one in five of all the birds in the world live in the rainforests of the Amazon. To date, some 438,000 species of plants of economic and social interest have been registered in the region, and many more have yet to be catalogued or even discovered.

Once a vast sea of tropical forest, the Amazon rainforest today is scarred by roads, farms, ranches, and dams. Brazil is gifted with a full third of the world's remaining rainforests; unfortunately, it is also one of the world's great rainforest destroyers, burning or felling over 2.7 million acres each year. More than 20 percent of rainforest in the Amazon has been razed and is gone forever. This ocean of green, nearly as large as Australia, is the

> This century—considered to many to be an age of enlightenment, progress, and development—has witnessed more genocides, ethnocides, and extinctions of indigenous peoples than any other in history. In recent years, no groups have been more threatened than those living in the rainforests. In Brazil alone, an average of one Indian culture per year has disappeared since the turn of the century. The survival of such groups depends on the survival of the forests, and the policies and lifestyles of dominant cultures are destroying both.
>
> —Jason W. Clay,
> *Indigenous Peoples*

last great rainforest in the known universe and it is being decimated like the others before it. Why? Like other rainforests already lost forever, the land is being cleared for logging timber,
large-scale cattle ranching, mining operations, government road
building and hydroelectric schemes, military operations, and the
subsistence agriculture of peasants and landless settlers. Sadder
still, in many places the rainforests are burnt simply to provide
charcoal to power industrial plants in the area.

THE DRIVING FORCES OF DESTRUCTION

COMMERCIAL LOGGING IS the single largest cause of rainforest
destruction, both directly and indirectly. The simple fact is that
people are destroying the Amazon rainforest and the rest of the
rainforests of the world because "they can't see the forest for
the trees." Logging tropical hardwoods like teak, mahogany,
rosewood, and other timber for furniture, building materials,
charcoal, and other wood products is big business and big profits. Several species of tropical hardwoods are imported by developed counties, including the United States, just to build coffins
that are then buried or burned. The demand, extraction, and
consumption of tropical hardwoods has been so massive that
some countries that have been traditional exporters of tropical
hardwoods are now importing them because they have already
exhausted their supply by destroying their native rainforests in
slash and burn operations. It is anticipated that the Philippines,
Malaysia, the Ivory Coast, Nigeria, and Thailand will soon follow as all these countries will run out of rainforest hardwood
timber for export in less than five years. Japan is the largest im-
porter of tropical woods. Despite recent reductions, Japan's 1995
tropical timber import total of 11,695,000 cubic meters is still
gluttonous; damaging to the ecological, biological, and social
fabric of tropical lands; and clearly unsustainable for any length
of time.

Behind the hardwood logger come others down the same roads built to transport the timber. The cardboard packing and the wood chipboard industries use 15-ton machines that gobble up the rainforest with 8-foot cutting discs that have eight blades revolving 320 times a minute that cut entire trees into chips half the size of a matchbox. More than 200 species of trees can be gobbled up by these machines in mere minutes.

Logging rainforest timber is a large economic source, and in many cases the main source of revenues for servicing the national debt of developing countries. Logging profits are real to these countries who must service their debts, but they are fleeting. Governments are selling their assets too cheaply, and once the rainforest is gone, their source of income is gone. Sadly, most of the real profits of the timber trade are made not by the developing countries, but by multinational companies and industrialists of the Northern Hemisphere. These huge, profit-driven companies pay governments a fraction of the timber's worth for large logging concessions on immense tracts of rainforest land and reap huge profits by harvesting the timber in the most economical manner feasible with little regard to the destruction left in their wake. Logging concessions in the Amazon are sold for as little as $2 per acre, with logging companies felling timber worth thousands of dollars per acre. Governments are selling their natural resources, hawking for pennies resources that soon will be worth billions of dollars. Some of these government concessions and land deals made with industrialists make the sale of Manhattan for $24 worth of trinkets look shrewd. In 1986 a huge industrial timber corporation bought thousands of acres in the Borneo rainforest by giving 2,000 Malaysian dollars to twelve longhouses of local tribes. This sum amounted to the price of two bottles of beer for each member of the community. Since then, this company and others have managed to extract and destroy about a third of the

> **Logging companies reap huge profits by harvesting the timber in the most economical manner feasible with little regard to the destruction left in their wake.**

Borneo rainforest—about 6.9 million acres—and the local tribes have been evicted from the area or forced to work for the logging companies at slave wages.

In addition to being logged for exportation, rainforest wood stays in developing countries for fuel wood and charcoal. One single steel plant in Brazil making steel for Japanese cars needs millions of tons of wood each year to produce charcoal that can be used in the manufacture of steel. Then there is the paper industry. A pulpwood project in the Brazilian Amazon consists of a Japanese power plant and pulp mill. To set up this single plant operation, 5,600 square miles of Amazon rainforest was burned to the ground and replanted with pulpwood trees. This single manufacturing plant consumes 2,000 tons of surrounding rainforest wood every day to produce 55 megawatts of electricity to run the plant. The plant, which has been in operation since 1978, produces over 750 tons of pulp for paper every 24 hours, worth approximately $500,000, and has built 2,800 miles of roads through the Amazon rainforest to be used by its 700 vehicles. In addition to this pulp mill, the world's biggest pulp mill is the Aracruz mill in Brazil. Its two units produce 1 million tons of pulp a year and displaced thousands of indigenous tribes harvesting the rainforest to keep the plant in business. Where does all this pulp go? Aracruz's biggest customers are the United States, Belgium, Great Britain, and Japan. More and more rainforest is destroyed to meet the demand of the developed world's paper industry, which requires a staggering 200 million tons of wood each year simply to make paper. If the world continues at the present rate, 4 billion tons of wood is estimated to be consumed annually by the year 2020 in the paper industry alone.

Once an area of rainforest has been logged, even if given the rare chance to regrow, it can never become what it once was. The intricate ecosystem nature devised is lost forever. Only 1 to 2 percent of light at the top of a rainforest canopy manages to reach the forest floor below. Most times when timber is harvested, the plants and animals of the original forest become extinct; trees and other plants that have evolved over centuries to grow in the dark, humid environment below the canopy simply cannot live out in the open. Even if only sections of land throughout an area are destroyed, these remnants change drastically. Birds and other animals cannot cross from one remnant of land to another in the canopy, so plants are not pollinated, seeds are not dispersed by the animals, and the plants around the edges are not surrounded by the high jungle humidity they need to grow properly. As a result, the remnants slowly become degraded and die. Rains come and wash away the thin topsoil that was previously protected by the canopy, and this barren, infertile land results in erosion. Sometimes the land is replanted in African grasses for cattle operations; other times more virgin rainforest is destroyed for cattle operations because grass planted on recently burned land has a better chance to grow.

As the demand in the Western world for cheap meat increases, more and more rainforest is destroyed to provide grazing land for animals. In Brazil alone there are an estimated 220 million head of cattle, 20 million goats, 60 million pigs, and 700 million chickens. Most of Central and Latin America's tropical and temperate rainforests have been lost to cattle operations to meet the world demand, and still the cattle operations continue to move southward into the heart of the South American rainforests. To graze one steer in Amazonia takes two full acres. Most of the ranchers in the Amazon operate at a loss, yielding only paper profits purely as tax shelters. Ranchers' fortunes are made only when ranching is supported by government giveaways. A banker or rich land owner in Brazil can slash and burn a huge tract of land in the Amazon rainforest, seed it with grass for cattle, and realize millions of dollars worth of government-subsidized loans, tax credits, and write-offs in return for developing the land. These government development schemes

As the Western world's demand for cheap meat increases, more and more rainforest is destroyed to provide grazing land for animals.

rarely make a profit, actually selling cheap beef to industrialized nations. One single cattle operation in Brazil that was co-owned by British Barclays Bank and one of Brazil's wealthiest families was responsible for the destruction of almost 500,000 acres of virgin rainforest. The cattle operation never made a profit, but government write-offs sheltered huge logging profits earned off of logging other land in the Brazilian rainforest owned by the same investors. These generous tax and credit incentives have created over 29 million acres of large cattle ranches in the Brazilian Amazon, even though the typical ranch could cover less than half its costs without these subsidies.

This type of government-driven destruction of rainforest land is promoted by a common attitude among governments in rainforest regions that the forest is an economic resource to be harnessed to aid in the development of their countries. The same attitudes that accompanied the colonization of our own frontier are found today in Brazil and other countries with wild, unharnessed rainforest wilderness. These beliefs are exemplified by one Brazilian official's public statement that "not until all Amazonas is colonized by real Brazilians, not Indians, can we truly say we own it." Were we Americans any different with our own colonization, decimating the North American Indian tribes? Like Brazil, we sent out a call to all the world that America had land for the landless in an effort to increase colonization of our country at the expense of our indigenous Indian tribes. And like the first American colonists, colonization in the rainforest really means subsistence farming.

Subsistence farming has for centuries been a driving force in the loss of rainforest land. And as populations explode in third-world countries in South America and the Far East, the impact has been profound. By tradition, wildlands and unsettled lands in the rainforest are free to those who clear the forest and till the soil. "Squatter's rights" still prevail, and poor, hungry people show little enthusiasm for arguments about the value of biodiversity or the plight of endangered species when they struggle daily to feed their families. The present approach to rainforest cultivation produces wealth for a few, for a short time, because farming burned-off tracts of Amazon rainforest seldom works for long. Less than 10 percent of Amazonian soils are suitable for sustained conventional agriculture. However lush they look, rainforests often flourish on such nutrient-poor soils that they are essentially "wet deserts," easier to damage and harder to cultivate than any other soil. Most are exhausted by the time they have produced three or four crops. Many of the thousands of homesteaders who migrated from Brazil's cities to the wilds of the rainforest, responding to the government's call of "land without men for men without land," have already had to abandon their depleted farms and move on, leaving behind fields of baked clay dotted with stagnant pools of polluted water. Experts agree that the path to conservation begins with helping these local residents meet their own daily needs. Because of the infertility of the soil, and the lack of knowledge of sustainable cultivation practices, this type of agriculture strips the soil of nutrients within a few harvests and the farmers continue to move farther into the rainforest in search of new land. They must be helped and educated to break free of the need to continually clear rainforest in search of fresh, fertile land if the rainforest is to be saved.

Directly and indirectly, the leading threats to rainforest ecosystems are governments and their unbridled, unplanned, and uncoordinated development of natural resources. Rainforest timber exports and large-scale development projects go a long way in servicing national debt in many developing countries, which is why governments and international aid-lending institutions like the World Bank support them. In the tropics governments own or control nearly 80 percent of tropical forests, so these forests stand or fall according to government policy; and in many countries, government policies lie behind the wastage of forest resources. Besides the tax incentives and credit subsidies that guarantee large profits to private investors who convert forests to pastures and farms, governments allow private concessionaires to log the national forests on terms that induce uneconomic or wasteful uses of the public domain. Massive public expenditures on highways, dams, plantations, and agricultural settlements, too often supported by multilateral development lending, convert or destroy large areas of forest for projects of questionable economic worth.

Tropical countries are among the poorest countries on Earth. Brazil alone spends 40 percent of its annual income simply servicing its loans, and the per capita income of Brazil's people is less than $2,000 annually. Sadly, these numbers don't even represent an accurate picture in the Amazon because Brazil is one of the richer countries in South America. These struggling Amazonian countries must also manage the most complex, delicate, and valuable forests remaining on the planet, and the economic and technological resources available to them are limited. They must also endure a dramatic social and economic situation, as well as deeply adverse terms of trade and financial relationships with industrial countries. Under such conditions, the possibility of them reaching sustainable models of development alone is virtually nil.

There is a clear need for industrial countries to sincerely and effectively assist the tropics in a quest for sustainable forest management and development if the remaining rainforests are to be saved. The governments of these developing countries need help in learning how to manage and protect their natural resources for long-term profits while still managing to service their debts, and they must be given the incentives and tools to do so. Programs to redefine the timber concessions so concessionaires have greater incentives to guard the long-term health of the forest and programs to revive and expand community-based forestry schemes, which ensure more rational use of forests and a better life for the people who live near them, must be developed. First-world capital must seek out opportunities to partner with

...nizations that have the technical expertise to guide these ...grams of sustainable economic development. In addition, programs teaching techniques for sustainable harvesting practices and identifying profitable, yet sustainable, forest products can enable developing countries to improve the standard of living for its people, service national debt, and contribute meaningfully to the country's land use planning and conservation of natural resources.

RAINFORESTS, PHARMACY TO THE WORLD

IT IS ESTIMATED that nearly half of the world's estimated 10 million species of plants, animals, and microorganisms will be destroyed or severely threatened over the next quarter-century due to rainforest deforestation. Harvard's Pulitzer Prize–winning biologist Edward O. Wilson estimates that we are losing 137 plant, animal, and insect species every single day. That's 50,000 species a year! Again, why should we in the United States be concerned about the destruction of distant tropical rainforests? Because rainforest plants are complex chemical storehouses that contain many undiscovered biodynamic compounds with unrealized potential for use in modern medicine. We can gain access to these materials only if we study and conserve the species that contain them. Rainforests currently provide sources for one-fourth of today's medicines, and 70 percent of the plants found to have anticancer properties are found only in the rainforest. The rainforest and its immense undiscovered biodiversity hold the key to unlocking tomorrow's cures for devastating diseases. How many cures for devastating disease have we already lost?

> **Pulitzer Prize–winning biologist Edward O. Wilson estimates that we are losing 137 plant, animal, and insect species every single day. That's 50,000 species a year!**

Two drugs obtained from a rainforest plant known as the Madagascar periwinkle, now extinct in the wild due to deforestation of the Madagascar rainforest, have increased the chances of survival for children with leukemia from 20 percent to 80 percent. Think about it: eight out of ten children are now saved, rather than eight of ten children dying from leukemia. How many children have been spared and how many more will continue to be spared because of this single rainforest plant? What if we failed to discover this one important plant among millions before it was extinct due to human destruction? When our remaining rainforests are gone, the rare plants and animals will be lost forever, and so will their possible cures for diseases like cancer.

No one can challenge the fact that we are still largely dependent on plants for treating our ailments. Almost 90 percent of people in developing countries still rely on traditional medicine—based largely on species of plants and animals—for their primary health care. In the United States some 25 percent of prescriptions are filled with drugs whose active ingredients are extracted or derived from plants. Sales of these plant-based drugs in the United States amounted to some $4.5 billion in 1980. Worldwide sales of these plant-based drugs were estimated at $40 billion in 1990. Still more drugs are derived from animals and microorganisms. Currently 121 prescription drugs sold worldwide come from plant-derived sources from only 90 species of plants.

The U.S. National Cancer Institute has identified over 3,000 plants that are active against cancer cells, and 70 percent of these plants are found only in the rainforest. More than 25 percent of the active ingredients in today's cancer-fighting drugs come from organisms found only in the rainforest. Among the thousands of species of rainforest plants that have not been analyzed are many more thousands of unknown plant chemicals, many of which have evolved to protect the plants from diseases. These plant chemicals may well help us in our own ongoing struggle with constantly evolving pathogens such as bacteria-resistant pathogens in tuberculosis, measles, and HIV. Experts now believe that if there is a

More than 25 percent of the active ingredients in today's cancer-fighting drugs come from organisms found only in the rainforest.

cure for cancer and even AIDS, it will probably be found in the rainforest.

In 1983 there were no U.S. pharmaceutical manufacturers involved in research programs to discover new drugs or cures from plants. Today over 100 pharmaceutical companies and several branches of the U.S. government, including giants like Merck, Abbott, Bristol-Myers Squibb, Eli Lilly, Monsanto, Smith-Kline Beecham, and the National Cancer Institute are engaged in plant-based research projects for possible drugs and cures for viruses, infections, cancer, and AIDS. Most of this research is currently taking place in the rainforest in an industry that is now called "bioprospecting." This new pharmacological industry draws together an unlikely confederacy: plant collectors and anthropologists; ecologists and conservationists; natural product companies and nutritional supplement manufacturers; AIDS and cancer researchers; executives in the world's largest drug companies; and native indigenous shamans. They are part of a radical experiment: to preserve the world's rainforests by showing how much more valuable they are standing than cut down. And it is a race against a clock whose every tick means another acre of charred forest. Yet it is also a race that pits one explorer against another, for those who score the first big hit in chemical bio-prospecting will secure wealth and a piece of scientific immortality.

In November 1991 Merck Pharmaceutical Company announced a landmark agreement to obtain samples of wild plants and animals for drug-screening purposes from Costa Rica's National Biodiversity Institute (INBio). Spurred by this and other biodiversity prospecting ventures, interest in the commercial value of plant genetic and biochemical resources is burgeoning today. While the Merck–INBio agreement provides a fascinating example of a private partnership that contributes to rural economic development, rainforest conservation, and technology transfer, virtually no precedent exists for national policies and legislation to govern and regulate what amounts to a brand new industry.

Since wealth and technology are as contrated in the North as biodiversity and poverty are in the South, the question of equity is particularly hard to answer in ways that satisfy everyone with a stake in the outcome. The interests of bioprospecting corporations are not the same as those of people who live in a biodiversity "hot spot," many of them barely eking out a living. As the search for wild species whose genes can yield new medicines and better crops gathers momentum, these rich habitats also sport more and more bioprospectors. Like the nineteenth-century California gold rush or its present-day counterpart in Brazil, this "gene rush" could wreak havoc on ecosystems and the people living in or near them. Done properly, however, bioprospecting can bolster both economic and conservation goals while underpinning the medical and agricultural advances needed to combat disease and sustain growing populations.

The majority of our current plant-derived drugs were discovered through the traditional uses of plants by the indigenous people where they grew and flourished. History has shown that the situation with the rainforest is no different, and bioprospectors now are working side by side with rainforest tribal shamans and herbal healers to learn the wealth of their plant knowledge and many uses of indigenous plants.

UNLOCKING THE SECRETS OF THE RAINFOREST

AFTER THE AMERINDIANS discovered America, about twenty millennia before Columbus, all their clothing, food, medicine, and shelter were derived from the forests. Those millennia gave the Indians time to discover and learn empirically the virtues and vices of the thousands of edible and medicinal species in the rainforest. More than 80 percent of the developed world's diet originated in the rainforest and from this empirical indigenous knowledge of the wealth of edible fruits, vegetables, and nuts. Of the estimated 3,000 edible fruits found in the rainforest, only 200 are cultivated for use today, despite the fact that the Indians use more than 1,500. Many secrets and untold treasures await discovery with the medicinal plants used by shamans, healers, and the indigenous people of the rainforest tribes. Long regarded as hocus-pocus by science, indigenous peoples' empirical plant knowledge is now thought by many to be the Amazon's new gold. This indigenous use of the plants provides the bioprospector with the necessary clues to target specific species to research in the race for time before the species are lost to deforestation. More often, the race is defined as being the first company to patent a new drug utilizing a newly discovered rainforest phytochemical—and, of course, profits for the pharmaceutical companies.

Laboratory syntheses of new medicines is increasingly costly and not as fruitful as companies would like. In the words of one major drug company: "Scientists may be able to make any molecule they can imagine on a computer, but Mother Nature . . . is an infinitely more ingenious and exciting chemist." Scientists have developed new technologies to assess the chemical makeup of plants, and they realize using medicinal plants identified by Indians makes research more efficient and less expensive. With these new trends, drug development has actually returned to its roots: traditional medicine. It is now understood by bioprospectors that tribal people of the rainforest represent the key to finding new and useful tropical forest plants. The degree to which they understand and are able sustainably to use this diversity is astounding. A single Amazonian tribe of Indians may use over 200 species of plants for medicinal purposes alone.

Of the 121 pharmaceutical drugs that are plant-derived today, 74 percent were discovered through follow-up research to verify the authenticity of information concerning the ethnic medical uses of the plant. Nevertheless, to this day, very few rainforest tribes have been subjected to a complete ethnobotanical analysis. Robert Goodland of the World Bank wrote, "Indigenous knowledge is

> Long regarded as hocus-pocus by science, indigenous peoples' empirical plant knowledge is now thought by many to be the Amazon's new gold.

essential for the use, identification and cataloguing of the [tropical] biota. As tribal groups disappear, their knowledge vanishes with them. The preservation of these groups is a significant economic opportunity for the [developing] nation, not a luxury."

Since Amazonian Indians are often the only ones who know both the properties of these plants and how they can best be used, their knowledge is now being considered an essential component of all efforts to conserve and develop the rainforest. Since failure to document this lore would represent a tremendous economic and scientific loss to the industrialized world, the bioprospectors are now are working side by side with the rainforest tribal shamans and herbal healers to learn the wealth of their plant knowledge. But bioprospecting has a dark side. Indian knowledge that has resisted the pressure of "modernization" is being used by bioprospectors who, like oil companies and loggers destroying the forests, threaten to leave no benefits behind them.

It's a noble idea, the ethnobotanist who works with the Indians seeking a cure for cancer or even AIDS, like Sean Connery in the movie *Medicine Man*. Yet behind this lurks a system that, at its worst, steals the Indian knowledge to benefit CEOs, stockholders, and academic careers and reputations. The real goal of these powerful bioprospectors is to target novel and active phytochemicals with medical applications, synthesize them in a laboratory, and have them patented for subsequent drug manufacture and resulting profits. In this process many active and beneficial plants have been found in the shaman's medicine chest, only to be discarded when it was found that the active ingredients of the plant numbered too many to be cost-effectively synthesized into a patentable drug. It doesn't matter how active or beneficial the plant is or how long the FDA process might take to patent and approve the new drug; if the bioprospector can't capitalize on it, the public will rarely hear about a newly discovered plant's benefits. The fact is, there is a lot of money at stake. In an article published in *Economic Botany*, Dr. Robert Mendelsohn, an economist at Yale

University, and Dr. Michael J. Balick, director of the Institute of Economic Botany at the New York Botanical Gardens, estimate the minimum number of pharmaceutical drugs potentially remaining to be extracted from the rainforests. It is staggering! They estimate that there are at least 328 new drugs that still await discovery in the rainforest, with a potential value of $3 billion to $4 billion to a private pharmaceutical company and as much as $147 billion to society as a whole.

While the indigenous Indian shamans go about their daily lives caring for the well-being of their tribe, thousands of miles away in U.S. laboratories, the shaman's rainforest medicines are being tested, synthesized, patented, and submitted for FDA approval. Soon children with viral infections, adults with herpes, cancer patients, and many others may benefit from new medicines from the Amazon rainforest. But what will the indigenous tribes see of these wonderful new medicines? As corporations rush to patent indigenous medicinal knowledge, the originating indigenous communities have received few, if any, benefits.

> **As corporations rush to patent indigenous medicinal knowledge, the originating indigenous communities have received few, if any, benefits.**

LOSING THE KNOWLEDGE

THE DESTRUCTION OF the rainforest has followed the pattern of seeing natural land and natural world peoples as resources to be used, and seeing wilderness as idle, empty, and unproductive. Destruction of our rainforests is not only causing the extinction of plant and animal species; it is also wiping out indigenous peoples who live in the rainforest. Obviously, rainforests are not idle land, nor are they uninhabited. Indigenous peoples have developed technologies and resource use systems that have allowed them to live on the land, farming, hunting, and gathering in a complex sustainable relationship with the forest. But when rainforests die, so do the indigenous peoples.

In 1500 there were an estimated 6 million to 9 million indigenous people inhabiting the rainforests in Brazil. When Western and European cultures were drawn to Brazil's Amazon in the hopes of finding riches beyond comprehension and artifacts from civilizations that have long since expired with the passage of time, they left behind decimated cultures in their ravenous wake. By 1900 there were only 1 million indigenous people left in Brazil's Amazon. Although the fabled Fountain of Youth was never discovered, many treasures in gold and gems were spirited away by the more successful invaders of the day, and the indigenous inhabitants of the rainforest bore the brunt of these marauding explorers and *conquistadores*.

Today there are less than 250,000 indigenous people of Brazil surviving this catastrophe, and still it continues. These surviving indigenous people still demonstrate the remarkable diversity of the rainforest because they comprise 215 ethnic groups with 170 different languages. They live in 526 territories nationwide, which together comprise an area of 190 million acres . . . twice the size of California. About 188 million acres of this land is inside the Brazilian Amazon, in the states of Acre, Amapa, Amazonas, Maranhao, Mato Grosso, Para, Rondonia, Roraima, and Tocantins. There may also be 50 or more indigenous groups still living in the depths of the rainforest that have never had contact with the outside world.

Throughout the rainforest, forest-dwelling peoples whose age-old traditions allow them to live in and off the forest without destroying it are losing out to cattle ranching, logging, hydroelectric projects, large-scale farms, mining, and colonization schemes. About half of the original Amazonian tribes have already been completely destroyed. The greatest threat to Brazil's remaining tribal people, most of whom live in the Amazon rainforest, is the invasion of their territory by these ranchers, miners, and land speculators and the conflicts that follow. In Amazonia thousands of peasants, rubber tappers, and indigenous tribes have been killed in the past decade in violent conflicts over forest resources and land.

As their homelands continue to be invaded and destroyed, rainforest people and their cultures are disappearing. When these indigenous peoples are lost forever, gone too will be their empirical knowledge representing centuries of accumulated knowledge of the medicinal value of rainforest plant and animal species. Very few tribes have been subjected to a complete ethnobotanical analysis of their plant knowledge, and most medicine men and shamans remaining in the rainforests today are seventy years old or more.

> **When a medicine man dies without passing his arts on to the next generation, the tribe and the world lose thousands of years of irreplaceable knowledge about medicinal plants.**

When a medicine man dies without passing his arts on to the next generation, the tribe and the world lose thousands of years of irreplaceable knowledge about medicinal plants. Each time a rainforest medicine man dies, it is as if a library has burned down.

THE SOLUTION: PROFITS WITHOUT PLUNDER

THE PROBLEM AND the solution of the destruction of the rainforest are both economic. Governments need money to service their debts, squatters and settlers need money to feed their families, and companies need to make profits. The simple fact is that the rainforest is being destroyed for the income and profits it yields, however fleeting. Money still makes the world go around . . . even in South America and even in the rainforest.

But this also means that if land owners, governments, and those living in the rainforest today were given a viable economic reason *not* to destroy the rainforest, it could and would be saved. And this viable economic alternative *does* exist, and it is working today. Many organizations have demonstrated that if the medicinal plants, fruits, nuts, oils, and other resources like rubber, chocolate, and chicle (used to make chewing gums) are harvested sustainably, rainforest land has much more economic value today and more long-term income and profits than if just timber is harvested or if it is burned down for cattle or farming operations. In fact, the latest statistics prove that rainforest land converted to cattle operations yields the land owner $60 per acre; if timber is harvested, the land is worth $400 per acre. However, if these renewable and sustainable resources are harvested, the land will yield the land owner $2,400 per acre. This value provides an income not only today, but year after year—for generations. These sustainable resources—not the trees—are the true wealth of the rainforest.

This is no longer a theory. It is a fact, and it is being implemented today. Just as important, to wild-harvest the wealth of sustainable rainforest resources effectively, local people and indigenous tribes must be employed. Today entire communities and tribes earn five to ten times more money in wild-harvesting medicinal plants, fruits, nuts, and oils than they can earn by chopping down the forest for subsistence crops. This much-needed income source creates the awareness and economic incentive for this population in the rainforest to protect and preserve the forests for long-term profits for themselves and their children and is an important solution in saving the rainforest from destruction.

Today entire communities and tribes earn five to ten times more money in wild-harvesting medicinal plants, fruits, nuts, and oils than they can earn by chopping down the forest for subsistence crops.

When the timber is harvested for short-term gain and profits, the medicinal plants, nuts, oils, and other important sustainable resources that thrive in this delicate ecosystem are destroyed. The real solution to saving the rainforest is to make its inhabitants see the forest *and* the trees by creating a consumer demand and consumer markets for these sustainable rainforest products . . . markets that are larger and louder than today's tropical timber market . . . markets that will put as much money in their pockets and government coffers as the timber companies do . . . markets that will give them the economic incentive to protect their sustainable resources for long-term profits rather than short-term gain.

This is the only solution that makes a real impact, and it can make a real difference. Each and every person here in America can take a part in this solution by helping to create this consumer market and demand for sustainable rainforest products. By purchasing renewable and sustainable rainforest products and resources and demanding sustainable harvesting of these resources utilizing local communities and indigenous tribes of the rainforests, we all can be part of the solution, and the rainforests of the world and their people can be saved.

Part Two

Medicinal Plants of the Rainforest

ABUTA

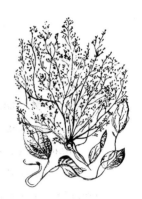

Family: Menispermaceae

Genus: *Cissampelos*

Species: *pareira*

Common Names: Abuta, abutua, barbasco, imchich masha, butua, false pareira, pareira, aristoloche lobee, bejuco de raton, feuille coeur, liane patte cheval, gasing-gasing

Parts Used: Whole vine, seed, bark, leaf

Medicinal Properties: Analgesic, anticarcinomic, anti-inflammatory, anti-leukemic, antiseptic, antispasmodic, aperient, diuretic, emmenagogue, expectorant, febrifuge, hepatoprotective, hypotensive, piscicide, purgative, stimulant, stomachic, tonic

BUTA IS A woody, climbing vine with leaves up to 30 cm long. It produces inedible, dark, grape-sized berries. It belongs to the genus *Cissampelos,* in which there are 30 to 40 species of vines. Abuta vine is blackish-brown and tough and when freshly cut has a waxy luster. Abuta is found throughout the Amazon in Peru, Brazil, Ecuador, and Colombia and is cultivated by many people to beautify their gardens.

Abuta is commonly referred to as the "midwives' herb" throughout South America due to its long history of use for all types of women's ailments. It has been used by indigenous peoples throughout the South American rainforest for thousands of years and is still in use today. The Palikur tribe in Guyana use a poultice of abuta leaves as a topical analgesic, and the Wayãpi Indians use the decoction of leaf and stem as an oral analgesic. Ecuadorean Ketchwa tribes use the leaf decoction for conjunctivitis and snakebite. Indigenous tribes in Peru use the seeds of abuta for snakebite, as a diuretic, as an expectorant, and for fevers and venereal disease. Amazonian herbal healers and shamans, called *curanderos,* toast the seeds of abuta and then brew it into tea to treat internal hemorrhages and external bleeding; they brew a leaf tea for rheumatism and a vine wood and bark tea to treat irregular heartbeat. In their book *Medical Botany,* Walter and Memory Lewis state, "*Cissampelos pareira* roots are used in tropical countries to prevent a threatened miscarriage. The herb is also used to stop uterine hemorrhages." Midwives in the Amazon still carry abuta with them for menstrual cramps and pre- and postnatal pain and uterine hemorrhaging. Abuta is widely employed in Brazilian herbal medicine today as a diuretic, tonic, and febrifuge used for menstrual cramps, difficult menstruation, pre- and postnatal pain, colic, constipation, blennorrhagia, poor digestion, and dyspepsia.

Midwives in the Amazon still carry abuta with them for menstrual cramps and pre- and postnatal pain and uterine hemorrhaging.

The genus *Cissampelos* contains alkaloids characteristic of other members of the family Menispermaceae. Saponins and sterols are common; occasional triterpenes, ethereal oils, polyterpenes, and polyphenols also are present. It is the alkaloids, however, that have received the most attention and research. Abuta contains the alkaloid tetrandrine, which has been documented to be an analgesic, anti-inflammatory, and febrifuge and has recently been shown to have antitumor and antileukemic properties as well.[1] It also contains an alkaloid called berberine, which has been documented to be hypotensive, antifungal, antitumorous, and antimicrobial and is used for the treatment of cardiac arrhythmia, cancer, candidiasis, diarrhea, and irritable bowel syndrome.[2] Cissampeline, another alkaloid found in abuta, is sold as a skeletal-muscle-relaxant drug in Ecuador; other alkaloids in abuta have documented neuromuscular blocking action.[3] In reviews of the alkaloids in general, the aporphine alkaloids and their role in the preparation of arrow poisons called *curares* have been well documented.[4-6]

Phytochemical analysis shows that abuta is a rich source of these alkaloids, which Western scientists began researching in the mid-1960s.[7–10] In addition to tetrandrine, abuta contains palmatine, hayatinin, and other berberine derivatives.[11] In more recent research, the bisbenzylisoquinoline alkaloids have demonstrated to be the anti-inflammatory constituents of abuta. In clinical experiments these alkaloids suppressed the production of nitric oxide, a critical mediator in inflammation, which explains some aspects of the anti-inflammatory mechanisms of abuta.[12] Additionally, according to two 1993 studies, abuta contains tropoloisoquinoline alkaloids, pareirubrines A and B, which have been isolated as alkaloids with antileukemic properties.[13, 14]

Today, abuta is still used in the Amazon and outlying areas for the same purposes for which it has been used traditionally. South and North American natural health practitioners still commonly rely on abuta as an excellent natural remedy to help relieve symptoms associated with menstruation, to help balance female hormones, and to help with high blood pressure. Documented uses in traditional medicine today show that abuta is used for diuretic, expectorant, emmenagogue, and febrifuge purposes. It is a common Brazilian remedy to prevent threatened abortion, relieve menorrhagia, and arrest uterine hemorrhages. It is also used in homeopathy in the form of a mother tincture. Other recent reported uses in herbal medicine in North America include relief for inflammation of the testicles and minor kidney problems.

> South and North American natural health practitioners still rely on abuta as a natural remedy to help relieve symptoms associated with menstruation, to help balance female hormones, and to help with high blood pressure.

Despite its strong taste, abuta has been traditionally prepared as leaf, vine, bark, and/or root decoctions and macerations mixed with other ingredients. It can be administered orally or applied topically directly to affected areas (for example, for snakebites).

The traditional natural remedy for menstrual disorders and pain is generally 1 to 2 g daily of the powdered vine or root, or 1 to 2 ml of a 4:1 tincture daily in divided doses.

WORLDWIDE USES

Region	Uses
Guatemala	Antidote, erysipelas, fever, snakebite
India	Boil, bronchitis, burn, chill, cholera, cold, convulsion, delirium, diarrhea, dog bite, dysentery, epilepsy, eye, gravel, hematuria, madness, pimples, rabies, stomachache
Mexico	Bladder, diuretic, dropsy, emmenagogue, expectorant, fever, jaundice, leucorrhea, nephritis, poultice, rheumatism, snakebite, tonic, urogenital
Panama	Snakebite
Trinidad	Boil, diabetes, hypertension, palpitation
Venezuela	Bladder, calculus, diuretic, kidney, snakebite
Elsewhere	Anabolic, antiecbolic, aphrodisiac, asthma, cough, cystitis, diarrhea, diuretic, dropsy, dyspepsia, emmenagogue, expectorant, febrifuge, hemorrhage, hypertension, itch, lithontriptic, malaria, menorrhagia, parturition, piscicide, purgative, snakebite, sore, stimulant, styptic, tonic, urogenital

PHYTOCHEMICALS

(+)-curine, (++)-curine-4'-methyl-ether, 4-O-methylcurine, alkaloids, berberine, cissamine, cissampareine, cyclanoline, cycleanine, D-quercitol, EO, hayatidine, hayatine, hayatinine, isochondodendrine, menismine, parierine, pelosine, quercitol, saponin, tetrandrine, tetrandrine-N-2'-oxide

ACEROLA

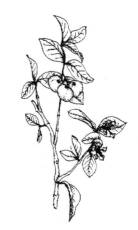

Family: Malpighiaceae

Genus: *Malpighia*

Species: *glabra*

Common Names: Acerola, cereso, Barbados cherry, Antilles cherry

Parts Used: Fruit, leaves

Medicinal Properties: Antioxidant, astringent, nutritive

CEROLA IS A small tree or shrub that grows up to 5 m high in the dry, deciduous forest. It produces an abundance of bright red fruit 1 to 2 cm in diameter, with several small seeds that look similar to the European cherry. For this reason, acerola is also known as Antilles cherry or Barbados cherry. The mature fruits are juicy and soft with a pleasant tart flavor. They contain about 80% juice and a large amount of vitamin C, as well as iron, calcium, and phosphorus. Acerola can be found growing wild and under cultivation on the sandy soils throughout northeastern Brazil. It is native to the West Indies and is also found in northern South America, Central America, and Jamaica.

The vitamin C content of acerola varies depending on ripeness, season, climate, and locality.[1, 2] As the fruit begins to ripen, it loses a great deal of its vitamin content; for this reason most commercially harvested acerola is harvested green. Until camu-camu appeared on the scene, acerola was considered the richest known source of natural vitamin C.[5] For example, oranges provide 500 to 4,000 ppm vitamin C or ascorbic acid, while acerola has assayed in a range of 16,000 to 172,000 ppm ascorbic acid.[3, 4]

Acerola can contain up to 4.5% vitamin C, compared to 0.05% in a peeled orange. Compared to oranges, acerola provides twice as much magnesium, pantothenic acid, and potassium. Other vitamins present include vitamin A (4,300 to 12,500 IU/100 g, compared to approximately 11,000 IU for raw carrots), thiamine, riboflavin, and niacin in concentrations comparable to those in other fruits.

> **Acerola can contain up to 4.5% vitamin C, compared to 0.05% in a peeled orange. Compared to oranges, acerola provides twice as much magnesium, pantothenic acid, and potassium.**

Acerola's Western use is mostly associated with its high content of vitamin C, which has come under a great deal of recent attention as a free radical scavenger due to its antioxidant properties. The leaves, bark, and fruit of acerola have also demonstrated active antifungal properties in laboratory tests.[5] Dried acerola fruit extracts can now be found in many over-the-counter

It has often been said that tropical rainforests are the richest ecosystems on Earth, but just how rich is only beginning to be appreciated. Terry Erwin, of the Smithsonian Institution, has investigated canopy communities and produced some amazing estimates for the number of Earth's insect species. Extrapolations from his quantitative collections suggest that between 10 million and 30 million yet-to-be-discovered insect species live in canopy trees. Presently, fewer than 2 million plant and animal species have been described by science. The rainforest contains up to 95 percent of the planet's species, two-thirds of which are in the canopy, but it remains a virtually unstudied ecosystem.

—Donald R. Perry, *Tropical Biology*

supplements in the United States as a natural form of vitamin C in multivitamins. Recent research in cosmetology indicates that vitamin C is a powerful antioxidant and free radical scavenger for the skin as well, and acerola extracts are now appearing in skin care products that fight cellular aging. In addition to its vitamin content, acerola contains mineral salts that have shown to aid in the remineralization of tired and stressed skin, while the mucilage and proteins have skin hydrating properties and promote capillary conditioning.

In the rainforest, acerola juice is used for fevers and dysentery, generally taken daily as 1/2 cup of juice or a handful of the fresh fruits 2 to 3 times daily. In North America, normally a dried juice powder extract is used for its natural vitamin C content.

WORLDWIDE USES

Region	Uses
Guatemala	Diarrhea, liqueur
Mexico	Astringent, fever
Venezuela	Breast, dysentery, tenesmus
Elsewhere	Astringent, diarrhea, dysentery, hepatitis

PHYTOCHEMICALS

ascorbic acid, calcium, dextrose, fructose, iron, l-malic acid, magnesium, niacin, pantothenic acid, phosphorus, potassium, protein, riboflavin, sucrose, thiamin

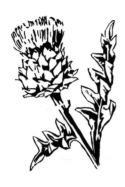

ALCACHOFRA Artichoke

Family: Asteraceae

Genus: *Cynara*

Species: *scolymus*

Common Names: Artichoke, alcachofra, alcachofera, artichaut, tyosen-azami

Part Used: Leaves

Medicinal Properties: Cholagogue, choleretic, choliokinetic, depurative, detoxifier, diuretic, hepatoprotective, hypocholesterolemic, hypotensive, stimulant, tonic

ALCACHOFRA IS THE Brazilian name for the globe artichoke. A member of the milk thistle family, it grows to a height of about 2 m and produces a large violet-green flower head. The flower petals and fleshy flower bottoms are eaten as a vegetable throughout the world, which has led to its commercial cultivation in many parts of South and North America as well as Europe. The artichoke was used as a food and medicine by the ancient Egyptians, Greeks, and Romans, and in Rome artichokes were an important menu item at feasts. It wasn't until the fifteenth century, however, that they made their appearance in Europe.

The artichoke is popular for its pleasant bitter taste, which is attributed to the phytochemicals cynaropicrin and cynarin found in the green parts of the plants. These chemicals are called sesquiterpene lactones, which have documented biologically active properties. The phytochemicals in alcachofra have been well documented,[1–5] and the leaves have been found to possess greater medicinal value than the flowers. The biological activity of the leaves is attributed to the presence of caffeoylquinic acids and acid derivatives, cynarin, and luteolin.[1] Artichoke leaf extracts have demonstrated a beneficial effect on the gallbladder and the ability to stimulate the secretion of bile in the liver, to detoxify the liver, and to lower the level of cholesterol in the blood.[6] In addition, other compounds in the leaves have been shown to possess a hypoglycemic effect.[7]

Cynarin, the main constituent in alcachofra, has shown highly specific properties as a cholagogue (increases bile production in the liver), choleretic (increases the flow of bile from the gallbladder), and choliokinetic (increases the contractive power of the bile duct).[8, 9] In animal studies its cholagogue effects are the most notable, demonstrating an ability to increase the flow of bile by 60%[10] to up to 400% in a 12-hour period.[8] In addition, artichoke has demonstrated lipid-producing and anticholesterolemic action by decreasing the rate of cholesterol synthesis in the liver and by mobilizing fat stores from the liver and other tissues, such as white adipose tissue.[8] Artichoke is also thought to reduce blood fats such as triglycerides.[8]

> **Artichoke leaf extracts have demonstrated a beneficial effect on the gallbladder and the ability to stimulate the secretion of bile in the liver, to detoxify the liver, and to lower the level of cholesterol in the blood.**

Alcachofra has been used in traditional medicine for centuries as a specific liver and gallbladder remedy, as well as a snakebite remedy.[11, 12] Its liver detoxifying and protective properties were the first to come to the attention of researchers in 1966, and investigations are still being conducted on alcachofra leaf's beneficial pharmacological effects on liver and gallbladder functions.[13–18] A French patent describes an artichoke extract for treating liver disease, high cholesterol levels, and kidney insufficiency.

Artichoke's current uses in natural medicine around the world include treatment of all types of liver and gallbladder disorders and prevention of gallstones, liver diseases (including those related to alcoholism), dyspepsia, chronic albuminuria, anemia, arteriosclerosis, diabetes, high cholesterol, and kidney disease.[8, 10]

Practitioners typically use 3 to 5 g daily of artichoke leaves as a natural remedy for digestive, gallbladder, and liver problems as well as high cholesterol. Relatively new in U.S. health food stores (and becoming more popular) are 4:1 extracts and concentrated extracts standardized to the cynarin content that are sold in capsules.

WORLDWIDE USES

Region	Uses
Dominican Republic	Cholagogue
Europe	Cancer
Haiti	Diuretic, hydropsy, hypertension, liver, uremia
Mexico	Calculus, cystitis, hypertension, liver
Elsewhere	Diabetes, diuretic, dropsy, rheumatism, tonic

PHYTOCHEMICALS

ascorbic acid, beta-carotene, beta-selinene, beta-sitosterol, boron, caffeic acid, caffeoyl-4-quinic acid, caffeoylquinic acids (7 types), calcium, caryophyllene, chlorogenic acid, cyanidol glucosides, cynaragenin, cynarapicrin, cynaratriol, cynarin, cynarolide, decanal, eugenol, ferulic acid, flavonoids, folacin, glyceric acid, glycolic acid, heteroside-B, inulin, iron, isoamerboin, lauric acid, linoleic acid, linolenic acid, luteolin glucosides, magnesium, manganese, mufa, myristic acid, neochlorogenic acid, niacin, oleic acid, palmitic acid, pantothenic acid, phenyl-acetaldehyde, phosphorus, potassium, protein, pseudotaraxasterol, pufa, riboflavin, scolymo-side, stearic acid, stigmasterol, tannin, taraxasterol, thiamin, vitamin B6, zinc

AMOR SECO

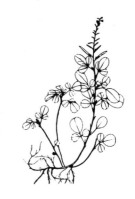

Family: Fabaceae

Genus: *Desmodium*

Species: *adscendens*

Common Names: Amor seco, strong back, carrapicho, pega pega, margarita, burbur, manayupa, hard man, hard stick, mundubirana, barba de boi, mundurana, owono-bocon, dipinda dimukuyi, dusa karnira

Parts Used: Aerial parts, leaves

Medicinal Properties: Antianaphylactic, antiasthmatic, antihistamine, anti–inflammatory, antispasmodic, bronchodilator, depurative, diuretic, laxative, vulnerary

A MOR SECO IS a multibranched, weedy, perennial herb that grows 50 cm tall and produces numerous light purple flowers and small, green fruits in 3-cm-long beanlike pods. It is indigenous to many tropical countries and grows in open forests, pastures, and yards and along roadsides.

Tribes in the Amazon rainforest use amor seco medicinally today much as they have for centuries. The plant is infused in water and given to people who suffer from nervousness, and it is used in baths to treat vaginal infections. Some tribes believe the plant has magic powers, and it is taken by lovers to rekindle a waning romance. Rio Pastaza natives in the Amazon brew a leaf tea and wash the breasts of dry mothers with it to promote lactation. Other Amazon tribes use amor seco as a contraceptive. Additional indigenous tribal uses include a leaf decoction for consumption, an application of pounded leaves and lime juice for wounds, and a leaf infusion for convulsions and venereal sores. An ethnobotanical survey interviewing over 8,000 natives in various parts of Brazil showed that a decoction of the dried roots of amor seco is a popular tribal remedy for malaria.[1] The indigenous Garifuna tribe in

Nicaragua uses a leaf decoction of amor seco internally for diarrhea, for venereal disease, and to aid digestion.[2]

Amor seco is also quite popular in herbal medicine throughout South and Central America. In Peruvian herbal medicine today, a leaf tea is used as a blood cleanser, to detoxify the body from environmental toxins and chemicals, as a urinary tract cleanser, and to treat ovarian and uterine problems such as inflammation and irritation, vaginal discharges, and hemorrhages. In Belize (where the plant is called "strong back") the entire plant is soaked in rum for 24 hours, and then 1/4 cup is taken 3 times daily for 7 to 10 days for backache. Alternatively, an entire plant is boiled in 3 cups of water for 10 minutes, and 1 cup of warm tea is taken before meals for 3 to 5 days for relief of backache, muscle pains, kidney ailments, and impotence. In Brazilian herbal medicine the dried leaves are used for the treatment of leucorrhea, body aches and pains, blennorrhagia, and diarrhea. In Ghana a leaf decoction is taken for constipation, dysentery, and colic and is also used to dress wounds. [3]

Herbalists in Ghana have long used amor seco leaves to treat bronchial asthma. The treatment has been so successful that scientists became interested in clinically testing this natural remedy.

> **Herbalists in Ghana have long used amor seco leaves to treat bronchial asthma. The treatment has been so successful that scientists became interested in clinically testing this natural remedy.**

In 1977 a small, open clinical observatory study on humans showed that 1 to 2 tsp of dried amor seco leaf powder given in 3 divided dosages daily produced improvement and remission in most asthma patients treated.[3, 4] In an effort to understand the mechanism of action of this effective natural remedy, scientists conducted animal studies to determine its antiasthmatic properties. Subsequent animal studies with guinea pigs showed that aqueous or ethanolic extracts of amor seco taken orally reduced anaphylactic contraction, interfered with histamine-induced contractions, and reduced the amount of smooth-muscle-stimulating substances released from lung tissue.[5–9] Further studies with guinea pigs showed that amor seco leaf extract caused a dose-dependent reduction in the amount of spasmogens released anaphylactically and an anaphylactic-induced contraction of ileal muscle.[10–13] These actions were cited as the basis for the beneficial effects observed in asthmatic patients treated, and researchers summarized the research by saying: "From the preliminary work cited above, it would seem that *D. adscendens* has a potential for being a useful antiasthmatic agent and warrants a thorough investigation."[3]

Whether or not scientists fully understand and explain amor seco's effectiveness or develop this plant into a proprietary asthma drug, natural health practitioners and herbalists will continue to use this wonderful herbal remedy effectively for asthma as well as allergies. With some of the newer published research linking arthritis and rheumatism to various allergic reactions and anaphylactic-induced chemical processes, the indigenous use of amor seco for back pain and arthritis just might be explained as well. Ease of administering amor seco in powdered capsules or in tea, highly effective results at low dosages, and no reported side effects or toxicity place amor seco in the first line of defense in the herbalist's medicine chest of natural remedies.

Generally, 1 to 3 cups of amor seco leaf tea (a standard infusion) daily, 4 to 6 ml of a standard tincture, or 4 to 5 g of powdered leaves in capsules are used by practitioners for most conditions.

WORLDWIDE USES

Region	Uses
Africa	Asthma, bronchitis, colic, ringworms, wounds
Amazonia	Consumption, contraceptive, convulsion, galactagogue, magic, nervousness
Belize	Ache (back, joint, muscle), headache, kidney disorders
Brazil	Ache (body), blennorrhagia, diarrhea, leucorrhea, malaria
Ghana	Asthma, colic, constipation, dysentery, wounds
Guinea	Anthelmintic, oxytoxic
Ivory Coast	Aphrodisiac, galactagogue
Liberia	Convulsion, sore, venereal disease
Nicaragua	Diarrhea, digestive, venereal disease
Peru	Blood, detoxifier, hemorrhage, inflammation, ovary, urinary, vaginitis
Trinidad	Depurative, marasmus, oliguria, venereal disease
Elsewhere	Cataplasm, consumption, convulsion, cough, fracture, laxative, sore, venereal disease, wound

PHYTOCHEMICALS

astragalin, beta-phenylethylamines, cosmosiin, cyanidin-3-o-sophoroside, dehydrosoyasaponin I, hordenine, pelargonidin-3-o-rhamnoside, salsoline, soyasaponin I, soyasaponin II, soyasaponin III, tectorigenin, tetrahydroisoquinolines, triterpenoid saponins, tyramine

ANDIROBA

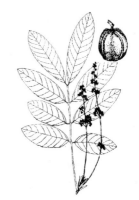

Family: Meliaceae

Genus: *Carapa*

Species: *guianensis*

Common Names: Andiroba, andiroba-saruba, iandirova, carapa, requia, Brazilian mahogany, bastard mahogany

Parts Used: Seed oil, bark, and leaves

Medicinal Properties: Analgesic, anti-inflammatory, antiparasitic, antiseptic, cicatrizant, emollient, febrifuge, insecticide, vermifuge

NDIROBA IS A huge rainforest tree that grows to a height of 130 m. It is in the same family as mahogany and has been called Brazilian mahogany or bastard mahogany due to its similarity. It is one of the large-leafed trees of the rainforest and can be identified by its distinctive textured leaves. It produces fragrant flowers and a brown, woody, four-cornered nut some 7 to 10 cm across that resembles a chestnut and contains an oil-rich kernel. The seeds contain pale yellow-colored oil. Andiroba can be found growing wild throughout the Amazon rainforest, usually on rich soils, in swamps, and in the alluvial flats, marshes, and uplands of the Amazon Basin. It can also be found wild or under cultivation in Brazil in the Islands region, in Tocantins, in Rio Solimoes, and near the seaside.

Andiroba wood is soft and much sought after by sawmills. It has in the past been shipped to the United States for utilization in the furniture industry, among other uses. Its durability and impalatability for insects have guaranteed commercial demand for the wood; as a result, the species has been rapidly devastated in all areas near major towns in Amazonia. It could, however, be easily cultivated either in the Amazon or other regions of Brazil.

The average nut yield of an andiroba tree is about 200 kg. The nuts contain seeds with an oil content averaging 63%. Some 6.25 kg of nuts are required to produce 1 kg of andiroba oil using the traditional extraction method. This traditional method is efficient, if somewhat primitive. The seeds are collected from rivers, where they float after being shed by the tree. They are then boiled and left for some two weeks until they have rotted; then they are squeezed (in a primitive press known as a *tipiti*) to extract the oil and sometimes fatty solids. One consequence of this extraction method is that crude andiroba oil is frequently associated with a red coloring that is derived from the skin of the seeds. The oil, which becomes rancid very quickly, requires rapid use; thus local usage is mostly limited to immediate use or the manufacture of soap.

Among the many properties attributed to andiroba oil by ethnopharmacological research, the most important are its anti-inflammatory qualities when applied to painful swellings and its use as an antirheumatic.

The tree bark, leaves, and seed oil of andiroba are most used medicinally. The indigenous Munduruku tribe traditionally used andiroba oil for the mummification of human heads taken as war trophies. The Wayãpi, Palikur, and Creole Indian tribes have used andiroba to remove ticks from their heads and for skin parasites. Indians have also used the oil as a solvent for extracting the plant colorants with which they paint their skin. Andiroba oil also burns well and is used as a natural lamp oil in the rainforest. Traditional forest-dwellers and river people called *caboclos* make a medicinal soap using crude andiroba oil, wood ash, and cocoa skin residue. This soap is especially recommended for the treatment of skin diseases and as an insect repellent.

Among the many properties attributed to andiroba oil by ethnopharmacological research, the most important are its anti-inflammatory qualities when applied to painful swellings and its use as an antirheumatic. The oil is also used as an insect repellent and for treating both insect bites and skin diseases. Information has recently been collected on the use of andiroba oil in gelatin capsules in the treatment of internal cancers in Brazil. The indigenous tribes of northwest Amazonia brew the bark, and sometimes leaves, into a febrifugal and vermifugal tea; they also apply this tea externally as a wash for ulcers and skin problems. Botanist James Duke reports that this same bark infusion may be useful in herpes, and that Native Americans trust the oil as an emollient and anti-inflammatory for skin rashes. Brazilians currently use the oil in soaps and sell the oil as an anti-inflammatory and antiarthritic. The fruit oil is also ingested in Brazil for coughs. *Curanderos* and herbalists in the Amazon use the leaves of andiroba in baths for skin irritations and itching; they use the oil for massages for muscle pain and for skin disorders.

Andiroba oil is used by Brazilian city dwellers either in pure form or mixed with other fatty oils or natural products. They apply it externally to wounds and bruises and use it as a massage oil. It is also applied to areas affected by skin diseases and psoriasis, to sore feet, or, when mixed with camphor, to the whole body in the case of a severe cold.[1] In Brazil 1/4 of a *cabacinha* (the fruit of *Luffa operculata*) is macerated in 250 ml of hot andiroba oil to yield an infusion that is rubbed into the skin to relieve arthritis and rheumatism and to cauterize wounds.

Andiroba oil is used by Brazilian city dwellers to treat wounds and bruises and as a massage oil.

Andiroba oil is also applied directly to the skin of dogs to treat wounds and relieve itchy skin conditions caused by tick bites. Andiroba oil has even been rubbed into other wood products to protect them from termites and other insects.[2]

The oil composition of andiroba is mostly represented by myristic and oleic acids and, to a lesser extent, palmitic and linoleic acids. Recent tests of crude andiroba oil by Brazilian pharmacologists have produced evidence of its anti-inflammatory and analgesic properties.[3] The anti-inflammatory properties of andiroba oil are probably due to the presence of a group of chemicals called limmonoids, which are soluble in the unsaturated fraction of the oil. Phytochemical studies have identified the presence of seven limmonoids.[4-6] The oil is rich in the limmonoid alkaloid called andirobin, which has demonstrated anti-inflammatory properties in laboratory tests.[7, 8] In addition, andiroba oil is rich in stearine and other unsaturated fatty acids (see Table A). Unsaponifiable matter is between 2% and 5%, and low free fatty acid content is up to 0.99%. It yields up to 65% in unsaturated fatty acids such as linoleic acid, which is currently being studied by Japanese cosmetology researchers.

North American practitioners are just beginning to learn of andiroba's wonderful healing properties. Andiroba oil can be applied topically several times daily to rashes, muscle/joint aches and injuries, wounds, boils, and herpes ulcers. It can also be used by itself or combined with other oils as a healing and anti-inflammatory massage oil.

Table A

FATTY ACID COMPOSITION OF ANDIROBA FILTERED OIL BY GAS CHROMATOGRAPHY

Fatty Acid	RT	%
C16:0 palmitic	6.33	28.1884
C16:1 palmitoleic	7.57	1.0490
C18:0 stearic	10.11	8.1134
C18:1 oleic	11.90	50.5035
C18:2 linoleic	14.96	8.5732
C20:0 arachidic	16.69	1.2201
C18:3 linolenic	19.59	10.3247

WORLDWIDE USES

Region	Uses
Brazil	Analgesic, arthritis, cancer, cough, fevers, insect repellent, muscle pain, parasites, psoriasis, skin, skin disease, skin rash, ulcers (skin), vermifuge
Guatemala	Insect repellent
Panama	Arthritis
Trinidad	Cold, feet, fever, flu, insectifuge, pediculicide
Venezuela	Itch, leprosy, malaria, parasiticide, skin
Elsewhere	Arthritis, herpes, insecticide, insectifuge, insect repellent, skin, soap, tetanus

PHYTOCHEMICALS

11-beta-acetoxy-gedunin, 6-alpha-acetoxy-epoxyazadiradione, 6-alpha-acetoxy-gedunin, 6-beta-acetoxy-gedunin, 6-alpha,11-beta-diacetoxy-gedunin, 6-alpha-hydroxygedunin, 6-beta, 11-beta-diacetoxy-gedunin, 7-deacetoxy-7-oxogedunin, 7-desacetoxy-7-ketogedunin, andirobin, epoxyazadiradione

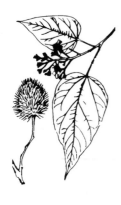

ANNATTO

Family: Bixaceae

Genus: *Bixa*

Species: *orellana*

Common Names: Annatto, achiote, achiotec, achiotl, achote, urucu, beni-no-ki, bija, onoto, orleanstrauch, roucou, roucouyer, uruku

Parts Used: Seeds, leaves, roots, shoots

Medicinal Properties: Antibacterial, antidysenteric, antigonorrheal, anti–inflammatory, antioxidant, antiseptic, antitussive, astringent, cicatrizant, depurative, diuretic, emollient, expectorant, febrifuge, hepatoprotective, hypoglycemic, hypotensive, nutritive, parasiticide, purgative, stomachic

B IXA IS A profusely fruiting shrub or small tree that grows 5 to 10 m in height. Approximately 50 seeds grow inside of prickly reddish-orange heart-shaped pods at the ends of the branches. The trees are literally covered by these brightly colored pods, and one small annatto tree can produce up to 270 kg of seeds. The seeds are covered with a reddish aril, which is the source of an orange-yellow dye. Annatto is known as *achiote* in Spanish and as *annatto* in Portuguese. It grows throughout South and Central America and the Caribbean and can be found in some parts of Mexico as well.

Traditionally, the crushed seeds are soaked in water that is allowed to evaporate. A brightly colored paste is then made and is added to soups, cheeses, and other foods to give them a bright yellow or orange color. Annatto seed paste produced in South America is exported to North America and Europe, where it becomes a food coloring for margarine, cheeses, microwave popcorn, and other yellow or orange foodstuffs. Many times, this food coloring replaces the very expensive saffron in recipes and dishes around the world. Annatto paste is also used as a natural dye for cloth and wool and is sometimes employed in the paint, varnish, lacquer, cosmetic, and soap industries.

Throughout the rainforest, indigenous tribes have used annatto seeds as a body paint and as a fabric dye. Although mostly only the seed paste or seed oil is used today, the rainforest tribes have used the entire plant as medicine for centuries. A tea made with the young shoots is used by the Piura tribe as an antidysenteric, aphrodisiac, and astringent and to treat skin problems, fevers, and hepatitis. The foliage has been used to treat skin problems, liver disease, and hepatitis; has been used as an aphrodisiac, antidysenteric, and antipyretic; and has been considered good for the digestive system. An infusion of the flowers is used by the Cojedes tribes as a purgative and to avoid phlegm in newborn babies. The seeds are believed to be an expectorant; the roots are thought to be a digestive as well as an antitussive. Annatto has been traced back to the ancient Mayan Indians, who employed it as a principal coloring agent in foods, for body paints, and as a coloring for arts, crafts, and murals.[1]

> Although mostly only the seed paste or seed oil is used today, the rainforest tribes have used the entire plant as medicine for centuries.

Today in Brazilian traditional medicine, annatto is used to treat heartburn and stomach distress caused by spicy foods, and as a mild diuretic and mild purgative. Traditional medicine in Peru recommends it as a vaginal antiseptic and cicatrizant, as a wash for skin infections, and for liver and stomach disorders. The leaves of *Bixa* are a common remedy in Peruvian herbal medicine today, and the dried leaves are called *achiotec*. Eight to 10 dried leaves of Annatto are boiled for 10 minutes in 1 l of water for this popular Peruvian remedy. One cup is drunk warm or cold 3 times daily after meals to treat prostate disorders and inflammation, to treat inflammation in the urinary tract, arterial hypertension, high cholesterol, cystitis, obesity, and renal insufficiency, and to eliminate uric acid in the urine. *Curanderos* in the Peruvian Amazon extract the juice from the leaves and stem and place it in the eye for inflammation, and they use the juice of 12 fruits taken twice daily for 5 days to "cure" epilepsy.

Annatto seeds contain 40% to 45% cellulose, 3.5% to 5.5% sucrose, 0.3% to 0.9% essential oil, 3% fixed oil, 4.5% to 5.5% pigments, and 13% to 16% protein, as well as alfa- and beta-carotenoids and other constituents.[2–5] In clinical experiments ethyl alcohol extracts of both the dried annatto fruit and the leaves have demonstrated an *in vitro* activity against *Escherichia coli* and *Staphylococcus aureus;* a water extract of the root demonstrated hypotensive activity in rats and smooth muscle–relaxant activity in guinea pigs; and a chloroform extract of dried seed demonstrated hypoglycemic activity in dogs.[6–8]

> **Bixin, a pigment extracted from annatto, is used as a colorant in foods, is believed to have UV protection capabilities, and has also demonstrated antioxidant and liver protective properties.**

Annatto also contains tannins, ethereal oils, saponins, mustard oil–like substances, and mono- and sesquiterpenes.[9] Annatto oil is extracted from the seeds and is the main source of the pigments bixin and norbixin, which are classified as carotenoids. Bixin is used as a colorant in foods, is believed to have UV protection capabilities, and has also demonstrated antioxidant and liver protective properties.[10–15] Annatto has also been documented as an aldose reductase inhibitor,[16] and a 1995 study demonstrated its antigonorrheal activity.[17]

Although its history of use as a food coloring is well established worldwide, current trends show that it is used increasingly in body care products. Annatto oil is an emollient, and its high carotenoid content provides antioxidant properties.[15] In body care products, annatto oil provides antioxidant benefits while adding a rich sunny color to creams, lotions, and shampoos.

Although not widely available in the United States, standard decoctions of annatto leaves are taken by the half cupful 2 to 3 times daily for prostate and urinary difficulties as well as high cholesterol and hypertension. Ground annatto seed powder is also used in small dosages of 1 to 20 mg daily for high cholesterol and hypertension. Higher dosages can cause a marked increase in urination. It has been noted that some individuals are highly sensitive to annatto seed and this diuretic effect can be caused at much lower doses, even by just eating a bag of popcorn in which annatto was used as a coloring or flavoring ingredient.

WORLDWIDE USES

Region	Uses
Brazil	Diuretic, excitant, heartburn, hepatitis, purgative, stomachache
Colombia	Aphrodisiac
Haiti	Douche, fever, insect repellent
Hawaii	Depurative, fainting, stomatitis
Mexico	Antidote, aphrodisiac, astringent, burn, diuretic, dysentery, epilepsy, erysipelas, fever, gonorrhea, headache, inflammation, insect repellent, malaria, purgative, refrigerant, stomachic, throat, tumor, unguent, vaginitis, venereal disease
Peru	Antiseptic, cholesterolemia, cicatrizant, conjunctivitis, cystitis, dye, epilepsy, hypertension, obesity, prostate, renal, urinary, urogenital
Trinidad	Dysentery, flu, jaundice, oliguria, venereal disease
Elsewhere	Antidote, aphrodisiac, astringent, cancer, coloring, cordial, cosmetic, diabetes, dysentery, fever, hair oil, kidney, parasiticide, skin disorders, styptic

PHYTOCHEMICALS

bixaghanene, bixein, bixin, bixol, crocetin, ellagic acid, ishwarane, isobixin, norbixin, phenylalanine, salicylic acid, threonine, tomentosic acid, tryptophan

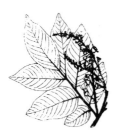

BALSAM OF TOLU, BALSAM OF PERU

Family: Fabaceae

Genus: *Myroxylon*

Species: *balsamum, pereirae*

Common Names: Balsam of Peru, balsam of Tolu, Peru balsam, balsam Peru, Tolu balsam, balsam of Tolu, balsamo de Peru, balsamo de Tolu, balsamo peruano, baume de Tolu, pau de balsamo, Tolu balsambaum, Tolu balsemboom

Parts Used: Resin, bark

Medicinal Properties: Antibacterial, antifungal, anti-inflammatory, antiparasitic, antiseptic, antitussive, cicatrizant, expectorant, respiratory, vulnerary

BALSAM OF TOLU *(Myroxylon balsamum)* is a tall tree native to northern South America, found predominantly in Colombia, Peru, and Venezuela and in some areas of Argentina, Paraguay, and Bolivia. A closely related species, called balsam Peru *(M. pereirae)*, is native to Central America farther north. (Balsam of Peru was named such because it was originally assembled and shipped to Europe from the ports of Callao and Lima, Peru, not because the species is indigenous to Peru.) Both trees grow 20 to 25 m high. They are tapped like rubber trees to extract the resin-like saps that are used medicinally.

The leaves and fruits of *M. pereirae* have been used by indigenous tribes of Mexico and Central America, which employ the bitter resin for asthma, catarrh, rheumatism, and external wounds.[1] The Choco Indians use the powdered bark as an underarm deodorant. The sap of *M. balsamum* has documented indigenous uses for colds and lung ailments, and the Amazon rainforest tribes have employed it for abscesses, asthma, bronchitis, catarrh, headache, rheumatism, sores, sprains, tuberculosis, venereal diseases, and wounds. The indigenous use of balsam of Peru led to its export to Europe in the seventeenth century, where it was first documented in the *German Pharmacopeia*,[2] and to its use as a bactericide, fungicide, and parasiticide in cases of scabies, ringworm, pediculosis, granulations, superficial ulcerations, wounds, bed sores, diaper rash, and chilblains.[3] Balsam of Peru has been in the *U.S. Pharmacopeia* since 1820, with documented uses for bronchitis, laryngitis, dysmenorrhea, diarrhea, dysentery, and leucorrhea. It is also used as a food flavoring and fragrance for its aromatic vanilla-like odor.[3] Today, it is used extensively in topical preparations for the treatment of wounds, ulcers, and scabies. It can be found in hair tonics, antidandruff preparations, and feminine hygiene sprays and as a natural fragrance in soaps, detergents, creams, lotions, and perfumes.[3] Balsam of Tolu was also included in the *U.S. Pharmacopeia* in 1820 and is used much like balsam of Peru. Additionally, it is shown to be an antitussive and respiratory aid used in cough lozenges and syrups, for sore throats, and as a vapor inhalant for respiratory ailments.[3] It has been documented as having antiseptic and expectorant properties.[3] The internal dosage is reported to be 1/2 to 1 g taken 3 times daily.

The sap of *M. balsamum* has documented indigenous uses for colds and lung ailments, and the Amazon rainforest tribes have employed it for abscesses, asthma, bronchitis, catarrh, headache, rheumatism, sores, sprains, tuberculosis, venereal diseases, and wounds.

Balsam of Peru contains 50% to 64% volatile oil and 20% to 28% resin. The volatile oil contains benzoic and cinnamic acid esters, small amounts of nerolidol, and free benzoic and cinnamic acids, which are believed to be the main active constituents.[4] Balsam of Peru has demonstrated antiseptic, antiparasitic, and antibacterial properties and has been shown to promote the growth of epithelial cells.[4] It is reported to be highly effective in cases of scabies, destroying the itch acarus and its eggs, and is preferred over other sulfur ointments. It is also reported to be useful in cases of prurigo and pruritus, and for later stages of acute eczema.[4]

WORLDWIDE USES

Region	Uses
Amazonia	Abscess, asthma, bronchitis, catarrh, headache, rheumatism, sore, sprain, tuberculosis, venereal disease, wound
Caledonia	Bronchitis, cough, perfume, skin, sore, wound
Dominican Republic	Expectorant, sore, stomachic, wound
Europe	Bactericide, cancer, chilblains, fungicide, parasiticide, pediculosis, scabies, skin rash, ulcers (skin), wounds
Mexico	Amenorrhea, asthma, bronchitis, catarrh, colic, diuretic, dysmenorrhea, freckle, gout, itch, osteomyelitis, parasiticide, rheumatism, ringworms, scabies, sore, spasm, stimulant, stomachache, tumor, venereal disease, vermifuge
South Africa	Antiseptic, bronchitis, cold, cough, expectorant, perfume
Elsewhere	Antiseptic, asthma, bactericide, catarrh, cough, deodorant, expectorant, fumigant, headache, pectoral, rheumatism, sclerosis, stimulant, stomachic, swelling, tonic, tuberculosis, umbilicus, venereal disease

PHYTOCHEMICALS

1(5),6-guaiadiene, 1,2-diaphenlyethane, 1,2-diphenylethane, 3-oxo-6-beta-hydroxyolean-12-en-28-oic acid, 6-hydroxy-3-oxyolean-12-en-28-oic acid, 20-r-24-xi-2-ocotillone, 20-r-hydroxy-dammarenone, 20-s-dammarendol, 20-s-hydroxydammarenone, alpha-bourbonene, alpha-cadinene, alpha-calacorene, alpha-copaene, alpha-curcumene, alpha-muurolene, alpha-pinene, benzaldehyde, benzoic, benzoic acid, benzyl alcohol, benzyl-benzoate, benzyl-cinnamate, benzyl-ferulate, benzyl-isoferulate, beta-bourbonene, beta-elemene, cadalene, calamenene, caryophyllene, cinnamaldehyde, cinnamein, cinnamic acid, cinnamic alcohol, cinnamyl-benzoate, cinnamyl-cinnamate, cis-ocimene, coumarin, D-cadinene, dammaradienone, delta-cadinene, dihydrobenzoic acid, dihydrocinnamic acid, dihydromandelic acid, EO, ethyl-benzoate, eugenol, farnesol, ferulic acid, gamma-muurolene, hydroxyhopanone, L-cadinol, methyl-cinnamate, nerolidol, oleanolic acid, P-cymene, peruresinotannol, peruviol, resin, styrene, sumaresinolic acid, tannin, toluresinotannol-cinnamate, urs-12-en-3-on-28-al, vanillin, wax

BOLDO

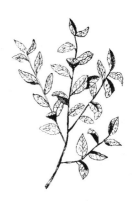

Family: Monimiaceae

Genus: *Peumus*

Species: *boldus*

Common Names: Boldo, boldina, baldina

Part Used: Leaves

Medicinal Properties: Anodyne, anthelmintic, antiseptic, cholagogue, choleretic, demulcent, depurative, detoxifier, diuretic, hepatic, hepatotonic, sedative, stimulant, stomachic, tonic, vermifuge

BOLDO IS A shrubby evergreen tree that grows 6 to 8 m in height and produces small, berry-like fruit. It is found in the Andean regions of Chile and Peru and is also indigenous to parts of Morocco. Boldo is cultivated in some parts of Italy, Brazil, and North Africa to meet the demand for its medicinal leaves in European and Canadian markets, where it is widely used.

> Indigenous uses were verified in the 1950s and 1960s by researchers, who showed that boldo leaves had diuretic, stomachic, and cholagogic properties.

Indigenous uses of boldo have been widely documented. For many years in Chile, the fruit has been eaten as a spice, the wood used for charcoal, and the bark used in tanning hides. It is also used in Chilean folk medicine as an anthelmintic against worms. This use has been attributed to the ascaridole content of the essential oil found in the leaves. In parts of Peru the leaves are used by indigenous tribes against liver diseases, to treat gallstones, and as a diuretic. The indigenous uses were verified in the 1950s and 1960s by researchers, who showed that boldo leaves had diuretic, stomachic, and cholagogic properties in animal studies.[1, 2]

A German therapeutic monograph shows the use of boldo leaves for mild gastrointestinal spasms and dyspeptic disorders.[3] A U.S. monograph reports that boldo causes clinically significant diuresis (increased urination).[4] Boldo's history in traditional medicine is well documented. The plant is used in homeopathy in the treatment of digestive disorders, as a laxative, choleretic, and diuretic, and for liver problems. The leaves are used against intestinal worms, and botanist James Duke reports its traditional use for urogenital inflammations like gonorrhea and syphilis, as well as for gout, jaundice, dyspepsia, rheumatism, head colds, and earaches.

Boldo is rich in phytochemicals, including at least 17 known alkaloids.[5–9] A total of at least 38 active phytochemical compounds have been identified. The choleretic activity of the plant has been attributed to an aporphine alkaloid called boldine,[8] which has demonstrated diuretic, uric acid excretory, antipyretic, anti-inflammatory, and weak hypnotic effects in laboratory tests.[10–12] In animal studies boldine has been shown to stimulate digestion, and specifically to stimulate the production of bile and its secretion from the gallbladder, and to stimulate the secretion of gastric juice.[13–15] Although its digestive and choleretic properties are largely attributed to boldine, one study indicated that an alcohol extract of boldo leaves caused higher choleretic activity in rats than boldine alone.[13] The antioxidant property of the leaves has also been documented.[16] A recent human study demonstrated that boldo relaxes smooth muscle and prolongs intestinal transit, which validated again its traditional medicinal uses.[17] The average therapeutic dose is reported to be 2 to 3 g daily.

> **Boldo is used throughout Europe, North America, South America, and Latin America as a specific treatment for gallstones and gallbladder inflammation and for many types of liver, stomach, and digestive disorders.**

In herbal medicine today, boldo is used extensively throughout Europe, North America, South America, and Latin America as a specific treatment for gallstones and gallbladder inflammation and for many types of liver, stomach, and digestive disorders.

WORLDWIDE USES

Region	Uses
Chile	Diuretic, earache, gallbladder, gallstones, jaundice, liver, stimulant, stomach
Latin America	Anodyne, antiseptic, choleretic, digestion, gallbladder, gallstones, gonorrhea, hepatotonic, liver, stimulant, stomachic, stomach, tonic, urogenital, vermifuge
Mexico	Anodyne, gallbladder, gallstones, liver, rheumatism, stomachic
Turkey	Antiseptic, diuretic, hepatotonic, rheumatism, sedative, stimulant, stomachic, tonic, vermifuge
Elsewhere	Cold, dyspepsia, gallbladder, gallstones, gastrointestinal disorders, gout, hepatosis, liver, rheumatism, stomach, syphilis, worms

PHYTOCHEMICALS

myrtenal,1,8-cineole,1-methyl-4-isopropenyl-benzene, 2-decanone, 2-heptaone, 2-nonanone, 2-octanone, alpha-3-carene, alpha-fenchol, alpha-hexylcinnamaldehyde, alpha-methylionone, alpha-pinene, alpha-terpineol, ascaridole, benzaldehyde, benzyl-benzoate, beta-pinene, boldine, boldoglucin, bornyl-acetate, camphene, camphor, choline, coumarin, cuminaldehyde, diethyl-phthalate, EO, eugenol, farnesol, fenchone, gamma-terpinene, isoboldine, isocorydine, isocory-dine-n-oxide, isorhamnetin-3-glucoside-7-rhamnoside, kaempferol-3-glucoside-7-rhamnoside, laurolitsine, laurotetanine, limonene, linalool, methyl-eugenol, norisocorydine, P-cymene, P-cymol, rhamnetin-3-arabinoside-3'-rhamnoside, sabinene, sparteine, tannin, terpinen-4-ol, terpinoline, 2-tridecanone, 2-undecanone, eta-isomethylionone, boldin, gum, isorhamnetin-3-alpha-l-arabinopyranosid\E-7-alpha-l-rhamn, N-methyllaurotetanine, pachycarpine, resin, reticuline

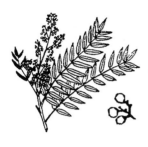

BRAZILIAN PEPPERTREE

Family: Anacardiaceae

Genus: *Schinus*

Species: *molle*

Common Names: Brazilian peppertree, aroeira, escobilla, Peruvian peppertree, Peruvian mastic tree, California peppertree, mastic-tree, aroeira salsa, aguaribay, American pepper, anacahuita, castilla, false pepper, gualeguay, Jesuit's balsam, molle del Peru, mulli, pepper tree, pimentero, pimientillo, pirul

Parts Used: Fruit, bark, leaf

Medicinal Properties: Analgesic, antibacterial, antidepressant, antifungal, antimicrobial, antispasmodic, antiviral, astringent, balsamic, cytotoxic, diuretic, expectorant, hypotensive, purgative, stomachic, tonic, uterine stimulant, vulnerary

BRAZILIAN PEPPERTREE IS a medium-sized to small shrubby tree with narrow, spiky leaves. It grows 4 to 8 m high and has a trunk 25 to 35 cm in diameter. It produces an abundance of small flowers formed in panicles and then bears a great many small flesh-colored berry-like fruits in December and January. It is indigenous to South and Central America and can be found in semi-tropical and tropical parts of the United States and Africa.

Virtually all parts of this tropical tree have been used medicinally throughout the tropics, including its leaves, bark, fruit, seeds, resin, and oleoresin or balsam. The plant has a very long history of use and shows up in ancient religious artifacts or idols among some of the Chilean Amerindians. All parts of the tree have a high oil and essential oil content that produces a spicy, aromatic scent. The leaves of Brazilian peppertree have such a high oil content that leaf pieces jerk and twist when placed in hot water as the oil is released. The berries, which have a peppery flavor, have been used in syrups, vinegar, and beverages in Peru, in Chilean wines, and are dried and ground up for a pepper substitute in Africa. The dried fruits have even been used as an adulterant of black pepper in some countries. The tree also produces a resin and oleoresin or balsam that is used medicinally.

Brazilian peppertree has a long history of uses throughout South and Central America and is reported to be an astringent, balsamic, collyrium, diuretic, emmenagogue, masticatory, piscicide, purgative, stomachic, tonic, antiviral, and vulnerary. Its uses by indigenous peoples in the countries where it grows are well documented. In Peru the sap is used as a purgative and a diuretic,[1] and the entire plant is used externally for fractures and as a topical antiseptic.[2] The oleoresin is used externally as a cicatrizant for wounds and for toothaches, and it is taken internally for rheumatism, a folk disease called suto, and as a purgative. In South Africa a leaf tea is used to treat colds, and a leaf decoction is inhaled for colds, hypertension, depression, and arrhythmia.[3] In the Brazilian Amazon a bark tea is used as a purgative,[4] and a bark and leaf tea is used as a stimulant and antidepressant.[5] In Argentina a decoction is made with the dried leaves and is taken for menstrual disorders[6] as well as for respiratory and urinary tract infections and disorders.[7] Throughout South America, the bark and leaves are used for menstrual disorders, as they are reported to have emmenagogue properties.

> **Throughout South America, the bark and leaves are used for menstrual disorders, as they are reported to have emmenagogue properties.**

Brazilian peppertree is still employed in herbal medicine today in many countries. It is used for many conditions in the tropics, including amenorrhea, apostemes, blennorrhagia, bronchitis, cataracts, dysmenorrhea, gingivitis, gonorrhea, gout, ophthalmia, rheumatism, sores, swellings, tuberculosis, ulcers, urethritis, urogenital and venereal disorders, warts, and wounds. In Brazilian herbal medicine today, the dried bark and leaves are employed for fevers, urinary tract disorders and pain, cystitis, urethritis, blennorrhagia, coughs, bronchitis and other upper respiratory problems, grippe, diarrhea, hemorrhages, and menstrual disorders with excessive bleeding, tumors, and general inflammation.

Phytochemical analysis of Brazilian peppertree reveals that the plant contains tannins, alkaloids, flavonoids, steroidal saponins, sterols, terpenes, gums, resins, and essential oils.[8–10] The essential oil, present in the leaves, bark, and fruit, is a rich source of triterpenes, sesquiterpenes, and monoterpenes, including several novel ones that scientists have not seen before. Many of the plant's documented biological activities are attributed to the essential oils found in the plant. The fruit can contain up to 5% essential oil, and the leaves can contain up to 2% essential oil.[8, 9] In laboratory tests the essential oil as well as a leaf extract demonstrated good to very strong antifungal actions against numerous fungi and even candida *in vitro*.[11–13] The essential oil and leaves have clinically demonstrated *in vitro* antibacterial and antimicrobial activity against numerous bacteria and pathogens in several studies.[12–14] In much earlier *in vitro* tests, a leaf extract of Brazilian peppertree demonstrated antiviral actions against several plant viruses[15] and was shown to be cytotoxic against 9kb cancer cells.[16]

> Many of the Brazilian peppertree's documented biological activities are attributed to the essential oils found in the plant. The fruit can contain up to 5% essential oil, and the leaves can contain up to 2% essential oil.

Over the years, several research groups have conducted animal studies on Brazilian peppertree that have substantiated some of its many traditional uses in herbal medicine. A fruit extract and a leaf extract were shown to produce hypotensive activity in dogs and rats,[17, 18] as well as uterine stimulant activity in guinea pigs and rabbits.[18, 19] Most recently, leaf extracts tested by other researchers between 1996 and 1997 demonstrated analgesic activity in mice[20] and antispasmodic properties in rats.[21] In 1996 the essential oil was also shown to be an effective insect repellent against the common housefly.[22]

Today, herbalists and natural health practitioners in both North and South America use Brazilian peppertree mostly for viral and bacterial infections like colds, flu, asthma, bronchitis, and other upper respiratory infections, as an aid to help lower high blood pressure, for fungal infections and candida, and as a female balancing herb for numerous menstrual disorders, menstrual cramps, PMS, and menopause. One to 3 cups daily of a standard leaf or bark infusion is generally used for this natural remedy. Alternatively, 2 to 3 g daily in capsules or combined with other herbs is used by practitioners as a natural remedy for many ailments of a bacterial, viral, or fungal nature.

The old ones teach an ancient lesson: The forest is the giver of all things. They teach as they were taught by those who came before them. The lesson reminds the People to walk barefoot and sit upon moist earth and know a mothering power. It reminds them why and how the forest rose from the earth, trees in every direction, a greenness broken only by great rivers, slow waters that flow to where they will again fall from the sky. The lesson is told through stories about the ancestors and their lives in the forest. The People know the stories are true. The stories are re-created each day with each fruit from the forest, with each sacred medicine from the forest, with each brilliant flickering of the firebug. The forest is all life.

—Robert Heinzman, *Visions of the Rainforest*

WORLDWIDE USES

Region	Uses
Argentina	Diarrhea, dysmenorrhea, emmenagogue, menstrual disorders, respiratory tract infections, urinary tract infections
Brazil	Astringent, balsamic, blennorrhagia, bronchitis, cough, cystitis, diarrhea, fever, inflammation, purgative, respiratory tract disorders, stimulant, tonic, tumor, urethritis, urinary tract disorders
Colombia	Diarrhea, hemoptysis, rheumatism
Lacadonia	Masticatory, purgative, spice, tea
Mexico	Aposteme, asthma, astringent, balsamic, blennorrhagia, bronchitis, cataract, colic, collyrium, conjunctivitis, cough, digestive disorders, foot, gonorrhea, grippe, gum, liqueur, masticatory, mouth, ophthalmia, preventative, purgative, rheumatism, sore, stomachache, toothache, tuberculosis, tumor, ulcer, urogenital, venereal disease, vulnerary, wound
Paraguay	Blennorrhagia, diuretic, emmenagogue, sore, urethritis, wound
Peru	Antiseptic, cicatrizant, diuretic, fractures, purgative, rheumatism, toothache, tumor, wart
South Africa	Antidepressant, arrhythmia, colds, gout, hypertension, rheumatism
Turkey	Diuretic, expectorant, gonorrhea, masticatory, purgative, stomachic, tonic
Uruguay	Amenorrhea, dysmenorrhea
Elsewhere	Amenorrhea, bronchitis, diuretic, dysmenorrhea, edema, emmenagogue, expectorant, eye, gingivitis, gout, hypertension, piscicide, poison, purgative, rheumatism, sore, stomachic, swelling, urogenital, venereal disease, viricide

PHYTOCHEMICALS

a-amyrin, behenic acid, a-bergamont-trans-ene, bourbonene, d-cadinene, a-cadinol, d-cadinol, t-cadinol, a-calacorene, g-calacorene, iso-calamenediol, calamenene, calcium, camphene, car-3-ene, carvacrol, b-caryophyllene, cerotic acid, a-copaene, croweacin, a-cubebene, cyanidin-3-o-alpha-l-galactoside, b-elemene, elemol, b-elemonic acid, a-eudesmol, b-eudesmol, g-eudesmol, fisetin, gallic acid, geraniol butyrate, germacrene D, b-guaiene, a-gurjunene, heptacosanoic acid, a-humulene, laccase, lignoceric acid, limonene, (+)limonene, linoleic acid, dihydro-malvalic acid, iso-masticadienoic acid, 3-epi-iso-masticadienolalic acid, iso-masticadienolic acid, menth-cis-2-en-1-ol, a-muurolene, g-muurolene, t-muurolol, myrcene, nerol hexanoate, octacosanoic acid, octanoic acid methyl ester, oleic acid, palmitic acid, para-cymene, penta-cosanoic acid, pentan-1-ol,3-methyl, peonidin-3-o-beta-d-glucoside, peroxidase, a-phellandrene, b-phellandrene, ortho-ethyl phenol, pinene, a-pinene, b-pinene, piperine, trans-piperitol, proto-catechuic acid, quercetin, quercetrin, quercitrin, iso-quercitrin, raffinose, rutin, sabinene, b-sitosterol, b-spathulene, tannin, a-terpinene, g-terpinene, a-terpineol, terpinolene, tricosanoic acid

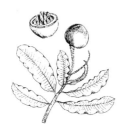

BRAZIL NUT

Family: Lecythidaceae

Genus: *Bertholletia*

Species: *excelsa*

Common Names: Brazil nut, castania, castanheiro do para, para-nut, creamnut, castana-de-para, castana-de-Brazil

Parts Used: Nut, seed oil

Medicinal Properties: Antioxidant, emollient, insecticide, nutritive

THE BRAZIL NUT tree is enormous, frequently attaining the height of 49 m or more. The fruit is a large, spherical woody capsule or pod that measures an average of 15 cm in diameter and weighs up to 2.25 kg. The tree is called *castanheiro do para* in Brazil and is found throughout the Amazon rainforest in Brazil, Peru, Colombia, Venezuela, and Ecuador. It is most prevalent in the Brazilian states of Maranhao, Mato Grosso, Acre, Para, Rondonia, and Amazonas.

The fruit pods grow at the ends of thick branches; they ripen and fall from the trees between January and June. Inside each fruit pod, wedged in like orange segments, are 12 to 25 Brazil nuts within their own individual shells. Brazil nut trees can produce approximately 300 or more of these fruit pods. The monetary value of Brazil nut exportation today from Amazonian Brazil, which began in the 1600s with Dutch traders, is second only to that of rubber. Although thousands of tons of Brazil nuts are exported each year from Brazil, virtually all Brazil nut production comes from wild forest trees

Although thousands of tons of Brazil nuts are exported each year from Brazil, virtually all Brazil nut production comes from wild forest trees and wild-harvesting.

and wild-harvesting. The trees grow very slowly, taking as long as 10 years before producing nuts; thus very few trees are actually cultivated. The United States alone imports more than 9 metric tons of Brazil nuts annually.[1]

A Brazil nut is a three-sided nut with white meat or flesh that consists of 70% fat or oil and 17% protein. The oil extracted from the nuts is commonly used in Peru and other South American countries to manufacture soap. In the Brazilian Amazon the tree bark is brewed into tea to treat liver ailments and diseases. For centuries the indigenous tribes of the rainforest have relied on Brazil nuts as an important and significant staple in their diet—so important, that it has even been used as a trade commodity, much like money. Indigenous tribes eat the nuts raw or grate them and mix them into gruels. In the Brazilian Amazon the nuts are grated with the thorny stilt roots of *socratea* palms into a white mush known as *leite de castanha* and then stirred into manioc flour. This food is a valuable source of calories, fat, and protein for much of the Amazon's rural and urban peoples.

> **In addition to protein and fat, Brazil nuts are a substantial source of selenium, an important antioxidant that has documented anticancer properties. One single Brazil nut exceeds the U.S. Recommended Daily Allowance of selenium.**

With such a high oil content, Brazil nuts will even burn like miniature candles when lit. The oil is extracted from the nuts and used by indigenous and rural people for cooking oil, lamps, soap, and livestock feed.[2] The empty seed pods, often called "monkey's pots," are used to carry around small smoky fires to discourage attacks of black flies and are also used as cups to collect rubber latex from tapped trees and as drinking cups. The husks of these seed pods have also been used in Brazilian folk medicine to brew into tea to treat stomachaches.

Brazil nut oil is a clear yellowish oil with a pleasant and sweet smell and taste. In addition to protein and fat, Brazil nuts are a substantial source of selenium, an important antioxidant that has documented anticancer properties.[3–6] One single Brazil nut exceeds the U.S. Recommended Daily Allowance of selenium. The proteins found in Brazil nuts are very high in sulfur-containing amino acids like cysteine (8%) and methionine (18%) and are also extremely rich in glutamine, glutamic acid, and arginine.[6-8]

Brazil nut oil contains mainly palmitic, oleic, and linoleic and alpha linolenic acids and small amounts of myristic and stearic acids and phytosterols. Today, Brazil nut oil is often used in soaps, shampoos, and hair conditioning/repair products. It is a wonderful hair conditioner, bringing shine, silkiness, malleability, and softness to hair and renewing dry, lifeless hair and split ends. It provides stabilizing detergent properties and helps clean the hair. Brazil nut oil in skin creams helps lubricate and moisturize the skin, provides antioxidant benefits, helps prevents dryness, and leaves skin soft, smooth, and hydrated.

WORLDWIDE USES

Region	Uses
Amazonia	Emollient, food, insect repellent, liver, soap
Venezuela	Insect repellent

PHYTOCHEMICALS

alpha-linolenic acid, antimony, cerium, cesium, europium, lanthanum, lutetium, samarium, scandium, selenoprotein, tantalum, tungsten, ytterbium

CAJUEIRO Cashew

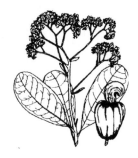

Family: Anacardiaceae

Genus: *Anacardium*

Species: *occidentale*

Common Names: Cajueiro, cashew, cashu, casho, acajuiba, caju, acajou, acaju, acajaiba, alcayoiba, anacarde, anacardier, anacardo, cacajuil, cajou, gajus, jocote maranon, maranon, merey, noix d'acajou, pomme cajou, pomme, jambu, jambu golok, jambu mete, jambu monyet, jambu terong

Parts Used: Fruit, leaves, bark, nut/seed

Medicinal Properties: Antidysenteric, anti-inflammatory, antitussive, aphrodisiac, astringent, diuretic, febrifuge, hypoglycemic, hypotensive, purgative, refrigerant, stomachic, tonic

CASHEW IS A multipurpose tree of the Amazon that grows up to 15 m high. It has a thick and tortuous trunk with branches so winding that they frequently reach the ground. Cashew trees are often found growing wild on the drier sandy soils in the central plains of Brazil and are cultivated in many parts of the Amazon rainforest.

The cashew tree produces many resources and products. The bark and leaves of the tree are used medicinally, and the cashew nut has international appeal and market value as a food. Even the shell around the nut is used medicinally and has industrial applications in the plastics and resin industries for its phenol content. Then there is the pseudo-fruit, a swollen peduncle that grows behind the *real* fruit, which yields the cashew nut. This large pulpy and juicy part has a fine, sweet flavor and is commonly referred to as the "cashew fruit" or the "cashew apple." Fresh or frozen cashew fruit concentrate is a common juice product found at food stores in South America, much like our orange juice.

The cashew nut is botanically defined as the fruit. It grows externally in its own kidney-shaped hard shell at the end of this pseudo-fruit, or peduncle. The nut kernel inside is covered with an inner shell, and between the two shells is a thick caustic toxic oil called cardol. Cashew nuts must be cleaned to remove the cardol and then roasted to remove the toxins before they can be eaten.

Native to the northeast coast of Brazil, cajueiro was domesticated long before the arrival of Europeans at the end of the fifteenth century. It was "discovered" by European traders and explorers and first recorded in 1578, and from Brazil was taken to India and East Africa, where it soon became naturalized. In sixteenth-century Brazil, cashew fruits and their juice were taken by Europeans to treat fever, sweeten breath, and "conserve the stomach." The cashew tree and its nuts and fruit have been used for centuries by the indigenous tribes of the rainforest, and it is a common cultivated plant in their gardens. The Tikuna tribe in northwest Amazonia considers the fruit juice to be medicinal against influenza, and they brew a tea of leaves and bark to treat diarrhea. The Wayãpi tribe in Guyana uses a bark tea for a diarrhea remedy or colic remedy for infants. Tribes in Suriname use the toxic seed oil as an external worm medicine to kill botfly larvae under the skin. In Brazil a bark tea is used as a douche for vaginal secretions and as an astringent to stop bleeding after a tooth extraction. Botanist James Duke reports that the green fruits are used to treat hemoptysis, the seed oil and fruit juice are used for warts, a leaf infusion is used for diarrhea, expectorants are made from the tender shoots, and wine made from the fruit is used as an antidysenteric in other parts of the Amazon rainforest. The fruit juice and bark tea are very common diarrhea remedies throughout the Amazon today, used by *curanderos* and local people alike.

In Peruvian herbal medicine today, cajueiro leaf tea (called *casho*) is employed as a common diarrhea remedy, a bark tea is

> **Cajueiro fruit juice and bark tea are very common diarrhea remedies throughout the Amazon today, used by *curanderos* and local people alike.**

used as an antiseptic vaginal douche, and the seeds are used for skin infections. In Brazilian herbal medicine the fruit is taken for syphilis and as a diuretic, stimulant, and aphrodisiac. A leaf tea is prepared as a mouthwash and gargle for mouth ulcers, tonsillitis, and throat problems and is used for washing wounds. An infusion and/or maceration of the bark is used to treat diabetes, asthenia, muscular debility, urinary disorders, and asthma. The leaves and/or the bark is also used in Brazil for eczema, psoriasis, scrofula, dyspepsia, genital problems, and venereal diseases, as well as impotence, bronchitis, cough, intestinal colic, leishmaniasis, and syphilis-related skin disorders. North American practitioners use cajueiro for diabetes, coughs, bronchitis, tonsillitis, intestinal colic, and diarrhea and as a general tonic.

Cajueiro and its many products, even its "fruit," cover a wide range of uses. In addition to being delicious, it is a rich source of vitamins, minerals, and other essential nutrients (it has up to five times more vitamin C than oranges and contains a high amount of mineral salts) and is used to make highly nutritive snacks and juices. Cashew fruit extracts are now being used in body care products. Because of the high amount of vitamin C and mineral salts, cashew fruit is used as a coadjutant in the treatment of premature aging of the skin and to remineralize the skin. It is also a good scalp conditioner and tonic and is often used in shampoos, lotions, and scalp creams due to the conditioning activity of its proteins and mucilage.

Because of the high amount of vitamin C and mineral salts, cashew fruit is used as a coadjutant in the treatment of premature aging of the skin and to remineralize the skin.

The bark and leaves of cajueiro are a rich source of tannins, a group of phytochemicals with documented physiological activities. These tannins have demonstrated an anti-inflammatory effect[1] and are astringent in nature, which may be one of the reasons cajueiro is effective in cases of diarrhea. Anacardic acids, another group of phytochemicals, are also found in cashew, with the highest concentration found in the nut shells. Several clinical studies have shown that these chemicals exhibit tyrosinase inhibitory activity, have molluscicide properties, and are cytotoxic to certain cancer cells.[2–6] Cashew's antimicrobial properties were documented in a 1982 *in vitro* study,[7] and its effectiveness against leishmanial ulcers was documented in two clinical studies.[8, 9]

The natural rainforest remedy for diarrhea is 1/2 cup of a standard decoction of leaves and twigs, taken 2 to 3 times daily.

WORLDWIDE USES

Region	Uses
Africa	Intoxicant, tattoo
Brazil	Analgesic, aphrodisiac, asthenia, asthma, bronchitis, callosity corn, cough, diabetes, diuretic, dyspepsia, eczema, fever, gargle, genital, impotence, intestinal colic, leishmaniasis, mouthwash, muscular debility, psoriasis, scrofula, stimulant, syphilis, throat, tonsillitis, ulcers (mouth), urinary, venereal disease, vesicant, wart, wounds
Haiti	Caries, diabetes, stomatitis, toothache, wart
Malaya	Catarrh, constipation, dermatosis, diarrhea, nausea, thrush
Mexico	Caustic, diabetes, diarrhea, freckle, leprosy, liqueur, poison, skin, swelling, syphilis, ulcer, wart
Panama	Asthma, cold, congestion, diabetes, diarrhea, hypertension, inflammation
Peru	Antiseptic, diarrhea, douche, flu, infection, skin infections
Trinidad	Asthma, cough, diarrhea, dysentery, dyspepsia, stomachache
Turkey	Diarrhea, fever, poison, wart
Venezuela	Dysentery, gargle, leprosy, sore throat
Elsewhere	Asthma, astringent, cold, colic, congestion, corn, cough, debility, diabetes, diuretic, dysentery, liqueur, piscicide, poison, purgative, scurvy, skin, tumor, vesicant, wart

PHYTOCHEMICALS

4-0-methylglucuronic acid, alanine, alpha-catechin, alpha-linolenic acid, aluminum, anacardic acid, anacardol, antimony, arabinose, arginine, arsenic, ascorbic acid, aspartic acid, barium, benzaldehyde, beta-carotene, beta-sitosterol, boron, bromine, cadmium, calcium, capric acid, caprylic acid, cardanol, cardol, cesium, cystine, europium, fluorine, folacin, gadoleic acid, galactose, gallic acid, gingkol, glucose, glucuronic acid, glutamic acid, glycine, hafnium, hexanal, histidine, hydroxybenzoic acid, iron, isoleucine, kaempferol-glycoside, L-epicatechin, lauric acid, leucine, leucocyanidin, leucopelargonidine, limonene, linoleic acid, lysine, magnesium, manganese, methionine, mufa, myristic acid, naringenin, niacin, oleic acid, oxalic acid, palmitic acid, palmitoleic acid, phenylalanine, phytosterols, potassium, proline, protein, pufa, quercetin-glycoside, riboflavin, salicylic acid, samarium, scandium, selenium, serine, SFA, silicon, squalene, stearic acid, strontium, sulfur, tannin, thiamin, threonine, titanium, tocopherol, trans-hex-2-enal tryptophan, tyrosine, valine, vanadium, zinc

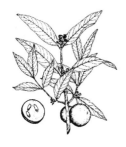

CAMU-CAMU

Family: Myrtaceae

Genus: *Myrciaria*

Species: *dubia*

Common Names: Camu-camu, rumberry

Part Used: Fruit

Medicinal Properties: Anti-inflammatory, antioxidant, astringent, emollient, nutritive

CAMU-CAMU IS A low-growing shrub found throughout the Amazon rainforest, mainly in swampy or flooded areas. It grows to a height of about 2 to 3 m and has large feathery leaves. It produces round, light-orange-colored fruits about the size of lemons that have the highest recorded source of natural vitamin C known on the planet. Oranges provide 500 to 4,000 ppm vitamin C, or ascorbic acid, while acerola has assayed 16,000 to 172,000 ppm ascorbic acid. Camu-camu provides 21,000 to 500,000 ppm ascorbic acid, or 2 to 3 grams per kilogram.[1] In comparison to oranges, camu-camu provides 30 times more vitamin C, 10 times more iron, 3 times more niacin, twice as much riboflavin, and 50% more phosphorus.[1]

> In comparison to oranges, camu-camu provides 30 times more vitamin C, 10 times more iron, 3 times more niacin, twice as much riboflavin, and 50% more phosphorus.

Its high vitamin C content has created a demand for camu-camu fruit. Some groups are now beginning to determine cultivation methods for this important new rainforest resource, which is still harvested wild throughout the Amazon region. Ethnobotanist Mark Plotkin notes in his book, *Tales of a Shaman's Apprentice*, that "a forest stand of camu-camu is worth twice the amount to be gained from cutting down the forest and replacing it with cattle," and he believes that it holds real economic promise for local economies. Usually, camu-camu fruit is wild-harvested in the rainforest in canoes because the fruits mature at high water or flooding seasons in the Amazon. The fruits are popular in Iquitos, Peru, where they are made into drinks and ice creams.

PHYTOCHEMICALS

ascorbic acid, beta-carotene, calcium, iron, niacin, phosphorus, protein, riboflavin, thiamin

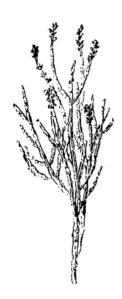

CARQUEJA

Family: Asteraceae

Genus: *Baccharis*

Species: *genistelloides*

Common Names: Carqueja, cacalia amara, caclia doce, carqueja amara, carqueja amarga, cuchi-cuchi, quinsu-cucho, tres-espigas, bacanta, bacárida, cacaia-amarga, cacália-amarga, cacália-amargosa, carqueja-do-mato, carquejinha, condamina, quina-de-condamiana, tiririca-de-balaio, vassoura

Parts Used: Aerial parts

Medicinal Properties: Analgesic, antacid, anthelmintic, antihepatotoxic, anti-inflammatory, antirheumatic, antiulcerogenic, aperient, depurative, digestive, diuretic, febrifuge, gastrotonic, hepatic, hepatoprotective, hepatotonic, hypoglycemic, laxative, refrigerant, stomachic, tonic, vermifuge

CARQUEJA IS A perennial green herb that grows almost straight up to a height of 46 cm and produces yellowish-orange flowers at the top of the plant. The bright green, flat, leafy stalks have a fleshy, succulent consistency. Carqueja is known by several botanical names, including *Baccharis genistelloides, B. triptera,* and *B. trimera.* It is found mostly in the swampy areas throughout the Amazon rainforest in Peru, Brazil, and Colombia, as well as in tropical parts of Argentina, Paraguay, and Uruguay.

Indigenous peoples of the rainforest have utilized this herb for centuries to cure common ailments. Its uses in herbal medicine were first recorded in Brazil in 1931 by Pio Correa, who wrote about an infusion of carqueja being used for sterility in women and impotency in men. Correa described carqueja as having the therapeutic properties of a tonic, bitter, febrifuge, and stomachic, with cited uses for dyspepsia, gastroenteritis, liver diseases, and diarrhea. Since that time, carqueja has long been used in Brazilian medicine to treat liver diseases, to strengthen stomach and intestinal function, and to help purge obstructions of the liver and gallbladder.[1–4] Almost every book published in South America on herbal medicine includes carqueja, since it has shown to be so effective for liver and stomach disorders as well as being a good blood cleanser and fever reducer. Other popular uses for carqueja in Brazilian herbal medicine today are to treat digestive disorders, malaria, diabetes, ulcers, sore throat and tonsillitis, angina, anemia, diarrhea, indigestion, hydropsy, urinary inflammation, kidney disorders, intestinal worms, leprosy, and poor blood circulation.

In Peruvian herbal medicine today, carqueja is used for liver ailments, gallstones, diabetes, allergies, gout, intestinal gas and bloating, and venereal diseases. Normally, the medicine is a simple tea brewed with 2 cups of the dried plant infused in 1 l of water; 1 cup of this infusion is drunk up to 3 times daily on an empty stomach. Herbalists and natural health practitioners in the United States are just learning of the many effective uses of carqueja. They document that it helps strengthen digestive, ileocecal valve, stomach, and liver functions; fortifies and cleanses the blood; expels intestinal worms; is helpful for poor digestion, liver disorders, anemia, or loss of blood; and removes obstructions in the gallbladder and liver.

Carqueja's many properties and uses recorded in herbal medicine have been studied by scientists and have been validated time and time again. Its hepatoprotective (liver-protective) properties have been demonstrated by scientists, which helps explain its almost century-long use against many types of liver disorders and diseases. In a study with mice in 1986, a crude water extract of carqueja protected against liver damage and increased the survival rate by 100% when the liver toxin phalliodin was administered.[2] Its digestive, antiulcer, and antacid properties were

> Almost every book published in South America on herbal medicine includes carqueja, since it has shown to be so effective for liver and stomach disorders as well as being a good blood cleanser and fever reducer.

verified in a 1991 clinical study, which showed that carqueja reduced gastric secretions and had an analgesic effect in rats. The study concluded that carqueja "may relieve gastrointestinal disorders by reducing acid secretion and gastrointestinal hyperactivity."[5] Scientists first studied carqueja for its hypoglycemic effects in 1967, demonstrating that it had the ability to lower sugar levels in the blood.[6] Several novel phytochemicals called diterpenoids were discovered in carqueja in 1977.[7] These phytochemicals were later tested, in 1994, and scientists showed they "exhibited maximum antifeedant and repellent activities" against worms (*Tenebrio molitor* larvae).[8] This validates carqueja's long history of use as an anthelmintic (to expel intestinal worms). A closely related Brazilian species, *B. gaudichaudiana*, which contains these diterpenoids and others, exhibited significant cytotoxic activity against cancer cells in another clinical study in 1994.[9] More recently, carqueja's anti-inflammatory, analgesic, and antiulcer effects were yet again proven in a 1996 clinical study that reported a protective effect against ulcers and that carqueja "shows strong anti-inflammatory and analgesic properties which seem to be due, at least partly, to the inhibition of prostaglandin biosynthesis."[10]

WORLDWIDE USES

Region	Uses
Brazil	Anemia, angina, antacid, anthelmintic, bitter, calculus, circulation, constipation, depurative, diabetes, diarrhea, digestive, dyspepsia, febrifuge, gastritis, gastroenteritis, grippe, hydropsy, impotence, indigestion, intestines, kidney, leprosy, liver, malaria, nausea, sore throat, sterility, stomach, stomachic, tonic, tonsillitis, ulcers, urinary, vermifuge
Peru	Allergies, bloating, diabetes, gallstones, gastritis, gout, grippe, intestinal gas, liver, urinary, venereal disease

Practitioners employ carqueja as a natural remedy for many conditions. Reported therapeutic dosages are generally 1 to 3 cups daily of a standard infusion or 3 to 4 g daily in capsules or tablets or combined with other herbs in liver, digestion, or antiparasite formulas.

PHYTOCHEMICALS

apigenin, camferol, carquejol, clerodane derivatives, diterpenoids, essential oils, flavonoids, glycosides, hispidium, hispidulin, luteolin, neptin, quercetin, resins, saponins, squalene

The annual world market value for medicines derived from medicinal plants discovered from indigenous peoples is $43 billion (U.S. dollars). Although no comparable figures are published for natural insecticides, insect repellents, and plant genetic materials acquired from native peoples, the annual potential for such products is easily that of medicinal plants. . . . Growing interest and catapulting markets in natural food, medicinal, agricultural, and body products signal increased research activities into traditional knowledge systems. Now, more than ever, the intellectual property rights of native peoples must be protected and just compensation for knowledge guaranteed. If something is not done now, mining of the riches of indigenous knowledge will become the latest—and ultimate—neocolonial form of exploitation of native peoples.

—Darrel A. Posey, *Traditional Knowledge,*
Conservation, and the Rain Forest Harvest

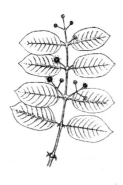

CAT'S CLAW Uña de gato

Family: Rubiaceae

Genus: *Uncaria*

Species: *tomentosa*

Common Names: Cat's claw, uña de gato, paraguayo, garabato, garbato casha, samento, toroñ, tambor huasca, uña huasca, uña de gavilan, hawk's claw

Parts Used: Bark, root, leaves

Medicinal Properties: Antibacterial, anti-inflammatory, antimutagenic, antioxidant, antitumorous, antiviral, cytostatic, depurative, diuretic, hypotensive, immunostimulant, vermifuge

CAT'S CLAW IS a large, woody vine that derives its name from hook-like thorns that grow along the vine and resemble the claw of a cat. Two closely related species of *Uncaria* are used almost interchangeably in the rainforests: *U. tomentosa* and *U. guianensis*. Both species can reach over 30 m high into the canopy; however, *U. tomentosa* has small, yellowish-white flowers, while *U. guianensis* has reddish-orange flowers and thorns that are more curved. Cat's claw is indigenous to the Amazon rainforest and other tropical areas of South and Central America, including Peru, Colombia, Ecuador, Guyana, Trinidad, Venezuela, Suriname, Costa Rica, Guatemala, and Panama.

Both *Uncaria* species are used by the indigenous peoples of the rainforest in very similar ways and have long histories of use. Cat's claw *(U. tomentosa)* has been used medicinally by the Aguaruna, Asháninka, Cashibo, Conibo, and Shipibo tribes of Peru for at least 2,000 years.[1] The Asháninka Indian tribe in central Peru has the longest recorded history of use of the plant, and they are also the largest commercial source of cat's claw from Peru today. The Asháninka use cat's claw to treat asthma and inflammations of the urinary tract; to recover from childbirth; as a kidney cleanser; to cure deep wounds; for arthritis, rheumatism, and bone pain; to control inflammation and gastric ulcers; and for cancer.[1-3] Indigenous tribes in Piura use cat's claw to treat tumors, inflammations, rheumatism, and gastric ulcers. Indian tribes in Colombia use the vine to treat gonorrhea and dysentery. Other Peruvian indigenous tribes use cat's claw to treat diabetes, urinary tract cancer in women, cirrhosis, gastritis, rheumatism, inflammations, and tumors.[4] The Cashibo tribe of eastern Peru believes that cat's claw "normalizes the

> **Cat's claw has been used medicinally by the Aguaruna, Asháninka, Cashibo, Conibo, and Shipibo tribes of Peru for at least 2,000 years.**

body," and they have used it since ancient times to treat fevers and abscesses and to cleanse the system. Other documented indigenous uses of this important vine in Peru include treatments for hemorrhages and impurities of the skin, as a blood cleanser, and for irregularity of the menstrual cycle.[1] Cat's claw has also been reportedly used as a contraceptive by several different tribes of Peru, but only in excessive amounts. Dr. Fernando Cabieses, M.D., a noted authority on Peruvian medicinal plants, explains that the Asháninka boil 5 to 6 kg of the root in water until it is reduced to a little more than 1 cup. This decoction is then taken daily during the period of menstruation for three consecutive months, which supposedly causes sterility for three to four years.[5]

With so many documented uses of this important rainforest plant, it is not surprising that it came to the attention of Western researchers and scientists. Cat's claw was first written about in the mid-1960s by a European teacher, Arturo Brell, and an American university professor, Eugene Whitworth. The ethnic uses began to be recorded, plant samples taken, and initial screening of active constituents performed.[3] Then, in the early 1970s, Klaus Keplinger, a journalist and self-taught ethnologist from Innnsbruck, Austria, organized the first definitive studies on cat's claw. Keplinger's work in the 1970s and 1980s led to several extracts of cat's claw being sold in Austria and Germany as prescription medicines,[5-7] as well as to three U.S. patents describing the alkaloid extraction methods and the immunostimulating actions of these alkaloids found in cat's claw.[8–10] It also fueled worldwide interest in the medicinal properties of this valuable vine of the rainforest. In May 1994 the World Health Organization sponsored the First International Conference on cat's claw in Geneva, Switzerland. At the conference, cat's claw received official recognition as a medicinal plant. There it was pointed out that not since quinine was discovered in the bark of a Peruvian tree in the seventeenth century had any other rainforest plant ever prompted such worldwide attention.[11]

Oxindole alkaloids found in the bark and roots of cat's claw have been documented to stimulate the immune system. Many studies indicate that at least six of these oxindole alkaloids can increase immune function by up to 50% in relatively small amounts.

The most attention to date has been given to the oxindole alkaloids found in the bark and roots of cat's claw, which have been documented to stimulate the immune system. Many studies indicate that at least six of these oxindole alkaloids can increase immune function by up to 50% in relatively small amounts.[3, 8–10, 12–21] This has led to its use around the world as an adjunctive treatment for cancer and AIDS, as well as other diseases that negatively impact the immunological system.[5–7, 22, 23] In addition to its immunostimulating activity for cancer patients, other anticancerous properties have been documented on these alkaloids and other constituents in cat's claw. Five of the oxindole alkaloids have been clinically documented with antileukemic properties,[24] and various root and bark extracts have demonstrated antitumorous and antimutagenic properties.[5, 25–28] Reports on observatory trials with cancer patients taking cat's claw in conjunction with traditional cancer therapies like chemotherapy and radiation noted fewer side effects to the traditional therapies (such as hair loss, weight loss, nausea, secondary infections, and skin problems).[5]

Another significant area of study has focused on cat's claw's anti-inflammatory properties. While plant sterols like beta-sitosterol, acids, and other antioxidants found in cat's claw account for some of these properties, new and novel phytochemicals called quinovic acid glycosides were found in the bark and roots and documented to be the most potent anti-inflammatory constituents found in the plant.[29] These studies indicated that cat's claw and some of its constituents could inhibit inflammation from 46% to up to 69% in various *in vivo* and *in vitro* tests.[29-36] The results of these studies validated its long history of indigenous use for arthritis and rheumatism, as well as for other types of inflammation associated with various stomach disorders and ulcers, where it was clinically shown to be effective.[37] This same group of chemicals also demonstrated *in vitro* antiviral properties in another study.[38] Cat's claw also contains the alkaloids rhynchophylline, hirsutine, and mitraphylline, which have demonstrated hypotensive and vasodilating properties.[39, 40] Rhynchophylline has also shown to inhibit platelet aggregation and thrombosis and may help prevent blood clots in blood vessels,[40, 41] as well as relax the blood vessels of endothelial cells, dilate peripheral blood vessels, lower the heart rate, and lower blood cholesterol.[42]

In herbal medicine today cat's claw is employed around the world for many different conditions. Dr. Donna Schwontkowski reports it being used for the treatment of immune disorders, gastritis, ulcers, cancer, arthritis, rheumatism, irregularities of the female cycle, acne, organic depression, wounds, fungus, fistulas, hemorrhoids, rheumatic disorders, neuralgias, chronic inflammation (vaginal or intestinal), and viral diseases like herpes zoster (shingles). Dr. Brent Davis refers to cat's claw as the "opener of the way" because of its ability to cleanse the entire intestinal tract and its effectiveness in treating stomach and bowel disorders such as Crohn's disease, leaky bowel syndrome, ulcers, gastritis, diverticulitis, and other inflammatory conditions of the bowel, stomach, and intestines.[43]

Dr. Julian Whitaker, M.D., reports using cat's claw for its immune-stimulating effects, for cancer, to help prevent strokes and heart attacks, to reduce blood clots, and for diverticulitis and irritable bowel syndrome.[44] Phillip Steinberg, certified nutritional consultant, reports cat's claw as beneficial in the treatment of cancer, arthritis, bursitis, rheumatism, genital herpes and herpes zoster, allergies, ulcers, systemic candidiasis, PMS and irregularities of the female cycle, environmental toxin poisoning, numerous bowel and intestinal disorders, organic depression, and HIV.[45] Kenneth Jones, in his book on cat's claw, cites its usefulness in treating diverticulitis, hemorrhoids, peptic ulcers, colitis, gastritis, parasites, and leaky bowel syndrome.[46] In Peruvian medicine today, cat's claw is even being used in veterinary practices to benefit dogs and cats with hip dysplasia, arthritis, cancers, Parvo virus, dermatitis and other skin disorders, tumors, FIV, and feline leukemia.[47] In Peruvian herbal medicine cat's claw is used for rheumatism, colic and stomach disorders, prostate inflammation, ulcers, skin disorders, fevers, and coughs, as well as for cancer and AIDS.

Cat's claw is even being used in veterinary practices to benefit dogs and cats with hip dysplasia, arthritis, cancers, Parvo virus, dermatitis and other skin disorders, tumors, FIV, and feline leukemia.

The most common forms used today are cat's claw capsules and tablets, which have become widely available. For general immune and health benefits, practitioners usually recommend 500 mg to 1 g daily. Therapeutic dosages of cat's claw can be as high as 10 g daily, but generally for arthritis, bowel, and digestive problems 3 to 4 g daily is sufficient if a good product is obtained.

WORLDWIDE USES

Region	Uses
Colombia	Dysentery, gonorrhea
Guiana	Dysentery
Peru	Abscesses, arthritis, asthma, blood cleanser, "bone pains," cancer, cirrhosis, contraceptive, cytostatic, diabetes, diarrhea, disease prevention, dysentery, fevers, gastric ulcers, gastritis, gonorrhea, hemorrhages, inflammations, intestinal affections, kidney cleanser, menstrual irregularity, rheumatism, skin disorders, stomach, urinary tract disorders, tumors, wounds
Suriname	Dysentery, intestinal affections, wounds

PHYTOCHEMICALS

3-beta,-6beta, 7-acetoxydihydronomiline SD CCO, 19alpha-trihydroxy-urs-12-en-28-oic acid, 5alpha-carboxystrictosidine, acetyluncaric acid PL JSG, adipic acid, alloisopteropodine, allopteropodine, angustine, campesterol, carboxystrictosidine, catechol BR AYL, D-catechin, DL-catechol, catechutannic acid, beta-sitosterol, corynantheine, corynoxeine, dihydrocorynantheine, dihydrocorynantheine-N-oxide, dihydrogambirtannine, ellagic acid, L-epicathechol, (-)-epicathechin, gallic acid, hanadamine, hirsutine, hirsuteine, hirsutine-N-oxide, hyperin, 3-iso-19-epi-ajmalicine, isocorynozeine, isomitraphylline, isopteropodine, isorhynchophylline, isorhynchophylline-N-oxide, isorotundifoline, ketouncaric acid, mitraphylline, 11-methoxyyohimbine, oleanolic acid, ourouparin, oxogambirtannine, pteropodine, quinovic-acid-3beta-o-(beta-d-glucopyranosyl -(1->3)beta-d- fucopyranosyl-(27->1)beta d-glucopyranosyl-ester, quinovic-acid-3beta-o-beta-d-fucopyranoside, quinovic-acid-3beta-o-beta-d-fucopyranosyl-(27->1) beta-d-glucopyranosylester, quinovic-acid- 3beta-o-beta-d-quinovopyranoside, rhynchophylline, rotundifoline, speciophylline, stigmasterol, uncarine, uncarine-f, ursolic acid

CATUABA

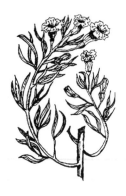

Family: Erythroxylaceae

Genus: *Erythroxylum*

Species: *catuaba*

Common Names: Catuaba, chuchuhuasha, tatuaba, pau de reposta, caramuru, piratancara

Part Used: Bark

Medicinal Properties: Antibacterial, antiviral, aphrodisiac, central nervous system stimulant, tonic

Catuaba has a long history in herbal medicine as an aphrodisiac. The Tupi Indians in Brazil first discovered the qualities of the plant, and over the past centuries they have composed many songs praising its wonders.

CATUABA IS A medium-sized, vigorous-growing tree. It produces pretty yellow and orange flowers and small, dark yellow, oval-shaped inedible fruit. It grows in the northern part of Brazil, the Amazon, Para, Pernambuco, Bahia, Maranhao, and Alagoas. Catuaba is known by two botanical names in Brazil, *Juniperus brasiliensis* and *Erythroxylum catuaba*. Catuaba belongs to the family Erythroxylaceae, whose principal genus, *Erythroxylon*, contains several species and varieties that are the source of cocaine. Catuaba, however, contains none of the active cocaine alkaloids.

Catuaba has a long history in herbal medicine as an aphrodisiac. The Tupi Indians in Brazil first discovered the qualities of the plant, and over the past centuries they have composed many songs praising its wonders. Indigenous people and local people have used catuaba for generations, and it is the most famous of all Brazilian aphrodisiac plants. In the state of Minas, there is a saying: "Until a father reaches 60, the son is his; after that, the son is catuaba's."

In Brazilian herbal medicine today, catuaba is considered a central nervous system stimulant with aphrodisiac properties; a bark decoction is used for sexual impotency, agitation, nervousness, neurasthenia, poor memory or forgetfulness, and sexual weakness. According to Dr. Meira Penna, catuaba "functions as a stimulant of the nervous system, above all when one deals with functional impotence of the male genital organs . . . it is an innocent aphrodisiac, used without any ill effects at all."[1] In Brazil it is regarded as an aphrodisiac with "proven efficacy," and in addition to treating impotence, it is employed for many types of nervous conditions including insomnia, hypochondria, and pain related to the central nervous system. In European herbal medicine catuaba is considered an aphrodisiac and a brain and nerve stimulant. A bark tea is used for sexual weakness, impotence, nervous debility, and exhaustion. Herbalists and health practitioners in the United States use catuaba in much the same way: as a tonic for the genitals as well as a central nervous system stimulant, for sexual impotence, general exhaustion and fatigue, insomnia related to hypertension, agitation, and poor memory. According to Michael van Straten, noted author and researcher of Brazilian plants, catuaba is beneficial to men and women as an aphrodisiac, but "it is in the area of male impotence that the most striking results have been reported" and "there is no evidence of side effects, even after long-term use."[2]

The constituents found in catuaba include alkaloids, tannins, aromatic oils and fatty resins, phytosterols, cyclolignans, and a

> Heirs to an oral tradition that stretches back deep into the mists of prehistory, the shamans are not only the critical link between the tropical rainforest and our neighborhood pharmacy; I believe they are our greatest hope for finding cures to currently incurable diseases (cancer, AIDS, the common cold), as well as diseases that will undoubtedly appear in the future.
>
> —Mark J. Plotkin, *Tales of a Shaman's Apprentice*

chemical Brazilian scientists named ioimbina.[3, 4] Clinical studies on catuaba have found very interesting results involving its antibacterial and antiviral properties. A clinical study conducted in 1992 indicated that an extract of catuaba was effective in protecting mice from lethal infections of *Escherichia coli* and *Staphlococcus aureus,* in addition to significantly inhibiting HIV.[5] The study found that catuaba's anti-HIV activity was shown to be induced, at least in part, via the inhibition of HIV absorption to the cells and suggested that catuaba extract has potential against opportunistic infections in HIV patients.[5]

The traditional method for this natural remedy is a standard infusion (bark tea), with 1 to 3 cups taken daily. However, an alcohol tincture can extract more of the active constituents and provide better results in some conditions at 2 to 3 ml per day.

WORLDWIDE USES

Region	Uses
Brazil	Aphrodisiac, central nervous system stimulant, fatigue, impotence, insomnia, neurasthenia, tonic
Peru	Skin cancer

PHYTOCHEMICALS

alkaloids, aromatic oils and fatty resins, cyclolignans, ioimbina, phytosterols, tannins

CHANCA PIEDRA

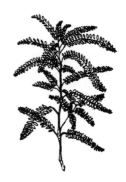

Family: Euphorbiaceae

Genus: *Phyllanthus*

Species: *niruri*

Common Names: Chanca piedra, quebra pedra, pitirishi, stone breaker, shatter stone, sasha foster, seed on the leaf, derriere dos, des dos, feuilles la fievre, quinina criolla, dukong anak (child pick-a-back), memeniran, meniran, rami buah, tamalaka, turi hutan

Parts Used: Aerial parts, whole herb

Medicinal Properties: Anodyne, antibacterial, antihepatotoxic, anti-inflammatory, antispasmodic, antiviral, aperitif, carminative, choleretic, digestive, diuretic, emmenagogue, febrifuge, hepatotonic, hypoglycemic, hypotensive, immunostimulant, laxative, stomachic, tonic, vermifuge

CHANCA PIEDRA IS a small, erect, annual herb that grows up to 30 to 40 cm in height. It is indigenous to the rainforests in the Amazon and other tropical areas, including the Bahamas, southern India, and China. The *Phyllanthus* genus contains over 600 species of shrubs, trees, and annual or biennial herbs distributed throughout the tropical and subtropical regions of both hemispheres. *P. niruri* is quite prevalent in the Amazon and other wet rainforests, growing and spreading freely, much like a weed. *P. amarus* and *P. sellowianus* are closely related to *P. niruri* in appearance, phytochemical structure, and history of use but are found in drier tropical climates in India, Brazil, and even Florida, where *P. amarus* is a common weed.

Chanca piedra, the Spanish name for *P. niruri*, means "stone breaker" or "shatter stone." It has been called stone breaker because it has been used for generations by the indigenous peoples of the Amazon as an effective remedy to

> Chanca piedra has been called "stone breaker" because it has been used by the indigenous peoples of the Amazon as an effective remedy to eliminate gallstones and kidney stones and for other kidney problems.

eliminate gallstones and kidney stones and for other kidney problems. The plant is employed for numerous other conditions, including blennorrhagia, colic, diabetes, dysentery, fever, flu, tumors, jaundice, vaginitis, and dyspepsia. It is little wonder that chanca piedra is used for so many purposes, since the plant has demonstrated antihepatotoxic, antispasmodic, antiviral, antibacterial, diuretic, febrifugal, and hypoglycemic activities.[1] It is also known as an anodyne, aperitif, carminative, digestive, emmenagogue, laxative, stomachic, tonic, and vermifuge, based on its long, documented history of uses.

Chanca piedra is still widely used in herbal medicine in South America, remaining the most popular remedy for gallstones and kidney stones throughout the continent. In Peruvian herbal medicine it is also used for hepatitis; urinary infections; calculus in the kidney, bladder, ovaries and liver; inflammation of the urinary tract system; diabetes; and as a diuretic, liver tonic, and blood purifier. In Brazilian herbal medicine it is called *quebra pedra* and is considered an excellent remedy for removing uric acid from the urine and eliminating stones. It is also used in Brazil for hydropsy, urinary and bladder infections and blockages, liver ailments, painful joints, cystitis, prostate disorders, kidney disorders, hepatitis, and diabetes and as an antispasmodic and muscle relaxant specific to the urinary tract system. Indigenous to India, where it is called *pitirishi* or *budhatri*, chanca piedra is a common household remedy for asthma and bronchitis and is used to treat coughing, extreme thirst, anemia, jaundice, and tuberculosis.[2] It is also indigenous to the Bahamas, where it is called hurricane weed or gale-wind grass. It is used in local herbal medicine there for poor appetite, constipation, typhoid fever, flu, and colds.[2]

Since the mid-1960s, chanca piedra has been the subject of much research to determine the active constituents and their pharmacological activities.[3] Indian and Brazilian research groups were the first to conduct these studies, since the plant was indigenous to their areas and had long histories of use by local inhabitants. In some of the published research, scientists make little or no distinction between *P. niruri* and *P. amarus* because of the very similar phytochemical makeup of both plants. In fact, some references are found in which scientists believe that it is one species of plant with two botanical names, but of course there are botanists who would argue this point. The antispasmodic activity of alkaloids in chanca piedra were documented by Brazilian researchers in the mid-1980s,[4] which explained the popular use of the plant for kidney and bladder stones. The alkaloid extract demonstrated smooth muscle relaxation specific to the urinary and biliary tract, which the researchers surmised facilitates the expulsion of kidney or bladder calculi. The antihepatotoxic (liver-protecting) activity of chanca piedra was attributed to two compounds in the plant, phyllanthin and hypophyllanthin, in a 1985 study by Indian researchers.[5] Glycosides found in chanca piedra demonstrated aldose reductase inhibitory activity in studies conducted by a Japanese research group in 1988 and 1989.[6,7] The analgesic activity of chanca piedra was demonstrated in 1994 and 1995 by another research group in Brazil.[8,9] The diuretic, hypotensive, and hypoglycemic effects of chanca piedra were documented in a small, open human study conducted in 1995. This study showed a significant diuretic effect, a significant reduction in systolic blood pressure in nondiabetic hypertensives and female subjects, and a significant reduction in blood glucose in diabetic patients taking chanca piedra for 10 days.[10]

> Chanca piedra gained worldwide attention in the late 1980s due to the plant's antiviral activity against hepatitis B.

Of particular note, chanca piedra gained worldwide attention in the late 1980s due to the plant's antiviral activity against hepatitis B. Preliminary clinical trials on children with infective hepatitis [11,12] using an Indian drug containing *P. niruri* as the main ingredient showed promising results that fueled the subsequent *in vitro* and *in vivo* studies. The *in vitro* inactivation of hepatitis B by chanca piedra was reported in India in 1982.[13] A study that followed indicated that *in vivo* chanca piedra eliminated hepatitis B in mammals within 3 to 6 weeks.[14] The subsequent clinical results concerning the use of chanca piedra for hepatitis have been conflicting, and this may have much to do with the extract standardization, species used, and harvest location, all of which may have affected the resulting levels of active constituents in the samples used. Several subsequent studies in the late 1980s and early 1990s failed to produce any effect against hepatitis, but other research, conducted from 1990 to 1995, has indicated that chanca piedra does demonstrate antiviral activity against hepatitis B.[15–17]

The most recent research on chanca piedra reveals that its antiviral activity extends to human immunodeficiency virus (HIV). A Japanese research group discovered *P. niruri*'s HIV-1 reverse transcriptase inhibition properties in 1992 with a simple water extract of the plant.[18] Bristol-Myers Squibb Pharmaceutical Research Institute isolated at least one of the constituents in the plant responsible for this activity—a novel compound that they named niruriside and described in a 1996 study.[19]

Certainly, much more research is needed before a new AIDS or hepatitis drug is developed from chanca piedra—if at all. In the meantime, chanca piedra, with its many effective uses for a wide range of indications, is one of the more important remedies coming from the rainforests and is gaining in popularity with herbalists and natural health practitioners worldwide. More important, there have been no side effects or toxicity reported in any of the clinical studies or in its many years of reported use in herbal medicine. Practitioners generally use 1 to 2 cups daily of standard infusion as a natural remedy for kidney stones and other urinary and liver problems.

WORLDWIDE USES

Region	Uses
Amazonia	Gallstones, kidney, kidney stones
Bahamas	Aperitif, cold, constipation, fever, flu, laxative, stomachache, typhoid
Brazil	Ache (joint), antispasmodic, bladder, cystitis, diabetes, diuretic, fever, gallbladder, gallstones, hepatitis, hydropsy, kidney, kidney stones, liver, prostate, urinary
Haiti	Carminative, colic, digestive, diuretic, fever, malaria, stomachache, stomachic, tenesmus
India	Anemia, asthma, bronchitis, cough, diuretic, dysentery, gonorrhea, hepatitis, jaundice, thirst, tuberculosis, tumor (abdomen)
Java	Cough, gonorrhea, stomachache
Malaya	Caterpillar sting, dermatosis, diarrhea, diuretic, itch, miscarriage, piscicide, renosis, syphilis, vertigo
Marianas	Dysentery, itch, rectitis, vaginitis
Peru	Calculus, diuretic, gallstones, hepatitis, kidney stones
Elsewhere	Blennorrhagia, diabetes, diarrhea, diuretic, dropsy, dysentery, dyspepsia, emmenagogue, fever, gallstones, gonorrhea, kidney stones, malaria, poultice, tonic

PHYTOCHEMICALS

3,5,7-trihydroxyflavonal-4'-o-alpha-l-(-)-rhamnopyranoside, 4-methoxy-norsecurinine, 4-methoxy-securinine, 5,3',4'-trihydroxyflavonone-7-o-alpha-l-(-)-rhamnopyranoside, astragalin, brevifolin-carboxylic-acid, cymene, hypophyllanthin, limonene, lintetralin, lupa-20(29)-ene-3-beta-ol, lupa-20(29)-ene-3-beta-ol-acetate, lupeol, methyl-salicylate, niranthin, nirtetralin, niruretin, nirurin, niruriside, phyllanthin, phyllochrysine, phyltetralin, quercetin, quercetin-heteroside, quercetol, quercitrin, rutin, saponins, triacontanal, tricontanol

CHUCHUHUASI

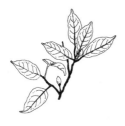

Family: Celastraceae

Genus: *Maytenus*

Species: *krukovit, laevis, macrocarpa, ebenifolia*

Common Names: Chuchuhuasi, chucchu huashu, chuchuasi, chuchasha

Part Used: Bark

Medicinal Properties: Adrenal supportive, analgesic, anodyne, antiarthritic, antidiarrheic, anti-inflammatory, antirheumatic, antitumor, aphrodisiac, immunostimulant, muscle relaxant, stimulant, stomachic, tonic

CHUCHUHUASI IS AN enormous canopy tree of the Amazon rainforest that grows up to 30 m high. Several botanical names have been given to this one species of tree, including *Maytenus krukovit*, M. *laevis*, M. *macrocarpa*, and M. *ebenifolia*.[1] It has large leaves that can reach lengths of between 10 and 30 cm, small, white flowers, and extremely tough, heavy, reddish-brown bark.

Indigenous people of the Amazon rainforest have been using the bark of chuchuhuasi medicinally for centuries. Its name means "trembling back," which describes its long history of use for arthritis, rheumatism, and back pain. One local arthritis and rheumatism remedy prescribes 1 cup of the decoction taken 3 times a day for more than a week. In addition, chuchuhuasi is also used as a muscle relaxant, aphrodisiac, and pain reliever, for adrenal support, as an insect repellent, as an immune stimulant, and for menstrual balance and regulation. People along the Amazon believe that chuchuhuasi is an aphrodisiac and tonic, and the bark soaked in the local rum (*aguardiente*) is a popular jungle drink that is even served to tourists. In Peru chuchuhuasi is still considered the "best remedy" for arthritis among both city and forest dwellers. In Colombia the Siona Indians boil a small piece of the bark (5 cm) in 2 l of water until 1 l remains, and then drink it for arthritis and rheumatism. In Peruvian herbal medicine today, chuchuhuasi is used to treat osteoarthritis, rheumatoid arthritis, bronchitis, diarrhea, hemorrhoids, and menstrual irregularities and pain. Local healers and *curanderos* in the Amazon use chuchuhuasi as a general tonic, to speed healing, and as a synergist combined with other medicinal plants for many types of illnesses.

> **Local healers and *curanderos* in the Amazon use chuchuhuasi as a general tonic, to speed healing, and as a synergist combined with other medicinal plants for many types of illnesses.**

Due to its long history of use and its incredible effectiveness, there has been much clinical interest in determining why chuchuhuasi works. In the 1960s an American pharmaceutical company discovered its potent immune-stimulating properties, finding that it dramatically increased phagocytosis in mice.[2] In the mid-1970s Italian researchers studying a chuchuhuasi extract used effectively to treat skin cancers identified its antitumor properties.[3] Its anti-inflammatory properties were discovered in the 1980s by another Italian research group. They discovered that its anti-inflammatory properties, radiation protectant action, and antitumor properties were at least partially linked to triterpenes and antioxidants isolated in the trunk bark.[4] In 1993 a Japanese research group isolated a group of novel alkaloids in chuchuhuasi that may be responsible for its effectiveness in treating arthritis and rheumatism.[5] In the United States a pharmaceutical company studying chuchuhuasi's anti-inflammatory and anti-arthritic properties has determined that these alkaloids can effectively inhibit enzyme production of protein kinase C (PKC).[6] PKC inhibitors have been of much interest worldwide because there is evidence that too much of this enzyme is involved in a wide variety of disease processes, including arthritis, asthma, brain tumors, cancer, and cardiovascular disease.[7] It is expected that if the constituents in chuchuhuasi that are responsible for inhibiting PKC can be synthesized, a new arthritis drug will be developed. Meantime, the natural bark of this important Amazon rainforest tree will continue to be one of the most effective natural remedies for arthritis, as it has been for centuries. Traditionally, 1 to 2 cups daily of a standard bark decoction or 3 to 6 ml of a standard tincture is used for this rainforest remedy.

WORLDWIDE USES

Region	Uses
Colombia	Analgesic, arthritis, rheumatism
Ecuador	Ache (menstrual, muscles), analgesic, aphrodisiac, arthritis, fever, rheumatism, stomachache, tumors (skin)
Peru	Ache (back, muscles), analgesic, aphrodisiac, arthritis, bronchitis, cancer, hemorrhoids, impotency, menstrual disorders, osteoarthritis, rheumatism, tumors (skin), virility

PHYTOCHEMICALS

22-hydroxytingenone, 6-benzoyl-6-deacetylmayteine, catechin tannins, maytansine, mayteine, maytenin, mebeverine, phenoldienones, pristimeran, proanthocyanidins, tingenone

COPAIBA

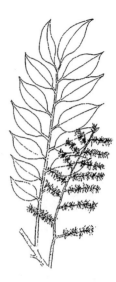

Family: Fabaceae

Genus: *Copaifera*

Species: *officinalis, reticulata*

Common Names: Copaiba, copal, balsam copaiba, copaiva, Jesuit's balsam, copaibeura-de-Minas, mal-dos-sete-dias

Part Used: Resin

Medicinal Properties: Antibacterial, anti-inflammatory, antimicrobial, astringent, cicatrizant, disinfectant, diuretic, emollient, expectorant, laxative, stimulant, vulnerary

COPAIBA TREES ARE considerably branched and grow up to 18 to 30 m high. The trees of *Copaifera* are found mainly in the South American rainforests, particularly Brazil, Colombia, Peru, and Venezuela.

The part of the tree that is most used medicinally is the oleoresin that accumulates in cavities within the tree trunk. It is harvested by tapping or drilling holes into the wood of the trunk and collecting the resin that drips out, much as rubber trees are tapped. Although this resin is often referred to as balsam, it is not a true balsam. Copaiba oil is obtained by direct vacuum distillation of the oleoresin containing large amounts of the volatile oil (60% to 90%).

The resin is a thick, clear liquid with a color that changes from pale yellow to golden light brown. Copaiba oil and/or resin has been used for several centuries in Europe and Latin America in the treatment of chronic cystitis, bronchitis, and diarrhea and as a treatment for hemorrhoids. On the Rio Solimoes in northwest Amazonia, copaiba resin is used topically by indigenous tribes as a cicatrizant, for skin sores, for psoriasis, and to treat gonorrhea. In the Peruvian Andes the resin is taken internally for urinary incontinence, syphilis, and catarrh. Traditional medicine in Brazil recommends copaiba oil today as an anti-inflammatory agent, for dandruff treatment, for all types of skin disorders, and for stomach ulcers. In Peruvian traditional medicine copaiba oil is used as an anti-inflammatory agent and for stomach ulcers; healers also combine it with andiroba oil for treating herpes. Noted ethnobotanist and author Mark Plotkin reports that copaiba oil is used in the United States as a disinfectant, diuretic, laxative, and stimulant, in addition to being used in cosmetics and soaps. Healers and *curanderos* in the Amazon today use copaiba for all types of pain and to cool inflammation.

> **Traditional medicine in Brazil recommends copaiba oil as an anti-inflammatory agent, for dandruff treatment, for all types of skin disorders, and for stomach ulcers.**

In addition to its traditional uses, copaiba is believed to have diuretic, expectorant, disinfectant, and stimulant properties.[1] The oil has been documented to have antibacterial activity.[2,3] The oleoresin has demonstrated marked anti-inflammatory activity in various animal experimental models, which has validated its traditional uses.[4] Research indicates that copaiba oil taken internally is nontoxic at traditional dosages, although in very large dosages it can cause diarrhea, vomiting, and/or a measles-like rash.[1,2,5]

Copaiba resin contains 30% to 90% volatile oil; the remaining material is resins and acids.[2] Active constituents are mainly attributed to the sesquiterpenes and diterpenes (up to 50% to 90% of the resin may be sesquiterpenes).[6] The resin contains two sesquiterpenes, caryophyllene and calamenene, which have clinically demonstrated anti-inflammatory, spasmoylitic, antimicrobial, and/or antibacterial properties.[7,8] It also contains copaibic or paracopaibic acid, copalic, copaiferic, and copaiferolic acids from the group of terpene-resins and acids that have been demonstrated as active constituents.[8–12] It also contains a true and yellow resin, made by the oxygenation of the essence exposed to the air.

In the United States copaiba oil is currently approved for food use and is used occasionally as a flavor component. In addition, it is commonly used as a fragrance component in perfumes, and it is widely used in cosmetic preparations (including soaps, bubble baths, detergents, creams, and lotions) for its emollient, antibacterial, and anti-inflammatory properties. Copaiba oil can be applied topically several times daily to rashes, muscle/joint aches and injuries, wounds, boils, and herpes ulcers. It can be used by itself or combined with other oils as a wonderful healing and anti-inflammatory massage oil.

WORLDWIDE USES

Region	Uses
Amazonia	Cicatrizant, disinfectant, diuretic, gonorrhea, inflammation, psoriasis, sores (skin)
Brazil	Anti-inflammatory, cicatrizant, dandruff, dermatitis, incontinence, inflammation, skin disorders, syphilis, tumor (prostate), ulcers (stomach)
Europe	Bronchitis, cystitis, diarrhea, hemorrhoids
Peru	Anti-inflammatory, catarrh, herpes, syphilis, ulcers (stomach), urinary
United States	Anti-inflammatory, disinfectant, diuretic, laxative, stimulant

PHYTOCHEMICALS

(-)-16beta-kauran-19-carbonic acid, (-)-kaur-16-en-19-carbonic acid, 7-hydroxyhardwickic acid, alloaromadendrene, alpha-bergamotene, alpha-cubebene, alpha-multijugenol, alpha-selinene, ar-curcumene, beta-bisabolene, beta-cubebene, beta-elemene, beta-farnesene, beta-humulene, beta-metacopaibic acid, beta-muurolene, beta-selinene, calamenene, calamesene, carioazulene, caryophyllene, caryophyllene-oxide, coipaiferic acid, copaene, copaiferolic acid, copalic acid, cyperene, delta-cadinene, delta-elemene, enantio-agathic acid, eperu-8(20)-en-15,18-dioic acid, gamma-cadinene, gamma-elemene, gamma-humulene, hardwickic acid, homoparacopaibic acid, illurinic acid, maracaibobalsam, paracopaibic acid, polyalthic acid,trans-alpha-bergamotene

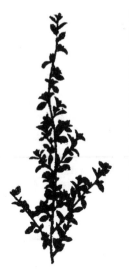

DAMIANA

Family: Turneraceae

Genus: *Turnera*

Species: *aphrodisiaca, diffusa*

Common Names: Damiana, damiane, oreganillo, the bourrique

Parts Used: Aerial parts, leaves

Medicinal Properties: Aphrodisiac, astringent, diuretic, emmenagogue, laxative, nervine, stimulant, stomachic, tonic

DAMIANA IS A small shrub with aromatic leaves that are lanceolate, are 10 to 25 mm long, and have three to six teeth along the margins. The plant is found throughout Mexico, Central and South America, and the West Indies.

The botanical name of the plant, *Turnera aphrodisiaca*, describes its ancient use as an aphrodisiac. Damiana was used as an aphrodisiac in the ancient Maya civilization, as well as for "giddiness and loss of balance."[1] From 1888 to 1947 damiana leaf and elixir were listed in the National Formulary (NF).[1] For more than a century damiana's use has been associated with improving sexual function in both males and females. Damiana is thought to act as an antidepressant, tonic, diuretic, cough treatment, and mild laxative. Dr. James Balch reports in his book *Prescription for Nutritional Healing* that damiana "relieves headaches, controls bed-wetting, and stimulates muscular contractions of the intestinal tract"; he also comments that "damiana interferes with iron absorption when taken internally." The leaves are used in Germany to relieve excess mental activity

> The botanical name of the plant, *Turnera aphrodisiaca*, describes its ancient use as an aphrodisiac.

and nervous debility and as a tonic for the hormonal and central nervous systems. E. F. Steinmetz states that in Holland, damiana is renowned for its sexual-enhancing qualities and positive effect on the reproductive organs. [2]

Damiana's chemical composition is complex, and components have not been completely identified. However, the known makeup is 0.5% to 1% volatile oil, gonzalitosin (cyanogic glycoside), arbutin, tannin, and damianin (a brown, bitter substance).[2, 3] The leaf also contains beta-sitosterol, which may account for the stimulant effect on the sexual organs. Therapeutic dosages for damiana are reported to be 3 to 4 g daily.

WORLDWIDE USES

Region	Uses
Bahamas	Enuresis, headache
France	Aphrodisiac
Haiti	Aphrodisiac, cold, intestine, liqueur, tonic, venereal disease
Mexico	Amaurosis, aphrodisiac, astringent, diabetes, diuretic, dysentery, dyspepsia, intestine, malaria, nerve, panacea, paralysis, renitis, stomachache, syphilis, tonic
United States	Aphrodisiac, astringent, dysmenorrhea, expectorant, laxative, stimulant, tonic
Elsewhere	Aphrodisiac, catarrh, laxative, nervine, stimulant, venereal disease

PHYTOCHEMICALS

8-cineole, 5-hydroxy-7,3',4-trimethoxyflavone, albuminoids, alpha-copaene, alpha-pinene, arbutin, ascorbic acid, beta-pinene, beta-sitosterol, calamenene, chlorophyll, chromium, damianin, gamma-cadinene, gonzalitosin-i, hexacosanol-1, magnesium, manganese, niacin, p-cymol, potassium, resin, riboflavin, selenium, silicon, tannins, thiamin, thymol, triacontane, zinc

ERVA TOSTÃO

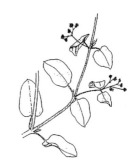

Family: Nyctaginaceae

Genus: *Boerhaavia*

Species: *diffusa, hirsuta*

Common Names: Erva tostão, erva toustao, pega-pinto, hog weed, pig weed, atikamaamidi, biskhapra, djambo, etiponia, fowl's lice, ganda'dar, ghetuli, katkatud, mahenshi, mamauri, ndandalida, oulouni niabo, paanbalibis, patal-jarh, pitasudu-pala, punar-nava, punerva, punnarnava, purnoi, samdelma, san, sant, santh, santi, satadi thikedi, satodi, spreading hog weed, tellaaku, thazhuthama, thikri, touri-touri, tshrana, yoegbe

Parts Used: Herb, roots

Medicinal Properties: Anthelmintic, antiamebic, antibacterial, anticonvulsant, antifibrinolytic, anti-inflammatory, antispasmodic, antiviral, choleretic, depurative, diuretic, hemostatic, hepatoprotective, hepatotonic, hypotensive, lactagogue, laxative, vermifuge

ERVA TOSTÃO IS a vigorous-growing weedy vine that grows up to 70 cm high. It has a large root system and produces yellow and white flowers. It can be found in many tropical and warm-climate countries. Indigenous to Brazil, it is found in abundance along roadsides and in the forests in and near São Paulo, Rio de Janeiro, and Minas Gerais. Erva tostão is also indigenous to India, where it is found in abundance in the warmer parts of the country.

The roots of erva tostão have held an important place in herbal medicine in both Brazil and India for many years. In Brazil G. L. Cruz reports erva tostão is "a plant medicine of great importance, extraordinarily beneficial in the treatment of liver disorders." It is employed in Brazilian herbal medicine as a cholagogue and diuretic, for all types of liver disorders (including jaundice and hepatitis), gallbladder pain and stones, urinary tract and renal disorders and calculi, and cystitis. Erva tostão is called *punar-nava* or *punarnava* in India, where it has a long history of use by indigenous and tribal people and in ayurvedic or natural/herbal medicine. There, the roots are employed for many purposes including liver, gallbladder, kidney, renal, and urinary disorders.[1-6] Throughout the tropics erva tostão is considered an excellent natural remedy for guinea worms, a bothersome tropical parasite that lays its eggs underneath the skin of humans and livestock; the eggs later hatch into larvae or worms that eat the underlying tissues. The roots of the plant are normally softened in boiling water and then mashed up and applied as a paste or poultice to the affected areas to kill the worms and express them from the skin.

> Erva tostão is called *punarnava* or *punarnava* in India, where it has a long history of use by indigenous and tribal people and in ayurvedic or natural/herbal medicine.

The diuretic action of erva tostão has been studied and validated by scientists in several studies, which helps to explain the vine's long history of use in various kidney and urinary conditions. Researchers showed in the mid-1950s that low dosages (10 mg/kg to 300 mg/kg) produced strong diuretic effects, while higher dosages (>300 mg/kg) produced the opposite effect, reducing urine output.[7] Other researchers who followed verified these diuretic and antidiuretic properties, as well as the beneficial kidney and renal effects of erva tostão roots in animals and humans.[5-10] Research indicates that a root extract can increase urine output by as much as 100% in a 24-hour period at dosages as low as 10 mg/kg of body weight.[5]

The worldwide use of erva tostão roots for various liver complaints and disorders was validated when researchers demonstrated in 1980 and again in 1991 that a root extract provided antihepatotoxic properties in animals, protecting the liver from numerous introduced toxins.[10, 11] In other clinical studies with animals, a root extract demonstrated smooth muscle and skeletal muscle stimulant activity in frogs and guinea pigs;[12] hypotensive actions in dogs[12] as well as *in vitro* hypotensive actions;[13] anti-spasmodic actions in frogs and guinea pigs;[12, 14] antiamebic actions in rats;[15] and hemostatic or antihemorrhaging properties in monkeys with IUDs.[16] The traditional use of erva tostão for convulsions and epilepsy was verified by scientists in two studies demonstrating that a root extract provided anticonvulsant action in mice.[17, 18] *In vitro* testing of erva tostão root extract shows it has antibacterial properties,[19, 20] including against gonorrhea,[20] antinematodal[21] properties, and antiviral actions against several viral plant pathogens.[22]

> **The traditional use of erva tostão for convulsions and epilepsy was verified by scientists in two studies demonstrating that a root extract provided anti-convulsant action in mice.**

With much of the clinical research validating erva tostão's long history of different uses in natural medicine, it is easy to understand why it has played such an important role in the herbal practitioner's medicine chest of natural remedies. It is an important and effective tropical plant resource that is deserving of much more use and interest here in the United States. Therapeutic dosages of erva tostão are reported to be 1 to 2 g daily in tablets or capsules or 1 to 2 cups daily of a standard decoction.

WORLDWIDE USES

Region	Uses
Brazil	Albuminuria, beri-beri, blennorrhagia, calculi, cholagogue, cystitis, diuretic, gallbladder, hepatitis, hepatoprotective, hepatotonic, hydropsy, liver, nephritis, sclerosis (liver), spleen (enlarged), urinary disorders
Guatemala	Erysipelas, guinea worms

(continues)

WORLDWIDE USES *(continued)*

Region	Uses
India	Abdomen, abdominal pain, anemia, anthelmintic, anti-inflammatory, ascites, asthma, blood purifier, calculi, cancer (abdominal), cataract, childbirth, cholera, cough, debility, diuretic, dropsy, dyspepsia, edema, emetic, expectorant, eye, fever, food, gonorrhea, guinea worms, heart ailments, heart disease, hemorrhages (childbirth), hemorrhages (thoracic), hemorrhoids, hepatoprotective, inflammation (internal), jaundice, kidney disorders, lactagogue, laxative, liver, menstrual, ophthalmic, renal, rheumatism, snakebite, spleen (enlarged), stomachic, urinary disorders, weakness
Iran	Antiflatulent, appetite stimulant, diuretic, edema, expectorant, gonorrhea, jaundice, joint pain, lumbago, nephritis, tonic, urticaria
Nigeria	Abscess, anticonvulsant, asthma, boil, convulsions, emetic, epilepsy, expectorant, febrifuge, guinea worms, laxative
West Africa	Abortifacient, aphrodisiac, dysmenorrhagia
Elsewhere	Childbirth, guinea worms, jaundice, sterility, yaws

PHYTOCHEMICALS

alanine, arachidic acid, aspartic acid, behenic acid, beta-sitosterol, boeravinone A-F, boerhaavic acid, borhavine, borhavone, campesterol, daucosterol, beta-ecdysone, flavone,5-7-dihydroxy-3'-4'-dimetho, xy-6-8-dimethyl, galactose, glutamic acid, glutamine, glycerol, glycine, hentriacontane,N, heptadecyclic acid, histidine, hydroxy-proline, hypoxanthine-9-l-arabinofuranoside, leucine, liriodendrin, methionine, oleaic acid, oxalic acid, palmitic acid, proline, punarnavine, serine, sitosterol oleate, sitosterol palmitate, stearic acid, stigmasterol, syringaresinol-mono-beta-d-glucoside, threonine, triacontan-1-OL, tyrosine, ursolic acid, valine, xylose

ESPINHEIRA SANTA

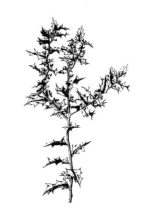

Family: Celastraceae

Genus: *Maytenus*

Species: *ilicifolia*

Common Names: Espinheira santa, cancerosa, cancrosa, chuchuwasi, maiteno, limaosinho

Parts Used: Leaves, bark, roots

Medicinal Properties: Analgesic, antacid, antiasthmatic, antibiotic, antileukemic, antiseptic, antitumorous, antiulcerogenic, cicatrizant, detoxifier, disinfectant, diuretic, laxative, stomachic, tonic

ESPINHEIRA SANTA IS a small, shrubby evergreen tree growing to 5 m high, with leaves and berries that resemble those of holly. It is native to many parts of South America and southern Brazil, and it is even grown in city landscapes for its attractive appearance. With over 200 species of *Maytenus* distributed in temperate and tropical regions throughout South America and the West Indies, many *Maytenus* species indigenous to the Amazon region have been used medicinally by indigenous tribes.

Espinheira santa has a much longer and better documented history of use in urban areas and in South American herbal medicine practices than in tribal areas, probably because of the types of illnesses that it treats. It has been the subject of many clinical studies, fueled by its effectiveness in treating ulcers and even cancer, with research beginning as early as the mid-1960s.[1,2] Early research revealed that espinheira santa, as well as a few other species in the *Maytenus* family, contains antibiotic compounds that showed potent antitumor and antileukemic activities *in vivo* and *in vitro* at very low dosages.[3–7] Two of these compounds, maytansine and mayteine, were tested in cancer patients in the

United States and South America in the 1970s.[8-12] Although there were some significant regressions in ovarian carcinoma and some lymphomas with maytansine,[10] further research was not continued due to the toxicity at the dosages used.[13] Research with the compound mayteine revealed little to no toxicity[5, 8, 9] and validated its uses in traditional and folk medicine for various types of skin cancers;[2, 14] cancer research is still ongoing in South America with this compound. In traditional medicine today, an application of the leaves of espinheira santa is employed as an ointment for treating skin cancer and a decoction is used as a wash for cancers.[15]

> Although espinheira santa is still used in traditional medicine for various types of cancer, its most popular use has been for the treatment of ulcers, indigestion, chronic gastritis, and dyspepsia.

Although espinheira santa is still used in traditional medicine for various types of cancer, its most popular use has been for the treatment of ulcers, indigestion, chronic gastritis, and dyspepsia, with a long recorded history of use for these purposes dating back to the 1930s.[16] In Brazilian traditional medicine espinheira santa is described as an excellent analgesic, disinfectant, tonic, and cicatrizant and as the leading remedy for gastritis, ulcers, and other stomach disorders. Western researchers have once again validated these traditional uses within the last ten years. Its potent antiulcerogenic abilities were demonstrated in a 1991 study that showed that a simple hot water extract of espinheira santa leaves was as effective as two of the leading antiulcer drugs, Ranitidine and Cimetidine. The same study showed that espinheira santa caused an increase in volume and pH of gastric juice.[17] Toxicological studies were also published in 1991 that demonstrated the plant's safety of use without side effects.[18]

Health practitioners in Brazil and other parts of South America utilize espinheira santa for acne, anemia, stomach ulcers, gastric ulcers, cancers, constipation, gastritis, dyspepsia, liver disorders, and many types of stomach disorders. With its popularity and beneficial results in South America, as well as its recent Western research, espinheira santa is slowly becoming more popular and known to health practitioners in the United States. The leaf extract is currently being used for ulcers, for restoring intestinal flora and inhibiting pathogenic bacteria, as a laxative, as a colic remedy, to eliminate toxins through the kidneys and skin, to regulate hydrochloric acid production in the stomach, for nervous disorders, and to support kidney, adrenal gland, digestive, and immune functions. While research continues on espinheira santa's anticancer and antitumor properties,[19] natural health practitioners around the world will still have an important and highly effective natural remedy for many types of stomach and intestinal disorders at their disposal. Generally, a leaf tea (infusion) is recommended with or shortly after meals for this natural digestion remedy, or 500 mg to 1 g daily in capsules or tablets for other digestion difficulties.

WORLDWIDE USES

Region	Uses
Argentina	Cancer, tea
Brazil	Acne, analgesic, anemia, antacid, aperitif, aphrodisiac, astringent, cancer, cicatrizant, dyspepsia, gastritis, indigestion, intestine, stomachic, tea, tonic, ulcers
Paraguay	Antifertility, aphrodisiac, contraceptive
Elsewhere	Antiarthritic, antirheumatic, aphrodisiac, cancer, diuretic, tea, tonic

PHYTOCHEMICALS

4'-methyl-(-)-epigallocatechin, 6-benzoyl-6-deacetylmayteine, 22-hydroxytingenone, maytansine, maytenin, phenoldienones, pristimerine, proanthocyanidins (ouratea-proanthocyanidins A and B), tingenone

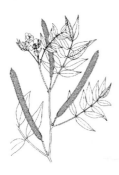

FEDEGOSO

Family: Leguminosae

Genus: *Cassia*

Species: *occidentalis*

Common Names: Fedegoso, fedegosa, yerba hedionda, brusca, guanina, martinica, platanillo, manjerioba, peieriaba, retama, achupa poroto, heduibda, folha-de-pajé, kasiah, khiyar shember, pois piante, shih chueh ming, sinamekki, tlalhoaxin, wang chiang nan, senting, kachang kota, menting

Parts Used: Roots, leaves, seeds, bark, flowers

Medicinal Properties: Analgesic, antibacterial, antifungal, antihepatotoxic, anti-inflammatory, antiparasitic, antiseptic, antispasmodic, antiviral, carminative, diaphoretic, emmenagogue, febrifuge, hepatoprotective, hepatotonic, insecticidal, laxative, parasiticide, purgative, stomachic, sudorific, vermifuge

FEDEGOSO IS A small tree that grows 5 to 8 m high and is found in many tropical areas of South America, including the Amazon. Indigenous to Brazil, it is also found in warmer climates and tropical areas of South, Central, and North America. It is in the same genus as senna *(C. senna)* and is sometimes called "coffee senna," since its seeds, found in long seed pods, are sometimes roasted and made into a coffee-like beverage. The *Cassia* genus has approximately 600 species of trees, shrubs, vines, and herbs, with numerous species growing in the South American rainforests and tropics. Many species have been used medicinally, and these tropical plants have a rich history in natural medicine. Various *Cassia* plants have been known since the ninth or tenth centuries as purgatives and laxatives, including C. *angustifolia* and C. *senna.*

Fedegoso has been used for natural medicine in the rainforest and other tropical areas for centuries. Its roots, leaves, flowers, and seeds have been employed in herbal medicine around the world. In Peru the roots are considered a diuretic, and a decoction is made for fevers. The seeds are brewed into a coffee-like beverage for asthma, and a flower infusion is used for bronchitis in the Peruvian Amazon. In Brazil the roots of fedegoso are considered a tonic, febrifuge, and diuretic and are used for fevers, tuberculosis, anemia, and liver complaints and as a reconstituent for general weakness and illness. The leaves and roots are also used in Brazil for gonorrhea, urinary tract disorders, hydropsy, erysclepias, and dysmenorrhea. The Miskito Indians of Nicaragua use a fresh plant decoction for general pain, menstrual and uterine pain, and constipation in babies.[1] In Panama a leaf tea is used for stomach colic, the crushed leaves are used in a poultice as an anti-inflammatory, and the crushed fresh leaves are taken internally to expel intestinal worms and parasites.[2]

Fedegoso has a long history of use in India by indigenous peoples for fever, malaria, liver problems, scabies, and skin disorders.[3] It is found in several formulas (mostly liver) in Indian ayurvedic medicine.[4] In many countries around the world, the fresh and/or dried leaves of fedegoso are crushed or brewed into a tea and applied externally for skin disorders, wounds, skin fungi, parasitic skin diseases, and abscesses and as a topical analgesic and anti-inflammatory natural medicine. Although the seeds of fedegoso are used in herbal medicine and even as a coffee substitute in some countries, several clinical studies have demonstrated the toxicity of the fresh and/or dried/roasted seeds. Ingestion of large amounts of the seeds by grazing animals has been reported to cause toxicity problems and even death in cows, horses, and goats.

Fedegoso has a long history of use in India by indigenous peoples for fever, malaria, liver problems, scabies, and skin disorders.

The best known species of *Cassia* is senna (*C. senna* or *C. acutifolia*), which is used as a purgative and strong laxative due to the action of chemicals called anthroquinones. While fedegoso does contain a small amount of these *Cassia* anthroquinones, it was shown in a rat study *not* to have the same purgative and laxative effects as senna.[5] In clinical research fedegoso leaves have demonstrated *in vitro* antibacterial, antifungal, antiparasitic, insecticidal, and antimalarial properties.[6–9] *In vivo* studies demonstrate that fedegoso leaves have anti-inflammatory, antihepatotoxic, hypotensive, smooth muscle–relaxant, spasmogenic, weak uterine stimulant, vasoconstrictor, hemolysis inhibition, and lipid peroxide formation inhibition activities.[10–12] In human studies, including one double-blind study, fedegoso has demonstrated antiviral properties against hepatitis B and antihepatotoxic properties.[13–15]

The clinical research on fedegoso has once again validated a plant's long history of effective uses in herbal and natural medicine. Natural health practitioners are now using fedegoso leaves for hepatitis, anemia, and other liver disorders, internal and external fungi and parasites, and inflammatory conditions, as a general tonic and specific liver tonic, and for various menstrual disorders and pain. Therapeutic dosages are reported to be 3 to 4 g daily or 1/2 cup twice daily of a standard leaf infusion.

WORLDWIDE USES

Region	Uses
Africa	Bilious, diuretic, dropsy, erysipelas, fever, jaundice, kidney, poultice, purgative, ringworms, sore throat, stomachache, sudorific, wound
Amazonia	Abdominal pain, antifertility, cholagogue, contraceptive, malaria
Brazil	Anemia, dysmenorrhea, energy, erysclepia, febrifuge, gonorrhea, liver, malaria, purgative, skin, tonic, tuberculosis, urinary disorders
Burkina Faso	Cataract, chancre, gonorrhea, leprosy, venereal disease

WORLDWIDE USES (*continued*)

Region	Uses
Central America	Abortifacient, antifertility, antifungal, antispasmodic, athlete's foot, coffee, constipation, diarrhea, diuretic, dysmenorrhea, emmenagogue, fungal disease (skin), headache, menstrual pain, pain, respiratory infections, ringworm, uterine pain, vermifuge
China/Malaysia	Eye, furuncle, headache, herpes, insecticide, sore, toothache
Ghana	Bronchitis, cataract, chancre, collyrium, fever, gonorrhea, guinea worms, headache, malaria, ophthalmia, rheumatism, swelling, syncope, tetanus, venereal disease, vermifuge
Haiti	Acne, asthma, burn, colic, diaphoretic, dropsy, erysipelas, eye, gonorrhea, headache, malaria, purgative, rheumatism, skin
India	Abscess, bite (scorpion), diabetes, febrifuge, itch, liver tonic, purgative, rheumatism, scabies, skin diseases, snakebite, swelling, wounds
Mexico	Anodyne, anthelmintic, astringent, chill, coffee, diuretic, dropsy, dyspepsia, earache, eczema, energy, fever, headache, inflammation (skin), leprosy, nausea, rash, rheumatism, ringworms, skin, sore, stomachache, stomachic, swelling, tonic, tumor, ulcer, venereal disease, yellow fever
Panama	Anthelmintic, anti-inflammatory, antiseptic, colic, spasm, stomach, vermifuge
Samoa	Asthma, stomach, typhoid
Trinidad	Abortifacient, cold, heart, heart attack, inflammation, palpitation, puerperium, purgative, womb
Venezuela	Asthma, carminative, cold, diuretic, emmenagogue, fever, malaria, skin
Zaire	Abscess, dysentery, hematuria, rheumatism, stomach
Elsewhere	Anthelmintic, bite (scorpion), cataract, childbirth, coffee, constipation, dermatosis, diuretic, dropsy, dysmenorrhea, eczema, febrifuge, gonorrhea, headache, hemorrhage, hypertension, liver, malaria, ophthalmia, parasiticide, purgative, rheumatism, ringworms, scabies, skin, snakebite, stomachic, tonic, vermifuge, yellow fever

PHYTOCHEMICALS

anthraquinones, aloe-emodin, anthrone, aurantiobtusin, chryso-obtusin, chrysophanic-acid-9-anthrone, chrysophanol, chrysophanol-1-beta- gentiobioside chrysoeriol-7-O-(2'-O-beta-D-mannopyranosyl)-beta-D-allopyranoside, emodin, kaempferol-3-sophoroside, lignoceric acid, linolenic acid, mannitol, myricylalcohol, nor-rubrofusarin, obtusifolin, obtusin, oleic acid, palmitic acid, physcion, rhamnetin-3-O-(2'-O-beta-D-mannopyranosyl)-beta-D-allopyranoside rhein, rubrofusarin, rubrofusarin-6-beta-gentiobioside, rubrofusarin-gentiobioside, sitosterol

GERVÃO

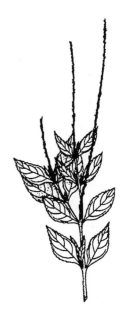

Family: Verbenaceae

Genus: *Stachytarpheta*

Species: *jamaicensis, cayennensis*

Common Names: Gervão, Brazilian tea, verbena cimarrona, bastard vervain, verbena azul, verbena, wild verbena, blue flower, rooster comb, jarbao, rat tail, vervain, verveine, porterweed

Parts Used: Plant, leaves

Medicinal Properties: Analgesic, antacid, anthelmintic, diuretic, emmenagogue, febrifuge, hypotensive, lactagogue, laxative, purgative, sedative, spasmogenic, stomachic, sudorific, tonic, vasodilator, vermifuge, vulnerary

ERVÃO IS A weedy annual and sometimes perennial herb that grows 60 to 120 cm high. It has pretty, reddish-purple flowers growing along long bracts, and it is indigenous to most parts of tropical America. It is in the Verbenaceae family with teak, vervain, and verbena; however, gervão is a different species of plant than true verbena or vervain. It is often referred to as "bastard vervain." Synonymous Latin binomials for this plant include *Stachytarpheta indica, S. marginata, S. pilosiuscula, S. urticifolia, S. villosa,* and *Verbena jamaicensis.* Another closely related species that is used interchangeably in the tropics is *S. cayennensis.*

In Brazilian herbal medicine a hot tea is prepared with the leaves or entire aerial parts for a stomach tonic, to stimulate the function of the gastrointestinal tract, for dyspepsia, for fevers, and to promote perspiration, as well as for chronic liver problems. Gervão is also used in Brazil for hepatitis, as a diuretic for various urinary complaints, and for constipation. In the West Indies it is largely employed as an anthelmintic and vermifuge, expelling intestinal worms and other parasites.[1] Gervão is a main ingredient in several commercial preparations sold in Jamaica for intestinal worms and parasites.[2] One popular preparation combines gervão with graviola *(Annona muricata)* and epazote *(Chenopodium ambrosioides)* into an effective leaf tea for parasites and intestinal worms.[3] Besides its long history of use as a vermifuge, which was documented as early as 1898,[4] gervão has also been used by women in Jamaica and in the West Indies as an emmenagogue and for dysmenorrhea.[2–6] In many parts of the West Indies, a leaf tea is drunk after childbirth to rebuild the health and to increase the supply of mother's milk.[5–7] In India a hot tea of gervão leaves has been used for dysentery, fevers, rheumatic inflammations, and it has been used externally for purulent ulcers.[8] In Belize a tea of the dried leaves and branches is drunk for nervousness, heart conditions, stomachache, neuralgia, cough, colds, fever, flu, and liver complaints. The mashed leaves are also used in Belize in a poultice for boils and infected sores, and the leaf juice is used for intestinal parasites.

Although the plant's chemical constituents have been screened and many identified, very little clinical research has taken place on gervão until just recently. In 1962 researchers did demonstrate spasmogenic and vasodilator activity of gervão in several small animal studies.[8] More recently, in 1990, other researchers demonstrated its anthelmintic and lavacidal properties in a small *in vitro* study.[9] In a 1995 Brazilian study, a gervão extract demonstrated an antidiarrheic effect in rats infected with enteropathogenic agents.[10] Another Brazilian study in 1997 demonstrated antacid, antiulcer, and laxative effects in rats.[11]

North American practitioners use gervão leaves as a natural remedy for parasite, liver, and digestive problems.

North American practitioners use gervão leaves as a natural remedy for parasite, liver, and digestive problems. A standard leaf infusion is often employed, with 1/2 cup taken 2 to 3 times daily with meals. Two to 3 g daily of the powdered leaves are used in tablets, capsules, and formulas for these types of conditions as well.

WORLDWIDE USES

Region	Uses
Bahamas	Abortifacient, asthma, bronchitis, chest cold, emetic, itch, puerperium, skin, sore, vermifuge
Belize	Boils, colds, cough, fever, flu, heart, intestinal parasites, liver, nervousness, neuralgia, sores, stomachache
Brazil	Cathartic, dropsy, dysentery, emetic, emmenagogue, erysipelas, sore, stomach, tea, tumor, venereal disease, vermifuge
Ghana	Cataract, sore
Haiti	Cathartic, dropsy, emetic, emmenagogue, erysipelas, nerve, sedative, sore, stomachic, tumor, vermifuge
India	Abortifacient, dysentery, fever, inflammation, rheumatism, ulcers (skin)
Jamaica	Emmenagogue, intestinal worms
Malaya	Abortive, malaria, rhinosis, sore
Mexico	Amenorrhea, anodyne, gonorrhea, nerve, sudorific, syphilis, yellow fever
Samoa	Boil, nausea, rhinitis, sore
South America	Anthelmintic, antifertility, emmenagogue, vermifuge
Trinidad	Boil, cough, depurative, eczema, fever, flu, lactagogue, purgative, rash, rectitis, stomach, vermifuge, vitiligo
West Indies	Anthelmintic, childbirth, dysmenorrhea, emmenagogue, lactagogue, parasites, vermifuge, worms
Elsewhere	Abortifacient, alopecia, boil, bruise, cardiac, diarrhea, dropsy, dysentery, dysmenorrhea, emmenagogue, erysipelas, fever, headache, inflammation, liver disease, poison, pressor, rheumatism, sore, sprain, stomach, venereal disease, vermifuge

PHYTOCHEMICALS

6-hydroxyluteolol-7-glucuronide, apigenol-7-glucuronide, alpha-spinasterol, butyric acid, chlorogenic acid, dopamine, dotriacontanen, friedelin, hentriacontane, hispidulin, ipolamide, luteolol-7-glucuronide, nonacosanen, pentriacontane, scutellarein, spinasterol, stachytarphine, stigmasterol, tarphetalin, tetratriancontane, triacontanen, tritriacontane, ursolic acid

GRAVIOLA

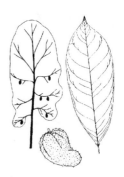

⟨ **Family:** Annonaceae

⟨ **Genus:** *Annona*

⟨ **Species:** *muricata*

⟨ **Common Names:** Graviola, soursop, guanabana, guanavana, corossolier, toge-banreisi, durian benggala, nangka blanda, nangka londa

⟨ **Parts Used:** Leaves, fruit, seeds, bark, roots

⟨ **Medicinal Properties:** Antibacterial, antiparasitic, antispasmodic, astringent, cytotoxic, febrifuge, hypotensive, insecticide, nervine, pectoral, piscicide, sedative, stomachic, vasodilator, vermifuge

RAVIOLA IS A small, upright evergreen tree, 5 to 6 m high, with large, glossy, dark green leaves. It produces a large, heart-shaped edible fruit that is 15 to 23 cm in diameter, is yellow-green in color, and has white flesh inside. Graviola is indigenous to most of the warmest tropical areas in South and North America, including the Amazon. The fruit is sold in local markets in the tropics, where it is called *guanabana* or Brazilian cherimoya. The fruit pulp is excellent for making drinks and sherbets and, though slightly sour-acid, can be eaten out of hand.

> **All parts of the graviola tree are used in natural medicine in the tropics, including the bark, leaves, roots, fruit, and fruit-seeds.**

All parts of the graviola tree are used in natural medicine in the tropics, including the bark, leaves, roots, fruit, and fruit-seeds. Different properties and uses are attributed to the different parts of the tree. Generally, the fruit and fruit juice are taken for worms and parasites, to cool fevers, to increase mother's milk after childbirth (lactagogue), and as an astringent for diarrhea and dysentery.

The crushed seeds are used as a vermifuge and anthelmintic against internal and external parasites and worms. The bark, leaves, and roots are considered sedative, antispasmodic, hypotensive, and nervine, and a tea is made for various disorders for those purposes.

Graviola has a long, rich history of use in herbal medicine as well as a long recorded indigenous use. In the Peruvian Andes a leaf tea is used for catarrh (inflammation of a mucous membrane), and the crushed seed is used to kill parasites. In the Peruvian Amazon the bark, roots, and leaves are used for diabetes and as a sedative and antispasmodic. Indigenous tribes in Guyana use a leaf and/or bark tea of graviola as a sedative and heart tonic. In the Brazilian Amazon a leaf tea is used for liver problems, and the oil of the leaves and unripe fruit is mixed with olive oil and used externally for neuralgia, rheumatism, and arthritis pain. In Jamaica, Haiti, and the West Indies, the fruit and/or fruit juice is used for fevers, parasites and diarrhea and as a lactagogue, while the bark or leaves are used as an antispasmodic, sedative, and nervine for heart conditions, coughs, grippe, difficult childbirth, asthma, asthenia, hypertension, and parasites.

Many bioactive compounds and phytochemicals have been found in graviola, as scientists have been studying its properties since the 1940s. Its many uses in natural medicine have been validated by this scientific research. The earliest studies were between 1941 and 1962. Several studies by different researchers demonstrated that the bark as well as the leaves had hypotensive, antispasmodic, vasodilator, smooth muscle–relaxant, and cardiodepressant activities in animals.[1, 2] Researchers reverified graviola leaf's hypotensive properties in rats again in 1991.[3] Several studies over the years have demonstrated that leaf, bark, root, stem, and seed extracts of graviola are antibacterial *in vitro* against numerous pathogens,[4–6] and that the bark has antifungal properties.[6, 7] Graviola seeds demonstrated active antiparasitic properties in a 1991 study,[8] and a leaf extract showed to be active against malaria in two other studies, in 1990 and 1993.[9, 10] The leaves, root, and seeds of graviola demonstrated insecticidal properties, with the seed demonstrating strong insecticidal activity in an early 1940 study.[11] In a 1997 clinical study, novel alkaloids found in graviola fruit exhibited antidepressive effects in animals.[12]

Much of the recent research on graviola has focused on a novel set of phytochemicals found in the leaves, seeds, and stem that are cytotoxic against various cancer cells. In a 1976 plant screening program by the National Cancer Institute, the leaves and stem of graviola showed active cytotoxicity against cancer cells, and researchers have been following up on this research ever since.[13] Two separate research groups have isolated novel compounds in the seeds and leaves of the plant that have demonstrated significant antitumorous, anticancerous, and selective toxicity activity against various types of cancer cells; the research groups have published eight clinical studies on their findings.[14–21] One study demonstrated that an isolated compound in graviola was selectively cytotoxic to colon adenocarcinoma cells, showing that it had 10,000 times the potency of adriamycin, a leading chemotherapy drug.[15]

> **Much of the recent research on graviola has focused on a novel set of phytochemicals found in the leaves, seeds, and stem that are cytotoxic against various cancer cells.**

Natural health practitioners use graviola bark and leaves for many natural remedies, especially as a heart tonic, as a nervine, and for disorders of a bacterial nature such as colds and flu, and even cancer. The therapeutic dosage is reported to be 3 to 4 g daily of the leaves and/or bark, and sometimes a standard infusion is used in 1/2-cup dosages 1 to 3 times daily.

WORLDWIDE USES

Region	Uses
Bahamas	Chill, fever, flu, nervousness, palpitation, rash, sedative, skin disease
Brazil	Analgesic, fever, neuralgia, parasites, rheumatism
Curacao	Childbirth, gallbladder, nervousness, parturition, sedative, tea, tranquilizer
Haiti	Asthenia, cataplasm, cicatrizant, cough, diarrhea, emetic, grippe, pediculicide, pellagra, soporific, sore, spasm, stomachic
Jamaica	Antispasmodic, diuretic, fevers, lactagogue, vermifuge
Malaya	Boil, cough, dermatosis, rheumatism
Mexico	Astringent, diarrhea, dysentery, fever, liqueur, pectoral, ringworm, scurvy
Panama	Anthelmintic, diarrhea, dyspepsia, kidney, piscicide, ulcer (stomach), vermifuge
Trinidad	Depurative, fainting, flu, galactagogue, high blood pressure, hypertension, insomnia, palpitation, ringworms
Venezuela	Bilious, diarrhea
West Indies	Childbirth, diarrhea, hypertension, lactagogue, worms
Elsewhere	Analgesic, antiphlogistic, arthritis, asthma, astringent, cyanogenetic, dysentery, febrifuge, insecticide, kidney, lactagogue, malaria, pectoral, pediculicide, piscicide, scurvy, stomach

PHYTOCHEMICALS

acetaldehyde, amyl-caproate, amyloid, annonain, anomuricine, anomuricinine, anomurine, anonol, atherospermine, beta-sitosterol, campesterol, cellobiose, citric acid, citrulline, co-claurine, coreximine, dextrose, ethanol, folacin, fructose, gaba, galactomannan, geranyl-caproate glucose, HCN, isocitric acid, lignoceric acid, malic acid, manganese, mericyl-alcohol, methanol, methyl-hex-2-enoate, methyl-hexanoate, muricine, muricinine, myristic acid, P-coumaric acid, paraffin, potassium-chloride, procyanidin, reticuline, scyllitol, stearic acid, stepharine, stigmasterol, sucrose, tannin, xylosyl-cellulose

GUARANA

Family: Sapindaceae

Genus: *Paullinia*

Species: *cupana*

Common Names: Guarana, guarana kletterstrauch, guaranastruik, quarana, quarane

Parts Used: Fruit, seed

Medicinal Properties: Analgesic, antibacterial, aphrodisiac, astringent, cardiotonic, diuretic, febrifuge, nervine, purgative, stimulant, tonic, vasodilator

GUARANA IS A creeping shrub native to the Amazon, most particularly the regions of Manaus and Parintins. In the lushness of the Brazilian Amazon where it originated, it often grows 12 m high. The fruit is small, round, and bright red in color and grows in clusters. As it ripens, the fruit splits and a black seed emerges, giving it the appearance of an eye the Indians tell legends about.

The uses of this medicinal plant by the Amerindians predates the discovery of Brazil. The South American Indian tribes (especially the Guaranis, from whence the name is derived) dry and roast the seeds and mix them into a paste with water. They then use it much the same way as chocolate, to prepare various foods, drinks, and medicines. The rainforest tribes have used guarana mainly as a stimulant, as an astringent, and in treating chronic diarrhea. Botanist James Duke cites past and present tribal use in the rainforest as a preventative for arteriosclerosis, as an effective cardiovascular drug, as an analgesic, astringent, febrifuge, stimulant, and tonic used to treat diarrhea, and for hypertension, migraine, neuralgia, and dysentery. Throughout the centuries the many secrets and benefits of guarana were passed on to explorers and settlers. European researchers began studying guarana in France and Germany in the 1940s, finding that the Indians' uses to cure fevers, headaches, and cramps and as an energy tonic were well founded.

Today the plant is known and used worldwide and is the main ingredient in the "national beverage" of Brazil, Guarana Soda. Eighty percent of the world's commercial production of guarana paste is in the middle of the Amazon rainforest in northern Brazil, still performed by the Guarani Indians, who wild-harvest the seeds and process them into paste by hand. The Brazilian government has become aware of the importance of the local production of guarana by traditional methods employed by indigenous inhabitants of the rainforest. FUNAI (National Indian Foundation) has set up a number of projects since 1980 to improve the local production of guarana. Now, under the direction of the FUNAI regional authority in Manaus, many cooperatives in the rainforest support indigenous tribal economies through the harvesting and production of guarana.[1]

> European researchers began studying guarana in France and Germany in the 1940s, finding that the Indians' uses to cure fevers, headaches, and cramps and as an energy tonic were well founded.

The first chemical examination on the guarana seeds was performed by the German botanist Theodore von Martius in the 1700s. He isolated a bitter, white crystalline substance with a remarkable physiological action. Von Martius named this substance guaranine, and it was later renamed caffeine. Guarana seeds contain up to 5% caffeine (25,000 to 75,000 ppm), as well as trace amounts of theophylline (500 to 750 ppm) and theobromine (300 to 500 ppm).[2] It also contains large quantities of tannins, starch, a saponin, and resinous substances.

Guarana is used and well known for its stimulant and thermogenic action. In the United States today, guarana is reputed to increase mental alertness, to fight fatigue, and to increase stamina and physical endurance. Presently, guarana is taken daily as a health tonic by millions of Brazilians, who believe it helps overcome heat fatigue, combats premature aging, detoxifies the blood, and is useful for flatulence, obesity, dyspepsia, fatigue, and arteriosclerosis. Guarana has been used in body care products for its tonifying and astringent properties. It has been used in the treatment of cellulite due to its lipolytic and vasodilation action. Guarana has also been used as an ingredient in shampoos for oily hair and as a coadjutant in hair loss treatments. Therapeutic dosages are reported to be 4 to 5 g daily. Relatively new to the U.S. market are guarana extracts, which are concentrated and standardized to the caffeine content (between 5% and 15%) sold in tablets and capsules.

While the Indians have been using guarana for centuries, Western science has been slowly but surely proving that the indigenous uses are well grounded in science. In 1989 a U.S. patent was filed on a guarana seed extract that was capable of inhibiting platelet aggregation in mammalian blood. The patent described guarana's ability to prevent the formation of blood clots and to help in the breakdown of clots that had already been formed. Clinical evidence was presented in conjunction with the patent in 1989, and again in 1991 by a Brazilian research group demonstrating these antiaggregation properties.[3, 4] Once again, scientific validation is given to a plant used for centuries by the Indians as a heart tonic and to "thin the blood." The use of guarana as an effective energy tonic and for mental acuity and long-term memory was just recently validated by scientists. In a 1997 *in vivo* study, Guarana increased physical activity of rats, increased physical endurance under stress, and increased memory with single doses as well as with chronic doses. Interestingly, the study revealed that a whole-guarana-seed extract performed better and more effectively than did a comparable dosage of caffeine or ginseng extract.[5] Another Brazilian research group has been studying guarana's apparent

> The use of guarana as an effective energy tonic and for mental acuity and long-term memory was just recently validated by scientists.

effect of increasing memory,[6, 7] which is thought to be linked to the essential oils found in the seed.[8] Its antibacterial properties against *Escherichia coli* and salmonella have been documented as well.[9]

WORLDWIDE USES

Region	Uses
Amazonia	Arteriosclerosis, astringent, cardiotonic, coffee, cramps, depurative, diarrhea, dyspepsia, fatigue, fever, flatulence, headache, obesity, stimulant
Europe	Cardiotonic, diarrhea, intoxicant, migraine, nervine, neuralgia, stimulant, tonic
Mexico	Coffee, diarrhea, stimulant

PHYTOCHEMICALS

adenine, caffeine, catechutannic acid, choline, D-catechin, guanine, guaranine, hypoxanthine, mucilage, saponin, tannins, theobromine, theophylline, timbonine, xanthine

GUAVA

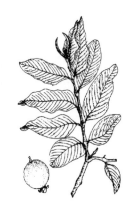

‖ **Family:** Myrtaceae

‖ **Genus:** *Psidium*

‖ **Species:** *guajava*

‖ **Common Names:** Guava, goiaba, guayaba, djamboe, djambu, goavier, gouyave, goyave, goyavier, perala, bayawas, dipajaya jambu, petokal, tokal

‖ **Parts Used:** Fruit, leaf, bark

‖ **Medicinal Properties:** Antibacterial, antimicrobial, antispasmodic, astringent, cicatrizant, emmenagogue, hypoglycemic, laxative, nutritive

IN THE RICHNESS of the Amazon, guava fruits often grow well beyond the size of tennis balls on well-branched trees or shrubs reaching up to 20 m high. Guava fruit today is considered minor in terms of world trade but is widely grown in the tropics, enriching the diet of hundreds of millions of people in the tropics of the world. Called *guayaba* in Spanish-speaking countries and *goiaba* in Brazil, guava is a common shade tree or shrub in door-yard gardens, providing shade while the guava fruits are eaten fresh and made into drinks, ice cream, and preserves. Guava has spread widely throughout the tropics with moderate to heavy rainfall because it thrives in a variety of soils, propagates easily, and bears fruit relatively quickly. The fruits contain numerous seeds that can produce a mature fruit-bearing plant within four years. In the Amazon rainforest the seeds of guava fruits are much enjoyed by birds and monkeys, which disperse guava seeds in their droppings and cause spontaneous clumps of guava trees to grow through the Amazon rainforest.

Guava may have been domesticated in Peru several thousand years ago. Peruvian archaeological sites have revealed guava seeds found stored with beans, corn, squash, and other cultivated plants. Centuries ago, European adventurers, traders, and missionaries in the Amazon Basin took the much enjoyed and tasty fruits to Africa, Asia, India, and the Pacific tropical regions, so that it is now cultivated throughout the tropical regions of the world.

Guava fruits have a distinctive, savory-fresh aroma that is thermostable and thus survives processing. Guava is higher in vitamin C than citrus and contains appreciable amounts of vitamin A as well. Guava fruits are also a good source of pectin, an enzyme used in making jam as well as promoting digestion. Guava fruit is still enjoyed as a sweet treat by indigenous peoples throughout the rainforest, and the leaves and bark of the guava tree have a long history of medicinal uses that are still employed today. A tea made from the leaves and/or bark has been used by many tribes for diarrhea and dysentery, and other tribes employ it for stomach upsets, for vertigo, and to regulate menstrual periods. Guava leaves still remain in the *Dutch Pharmacopoeia,* and the leaves are still used as a diarrhea treatment in Latin America, Central and West Africa, and Southeast Asia. The natural rainforest remedy for diarrhea or digestion difficulties is 1/2 cup of a standard decoction of leaves and twigs, taken 2 to 3 times daily with meals. This long history of use has led modern-day researchers to study guava leaf extracts, and its use as an effective treatment for gastrointestinal disorders has been validated in at least eight clinical studies.[1–10] Guava fruit has also demonstrated hypoglycemic properties.[11, 12]

> **Guava is higher in vitamin C than citrus and contains appreciable amounts of vitamin A as well. Guava fruits are also a good source of pectin.**

WORLDWIDE USES

Region	Uses
Amazonia	Diarrhea, dysentery, menstrual disorders, stomachache, vertigo
Cuba	Cold, dysentery, dyspepsia
Ghana	Astringent, cough, dentifrice, diarrhea, dysentery, laxative, toothache
Haiti	Antiseptic, astringent, cicatrizant, dysentery, diarrhea, epilepsy, itch, hemostat, pile, scabies, skin, sore, sore throat, stomachache
Malaya	Dermatosis, diarrhea, emmenagogue, epilepsy, hysteria
Mexico	Deafness, diarrhea, itch, scabies, stomachache, swelling, ulcer, vermifuge, vulnerary
Philippines	Astringent, sore, wound
Trinidad	Astringent, bactericide, depurative, diarrhea, dysentery
Elsewhere	Astringent, bactericide, bowel, bronchitis, cachexia, catarrh, cholera, chorea, colic, convulsion, diarrhea, dysentery, epilepsy, fattening, fever, gingivitis, jaundice, nausea, nephritis, respiratory, rheumatism, sore, spasm, tonic, toothache, wound

PHYTOCHEMICALS

alanine, alpha-humulene, alpha-linolenic acid, alpha-selinene, araban, arabinose, arginine, ascorbic acid, ascorbigen, aspartic acid, benzaldehyde, benzene, beta-bisabolene, beta-carotene, beta-caryophyllene, beta-copaene, beta-farnesene, beta-humulene, beta-ionone, beta-pinene, beta-selinene, butanal, calcium, cinnamylacetate, citral, citric acid, copper, D-galactose, D-galacturonic acid, delta-cadinene, ellagic acid, fructose, gallic acid, glutamic acid, glycine, histidine, iron, isoleucine, L-malic acid, lactic acid, leucine, leucocyanidins, limonene, linoleic acid, lysine, magnesium, manganese, mecocyanin, methylcinnamate, methylisopropylketone, mufa, myristic acid, niacin, oleic acid, oxalic acid, palmitic acid, palmitoleic acid, pantothenic acid, pectin, phenylalanine, phosphorus, phytin-phosphorus, potassium, proline, pufa, rhamnose, riboflavin, serine, SFA, stearic acid, sulfur, thiamin, threonine, tryptophan, tyrosine, valine, vitamin B6, xylose, zinc

IPORURU

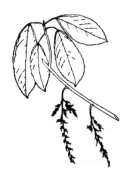

Family: Euphorbiaceae

Genus: *Alchornea*

Species: *castaneifolia, floribunda*

Common Names: Iporuru, iporoni, iporuro, ipururo, ipurosa, macochihua, niando

Parts Used: Leaves, bark, roots

Medicinal Properties: Analgesic, anodyne, antiarthritic, antibacterial, anti-inflammatory, antimicrobial, aphrodisiac, laxative

PORURU IS A medium-sized woody bush that grows in the lower elevations and flood plains of the Amazon River system in Peru. Iporuru can only be harvested in the Amazon's dry season because it spends the rainy season underwater. The active medicinal chemicals found in the bark are present only during the dry season. Iporuru belongs to the family Euphorbiaceae, or the spurge family, which contains about 5,000 species of trees, shrubs, and herbs. This family of plants is economically important in that it provides food, rubbers, medicinals, oils, dyes, and many other useful products.

The indigenous peoples of the Amazon have used the bark and roots of iporuru for many different purposes for centuries, preparing it in many different ways. One of the more popular preparations is an alcoholic bark maceration used to treat rheumatism, arthritis, colds, and muscle pains. It is well known to the indigenous peoples of Peru for relieving the symptoms of osteoarthritis and to help flexibility in movement and range of motion. The Candochi-Shapra and the Shipibo tribes use both the bark and roots for treating rheumatism. To prevent diarrhea, members of the Tikuna tribe take 1 tbsp of bark decoction before meals. The pain-relieving properties of iporuru are also employed topically by indigenous peoples. Crushed leaves are rubbed on painful joints as an analgesic and beaten into a paste and applied to painful stingray wounds.

Iporuru remedies and products are often sold in local markets and herbal pharmacies in Peru. In Peruvian herbal medicine iporuru is highly recommended for rheumatism. In addition to an arthritis and rheumatism remedy, local citizens of Pucallpa take the leaf decoction orally for coughs. The leaves of iporuru are used in the area around Piura to increase female fertility in cases where the male is relatively impotent. It is also used as an aphrodisiac and geriatric for males.

Currently, iporuru is gaining popularity among athletes and North American health practitioners due to properties that provide support of muscle and joint structure. Its analgesic and anti-inflammatory agents have also begun to make it popular for those suffering from arthritis and other joint problems. In addition to its anti-inflammatory and pain-relieving properties, an *in vitro* study in Argentina found that an extract of iporuru was antibacterial and effective against a penicillin G–resistant strain of *Staphylococcus aureus, Escherichia coli,* and *Aspergillus niger.*[1] The anti-inflammatory properties of iporuru are attributed to a group of alkaloids including alchorneine, which are found in the bark of iporuru as well as several other related species of *Alchornea.*[2]

Currently, iporuru is gaining popularity among athletes and North American health practitioners due to properties that provide support of muscle and joint structure.

Currently, in Peruvian herbal medicine iporuru is widely used to treat impotency and for reducing sugar in the blood and urine of diabetics. One cup of dried leaves is infused in 1/2 l of water for 1 day, and 2 to 3 doses (of 1/2 cup) are drunk daily for impotency. For diabetes, 1/2 cup of dried leaves is infused in 1 l of water, and 1 cup is drunk after each meal. Natural health practitioners also use iporuru bark for arthritis, inflammation, and pain, with the average therapeutic dose 2 to 3 g daily.

WORLDWIDE USES

Region	Uses
Amazonia	Aches (muscle), analgesic, anti-inflammatory, aphrodisiac, arthritis, colds, cough, diabetes, diarrhea, fertility, impotence, rheumatism
Venezuela	Wound

PHYTOCHEMICALS

alchorneine, alchorneinone, alkaloids, anthranilic acid, gentisinic acid, isoalchorneine, yohimbine

JABORANDI

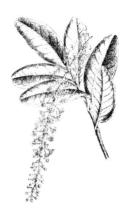

Family: Rutaceae

Genus: *Pilocarpus*

Species: *jaborandi*

Common Names: Jaborandi, Indian hemp, pernambuco jaborandi

Parts Used: Leaf, bark

Medicinal Properties: Anti-inflammatory, diaphoretic, diuretic, emetic, febrifuge, lactagogue

JABORANDI IS A 1- to 1.5-meter tall shrub with smooth gray bark and large, leathery leaves. It is native to the Brazilian Amazon. In 1570 Gabriel Soares de Souza, a European observer, noted the Guarani Indians using the plant to treat mouth ulcers. In the 1630s two Dutch West Indian Company scientists documented Brazilian Indians using it as a tonic or panacea, for colds and flu, as a remedy against gonorrhea and kidney stones, and as an antidote to various poisons or toxins due to its ability to promote sweating, urination, and salivation.[1] The indigenous tribes prized the diaphoretic properties of the plant, particularly since they viewed sweating as a treatment in many diseases. Jaborandi is a perfect example of a plant that made the transition from Amazonian indigenous tribal use and folklore to modern science and medicine.

Jaborandi leaves were introduced to Western medicine in 1873 when Symphronio Coutinho, a doctor from Bahia, Brazil, went to Paris for a European doctoral degree, taking with him samples of

> **In the 1630s two Dutch scientists documented Brazilian Indians using jaborandi as a tonic, for colds and flu, as a remedy against gonorrhea and kidney stones, and as an antidote to various poisons or toxins.**

the leaves. The copious sweating and salivation brought about by the leaves attracted the attention of French physicians, who began clinical research, publishing their first studies just one year later.[2] The studies showed that jaborandi leaves "increase enormously the perspiration and saliva, and, in a much less degree, the secretion from the mucous membranes of the nose, the bronchial tubes, and the stomach and intestines."[3] In 1875 two researchers independently discovered the alkaloid pilocarpine and its use to lower the intraocular pressure in glaucoma and act as a miotic. By 1876 jaborandi leaves were being employed in the treatment of many diseases, including "fever, stomatitis, enterocolitis, laryngitis and bronchitis, bronchiectasis, influenza, pneumonia, hydropericarditis, hydropsy, psoriasis, intoxications, neurosis, and renal disease—to mention only a few of the conditions for which they were valued."[4] M. Grieve, in *A Modern Herbal*, recorded almost a century later that jaborandi was still used for psoriasis, prurigo, baldness, tonsillitis, and dropsy.

An ophthalmological drug that contained the pilocarpine alkaloids extracted from jaborandi was introduced in 1876 by A. Weber. One year later it was used as a local drug to lower the intraocular pressure in glaucoma. The mixture of pilocarpine and another natural product, physostigmine, remains to this day one of the mainstays in ophthalmology. There are over 1,000 clinical studies on pilocarpine, but as with most plant-based drugs, the use of the whole natural plant fell out of disuse as a natural remedy in favor of the single isolated active ingredient that was used as the prescription drug.

Clinical research is still ongoing today on pilocarpine, the isolated alkaloid of jaborandi leaves. Some of the latest research is now focused on the topical applications of it as a transdermal penetration agent for other pharmacologic agents[5-7] since it has the ability to open skin pores and promote capillary blood circulation. These effects are also attributed to its use as a topical agent for baldness. Over the years, jaborandi and its constituents have been the subject of extensive research worldwide for their pharmacological properties and their uses in modern medicine.[8–21]

Jaborandi leaves and bark can cause copious amounts of sweating even at very low dosages of 20 to 30 mg. In higher dosages jaborandi may irritate the stomach and cause vomiting and nausea. Only experienced herbalists and practitioners should employ jaborandi as a natural remedy that is ingested. Employed externally in a decoction, tincture, or infusion, it is often used safely and effectively for skin problems and baldness.

WORLDWIDE USES

Region	Uses
Brazil	Colds, diaphoretic, emetic, febrifuge, flu, gonorrhea, kidney stones, tonic, ulcers (mouth)
Mexico	Bright's disease, dropsy, pleurisy, rheumatism
Peru	Diuretic, lactagogue
Elsewhere	Antidote (atropine, belladonna), baldness, bronchiectasis, bronchitis, diaphoretic, dropsy, enterocolitis, fever, glaucoma, hydropericarditis, hydropsy, influenza, intoxications, laryngitis, neurosis, pneumonia, prurigo, psoriasis, renal disease, renitis, stomatitis, tonsillitis

PHYTOCHEMICALS

2-undecanone, alpha-pinene, isopilocarpidine, isopilocarpine, limonene, myrcene, pilocarpidine, pilocarpine, sandaracopimaradiene, vinyl-dodecanoate

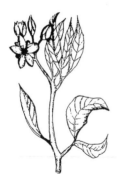

JATOBA

Family: Leguminosae

Genus: *Hymenaea*

Species: *courbaril*

Common Names: Jatoba, jatobá, algarrobo, azucar huayo, jataí, copal, Brazilian copal, courbaril, nazareno, cayenne copal, demarara copal, gomme animee, pois confiture, guapinol, guapinole, loksi, South American locust

Parts Used: Bark, resin, leaves

Medicinal Properties: Antibacterial, antifatigue, antifungal, anti-inflammatory, antioxidant, antispasmodic, astringent, decongestant, diuretic, expectorant, hemostatic, hepatoprotective, hypoglycemic, laxative, stimulant, stomachic, tonic, vermifuge

JATOBA IS A huge canopy tree that grows up to 30 m high. It has bright green leaves, small red flowers, and an edible, oblong, brown, pod-like fruit. Jatoba is indigenous to the Amazon rainforest and parts of tropical Central America. In the Peruvian Amazon it is called *azucar huayo,* and the Brazilian name is *jatobá.* An orange resinous gum that collects at the base of the tree is dug up and used to make incense and varnish. Indians in the Amazon have long used this gum to make lip plates and as a medicine for a variety of purposes.

Jatoba has a long history of use by the indigenous tribes of the rainforest as well as in South American traditional medicine. The Karaja tribe in Peru and Creole tribes in Guyana macerate the bark for diarrhea. The bark, sap or resin, and leaves are used medicinally in the Peruvian Amazon for cystitis, hepatitis, prostatitis, and cough. In the Brazilian Amazon the sap is used for coughs and bronchitis, and a bark tea is used for stomach problems as well as athlete's foot and foot fungus. Jatoba is still employed in traditional medicine throughout South America. It was first recorded in use in 1930. The bark was described by Dr. J. Monteiro Silva as being a carminative, sedative, and astringent and recommended for hematuria, diarrhea, dysentery, general fatigue, dyspepsia, constipation, bexiga, and hemoptysis; the resin was recommended for all types of upper respiratory and cardiopulmonary problems.[1] According to Dr. Silva, whoever drinks jatoba tea feels "strong and vigorous, with a good appetite, always ready to work."[1] In 1965 the traditional uses of jatoba were still being employed much as they had been since the 1930s, and a liquid extract called *vinho de jatoba* was widely sold throughout Brazil as a tonic and fortificant, for energy, and for numerous disorders.

> According to one doctor, whoever drinks jatoba tea feels "strong and vigorous, with a good appetite, always ready to work."

In Brazilian herbal medicine today, jatoba bark and resin are still recommended for the same indications and problems as they have since 1930 and are documented to be a tonic, stomachic, astringent, balsamic, vermifuge, and hemostatic. Today, jatoba bark tea is a quite popular drink of lumberjacks working in the forests in Brazil because it is a natural energy tonic that helps them work long hours without fatigue. Jatoba has also shown good results with acute and chronic cystitis and prostatitis. In traditional medicine in Panama the fruit is used to treat mouth ulcers, and the leaves and wood are used for diabetes.[2] In the United States jatoba is used as a natural energy tonic, for respiratory ailments like asthma, laryngitis, and bronchitis, as a decongestant and fungicide, and in the

> What the people of the city do not realize is that the roots of all living things are interconnected. When a mighty tree is felled, a star falls from the sky. Before one chops down a mahogany, one should ask permission of the guardian of the stars.
>
> —Chan K'in,
> Lacadon Mayan Patriarch

treatment of hemorrhage, bursitis, bladder infections, yeast and fungal infections, cystitis, arthritis, and prostatitis.

The leaves of jatoba contain a group of phytochemicals called terpenes and phenolics that are responsible for protecting the leaves of the tree from leaf fungus.[3, 4] These phytochemicals have been documented in several studies over the years, and the antifungal activity of jatoba is attributed to these chemicals found not only in the leaves, but in the bark as well.[5-7] Other clinical studies performed on the bark, leaves, and resin of jatoba since the early 1970s have shown that it has antimicrobial, antifungal, antibacterial, molluscicidal, and anti-yeast activities, which validates its long history of effective uses for numerous disorders.[8-12] In addition, a water extract of jatoba leaves demonstrated significant hypoglycemic activity, producing a significant reduction in plasma glucose levels.[12] Jatoba bark also contains a flavonoid called astilbin, which was shown to provide antioxidant and liver-protecting properties in a 1997 clinical study.[13, 14]

> **Clinical studies performed on the bark, leaves, and resin of jatoba have shown that it has antimicrobial, antifungal, antibacterial, molluscicidal, and anti-yeast properties.**

Natural health practitioners are using jatoba as an effective natural remedy for prostate disorders, reporting that in many cases it is more effective than saw palmetto. Therapeutic dosages are reported to be 2 to 3 cups daily of a standard bark infusion with some lemon juice added, or 4 to 5 ml of a standard tincture daily. It is also gaining popularity as a healthful tonic for added energy as well as for many fungal problems like candida and athlete's foot. A standard bark infusion or a standard tincture diluted with water and a small amount of cider vinegar is used topically for skin fungi or employed with reported success as a douche for candida and/or yeast infections.

WORLDWIDE USES

Region	Uses
Brazil	Arthritis, asthma, athlete's foot, bladder, bronchitis, bursitis, cough, cystitis, decongestant, energy, fever, fungicide, laryngitis, prostatitis, stomachache, tonic
Guatemala	Diuretic, fever, rheumatism, sudorific
Haiti	Antiseptic, arthritis, asthma, bruise, catarrh, diarrhea, emphysema, headache, intestine, kidney, laxative, respiratory, rheumatism, sore, spasm, stomach
Mexico	Asthma, catarrh, purgative, rheumatism, sedative, sore, venereal disease
Panama	Asthma, diabetes, diarrhea, hypoglycemia, stomach, ulcer (mouth)
Peru	Cough, cystitis, diarrhea, hepatitis, prostatitis
Venezuela	Fracture, lung, vermifuge
Elsewhere	Asthma, beri-beri, blennorrhagia, bronchitis, cystitis, dyspepsia, expectorant, indigestion, laryngitis, liqueur, malaria, rheumatism, stomachic

PHYTOCHEMICALS

1-beta-(2 -(3-furyl)-ethyl)-1-alpha-2-alpha-5 -alpha-trimethyl, 1-2-3-naphthalene-5-carboxylic acid-1-2-3(-)(A)-5-6-7-octahydro, 1-beta-(3-methyl-4-carboxy-butanyl)-1-alpha-naphthalene-5-carboxylic acid, 1-2-3-4-4-(A)-5-6-7- octahydro, 1-beta-(trans-3-methyl-4-carboxy-but-3-enyl)- 1-alpha-2-alpha-5-alpha- trimethyl, astilibin, beta-sitosterol, beta-bourbonene, alpha-cadinene, delta-cadinene, gamma-cadinene, caryophyllene, (-)epi catechin, iso-enantio communic acid, copacamphene, copaene, copalic acid, cubebene, copacamphene, alpha-copaene, beta-copaene, alpha-cubebene, cyclosativene, ent-eperua-7-13-dien- 15-oic acid, beta-gurjunene, hedychinene, alpha-himachalene, humulene, alpha-humulene, beta-humulene, beta-huurolene, ent-lab-13-en-8-beta-ol-15-oic acid, ent-labdan-8-beta-ol-15-oic acid, alpha-muurolene, gamma-muurolene, naphthalene-5-carboxylic acid,1-2-3 diterpene -4-4-(A)-5-6-7-octahydro, selina-4(14)-7-diene, alpha-selinene, beta-selinene, taxifolin-3-o-rhamnoside

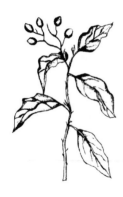

JURUBEBA

Family: Solanaceae

Genus: *Solanum*

Species: *paniculatum, insidiosum*

Common Names: Jurubeba, jubeba, juribeba, juripeba, jupela, juripeba, juuna, juvena, jurubebinha

Parts Used: Leaves, roots, fruit

Medicinal Properties: Anti-inflammatory, carminative, cholagogue, decongestive, digestive, diuretic, emmenagogue, febrifuge, gastrotonic, hepatotonic, hypotensive, stomachic, tonic

JURUBEBA IS A small tree that grows up to 3 m high, with heart-shaped leaves that are smooth on top and fuzzy underneath. There are both male and female jurubeba trees; the female species grows slightly taller, has larger leaves, and bears fruit. The leaves and roots of both the female and male specimens and the fruit are used interchangeably for medicinal purposes with equal effectiveness. Jurubeba is indigenous to the north of Brazil and other tropical parts of South America.

The indigenous uses of jurubeba are very poorly documented, but its use in Brazilian medicine has been described quite well. Jurubeba is listed as an official drug in the *Brazilian Pharmacopoeia* as a specific for anemia and for liver disorders. Jurubeba has long been used for liver and digestive disorders. In 1965 Dr. G. L. Cruz wrote that "the roots, leaves, and fruit are used as a tonic and decongestive. It stimulates the digestive functions and reduces the swelling of the liver and spleen. It is a good remedy against chronic hepatitis, intermittent fever, uterine tumors, and hydropsy." The leaves and roots are commonly used in Brazilian medicine today as a tonic and for fevers, anemia, erysipelas, hepatitis, liver and spleen disorders, urinary tumors, irritable bowel syndrome, chronic gastritis, and other digestive problems. Jurubeba leaf tea is a common household remedy throughout Brazil for hangovers and to relieve indigestion and bloating from too much alcohol and food consumption.

The active constituents of jurubeba were documented in the 1960s, when German researchers discovered novel plant steroids, saponins, glycosides, and alkaloids in the root, stem, and leaves.[1–3] The alkaloids are found in more abundance in the roots (0.25% to 0.96%), although they are present in the stem (0.28%) and leaves (0.20%).[3, 4] Solanidine and solasodine were discovered in the leaves and fruit of jurubeba, which accounted for its liver protective properties.[5, 6] The steroids and saponins were found in higher quantities in the roots, while the leaves had the greatest amount of glycosides.[2, 3, 7]

> **Jurubeba leaf tea is a common household remedy throughout Brazil for hangovers and indigestion**

The pharmacological properties documented from as early as 1940 to the present for jurubeba include stomachic, febrifuge, diuretic, emmenagogue, cholagogue, hepatoprotective, and tonic.[8–10] Animal studies have indicated that water as well as alcohol extracts of jurubeba lowered blood pressure while increasing respiration in cats, evidenced a stimulant action in the heart in toads, and had little to no toxicity in mice or fish.[11, 12]

While jurubeba is a very popular natural remedy, its use has mostly been confined to South America. It is a wonderful remedy for most types of digestive disorders, working quickly and efficiently, deserving of much more attention in the United States. A standard infusion (leaf tea) is taken with meals or shortly afterward, and the therapeutic dosage for other digestive difficulties is reported to be 1 to 3 g daily in capsules or tablets.

WORLDWIDE USES

Region	Uses
Brazil	Abscess (internal), anemia, bladder, boil, catarrh, decongestant, diuretic, fever, gastritis, hangover, hepatitis, hepatotonic, hydropsy, inappetence, liver, skin, spleen, stomachic, tumor (uterine)

PHYTOCHEMICALS

jurubepina, jurubilina, jurubina, muscilage, neochlorogenin, paniculidin, paniculogenin, paniculonin

MACA

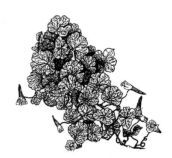

⟨⟨ **Family:** Brassicaceae

⟨⟨ **Genus:** *Lepidium*

⟨⟨ **Species:** *meyenii*

⟨⟨ **Common Names:** Maca, Peruvian ginseng, maka, maca-maca, maino, ayak chichira, ayuk willku

⟨⟨ **Part Used:** Roots

⟨⟨ **Medicinal Properties:** Antifatigue, aphrodisiac, immunostimulant, nutritive, steroidal, tonic

ACA IS A hardy perennial plant cultivated high in the Andean mountains, at altitudes from 11,000 to 14,500 feet.[1] It has one of the highest frost tolerances among native cultivated species. It has a low-growing, mat-like stem system, which at times goes unnoticed in a farmer's field. Its scalloped leaves lie close to the ground, and it produces small, self-fertile, off-white flowers typical of the mustard family to which it belongs. The part used is the tuberous root, which is pear shaped, up to 8 cm in diameter, and off-white in color. Unlike many other tuberous plants, maca is propagated by seed. Although it is a perennial, it is grown as an annual, and seven to nine months from planting is required to produce the harvested roots.

The area where maca is found, high in the Andes, is an inhospitable region of intense sunlight, violent winds, and below-freezing weather. With its extreme temperatures and poor rocky soil, the area rates among the world's worst farmland; yet over the centuries, maca evolved to flourish under these conditions. Maca was domesticated about 2,000 years ago by the Incas,[1, 2] and primitive cultivars of maca have been found in archaeological sites dating as far back as 1600 B.C.[3, 4]

To the Andean Indians, maca is a valuable commodity. Because so little else grows in the region, maca is often traded with communities at lower elevations for other staples like rice, corn, and beans. The dried roots can be stored for up to seven years. Native Peruvians have traditionally utilized maca since before the time of the Incas for both nutritional and medicinal purposes.[1] Maca is an important staple in the diets of the people indigenous to the region, since it has the highest nutritional value of any food crop grown there. It is rich in sugars, protein, starches, and essential minerals, especially iodine and iron. The tuber is consumed fresh or dried. The fresh roots are considered a treat and are baked or roasted in ashes, much like sweet potatoes. The dried roots are stored and later boiled in water or milk to make a porridge. In addition, they are often made into a popular sweet, fragrant, fermented drink called *maca chicha*. In Huancayo, Peru, even maca jam and pudding are popular. The tuberous roots have a tangy sweet taste and an aroma similar to that of butterscotch.

Maca has been used medicinally for centuries to enhance fertility in humans and animals.[2–6, 9] Soon after the Spanish conquest in South America, the Spanish found that their livestock were reproducing poorly in the highlands. The local Indians recommended feeding the animals maca, and so remarkable were the results that Spanish chroniclers gave in-depth reports.[3] Even colonial records of some 200 years ago indicate that payments of roughly nine tons of maca were demanded from one Andean area alone for this purpose.[4, 5] Its fertility-enhancing properties were supported clinically as early as 1961, when researchers discovered it increased the fertility of rats.[7] This energizing plant is also referred to as Peruvian ginseng,[1, 2, 4] although maca is not in the same family as ginseng.

Maca has been used medicinally for centuries to enhance fertility in humans and animals.

The nutritional value of dried maca root is high, resembling that of cereal grains such as maize, rice, and wheat. It has 59% carbohydrates, 10.2% protein, 8.5% fiber, and 2.2% lipids.[5] It has a large amount of essential amino acids and higher levels of iron and calcium than potatoes.[8] Maca contains important amounts of fatty acids including linolenic, palmitic, and oleic acids. It is rich in sterols and has a high mineral content as well.[5] In addition to its rich supply of essential nutrients, maca contains alkaloids, tannins, and saponins.[3, 8] A chemical analysis conducted in 1981 showed the presence of biologically active aromatic isothiocyanates, especially p-methoxybenzyl isothiocyanate, which have reputed aphrodisiac properties.[4] Initial analyses of maca indicate that the effects on fertility are a result of the glucosinolates.[3, 4, 8] Alkaloids are also present but have not yet been quantified.[8]

> Maca is growing in world popularity due to its energizing effects, fertility enhancement, and aphrodisiac qualities.

Maca is growing in world popularity due to its energizing effects, fertility enhancement, and aphrodisiac qualities. Other traditional uses include increasing energy, stamina, and endurance in athletes, promoting mental clarity, treating male impotence, and helping with menstrual irregularities, female hormonal imbalances, menopause, and chronic fatigue syndrome.[1, 10] It is used as an alternative to anabolic steroids by bodybuilders due to its richness in sterols.[10] Today, dried maca roots are ground to powder and sold in drugstores in capsules as a medicine and food supplement to increase stamina and fertility.[4, 11] In Peruvian herbal medicine, maca is also used as an immunostimulant and for anemia, tuberculosis, menstrual disorders, menopause symptoms, stomach cancer, sterility, and other reproductive and sexual disorders, as well as to enhance memory.[11] Therapeutic dosages are reported to be 5 to 20 g daily.

The cultivation of maca is increasing in the highlands of the Andes to meet the growing demand worldwide for medicinal uses.[4, 12] In this severely economically depressed region, the market created for maca will offer new and important sources of income for the indigenous peoples of the Andes. A new cultivar of maca, named *Lepidium peruvianum* Chacon sp.,[12] has been identified in the major growing regions of the highlands. It will supply much of this new demand.

WORLDWIDE USES

Region	Uses
Peru	Anemia, aphrodisiac, energy, fertility, impotence, memory, menopause, menstrual, tonic, tuberculosis

PHYTOCHEMICALS

alkaloids, amino acids, beta-ecdysone, calcium, carbohydrates, iron, magnesium, p-methoxy-benzyl isothiocyanate, phosphorus, protein, saponins, sitosterol, stigmasterol, tannins, vitamin B1, vitamin B2, vitamin B12, vitamin C, vitamin E, zinc

MACELA

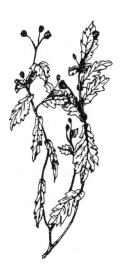

Family: Asteraceae

Genus: *Achyrocline*

Species: *satureoides*

Common Names: Macela, marcela, birabira, marcela del campo, hembra marcela, Juan blanco, macela-do-campo, marcela hembra, marcelita, mirabira, perpétua do mato suso, viravira, wira-wira, yatey-caa, yerba de chivo

Parts Used: Aerial parts, leaves, flowers

Medicinal Properties: Analgesic, anti-inflammatory, antimutagenic, antiseptic, antispasmodic, antitumorus, antiviral, cytotoxic, digestive, emmenagogue, genotoxic, hypoglycemic, immunostimulant, insecticidal, muscle relaxant, sudorific, vermifuge

MACELA IS A medium-sized aromatic annual herb that produces small white flowers with yellow centers and serrated green leaves. It is indigenous to much of tropical South and Central America and is found throughout Brazil, including in the Amazon rainforest.

Called macela or *marcela* in Brazil, it has been used in natural medicine for many years there. Using the flowers and/or the dried plant, a tea is prepared with 5 g of herb to 1 l of boiling water. It is used for nervous colic, epilepsy, and gastric problems. It is also used as an anti-inflammatory, antispasmodic, and analgesic for gastric disturbances, diarrhea, and dysentery, and as a sedative and emmenagogue in herbal medicine and by local people in Brazil.[1, 2] In Argentina 20 g of the flowers is infused in 1 l of hot water and taken to help regulate menstruation and for asthma.[3] In Uruguay it is used much the same way—for stomach, digestion, and gastrointestinal disorders, as an emmenagogue and menstrual regulator, and as a sedative and antispasmodic.[4]

> Phytochemical analysis of macela shows that it is a rich source of flavonoids, including novel ones never before seen in science.

> We are losing Earth's greatest biological treasures just as we are beginning to appreciate their true value. Rainforests once covered 14% of the Earth's land surface; now they cover a mere 6%, and experts estimate that the last remaining rainforests could be consumed in less than 50 years.

Phytochemical analysis of macela shows that it is a rich source of flavonoids, including novel ones never before seen in science. Many of its active properties are attributed to these flavonoids as well as to other sesquiterpenes and monoterpenes isolated in the plant.[5, 6] Macela has been of recent clinical interest, and its uses in natural medicine have been validated by science since the mid-1980s. In animal studies with mice and rats, macela demonstrated analgesic, anti-inflammatory, and smooth muscle–relaxant properties internally (gastrointestinal muscles) and externally without toxicity.[7, 8] This may well explain why macela has long been used effectively for many types of gastrointestinal difficulties as well as asthma. *In vitro* studies have demonstrated that macela is molluscicidal, and mutagenic against salmonella and *E. coli,* which could explain its uses against dysentery, diarrhea, and infections.[1, 9, 10]

Other research on macela has concentrated on its antitumorous, antiviral, and immunostimulant properties. It was shown to pass the initial anticrustacean screening test used to predict antitumor activity in 1993.[4] In the mid-1980s German researchers extracted the whole dried plant and demonstrated that in humans and mice it showed strong immunostimulant activity by increasing phagocytosis.[11, 12] They isolated a polysaccharide fraction in the macela extract that seemed to be responsible for this effect. In the mid-1990s Japanese researchers showed that an extract of macela flowers inhibited the growth of cancer cells by 67% *in vitro.*[13] In 1996 researchers in Texas found that a hot water extract of dried macela flowers demonstrated *in vitro* antiviral properties against T-lymphoblastoid cells infected with HIV.[14]

With its potential anti-HIV properties combined with its immunostimulant actions, macela could (and should) be the subject of further AIDS research. Until then, a simple macela tea (standard infusion) is still a highly effective natural remedy for many types of gastrointestinal complaints, especially where inflammation and spasms occur. Many practitioners in South and North America use macela in tea or capsules for spastic colon, Crohn's disease, colitis, and irritable bowel syndrome and as a general digestive aid. The therapeutic dosage is reported to be 3 to 4 g daily. Many natural health practitioners in South America still use macela to help regulate menstrual periods, as it has been used for many years with reported good results, although this effect has not yet been studied by scientists.

> **With its potential anti-HIV properties combined with its immunostimulant actions, macela could be the subject of further AIDS research.**

WORLDWIDE USES

Region	Uses
Argentina	Antidiabetic, asthma, digestive, emmenagogue, menstrual regulation
Bolivia	Carminative
Brazil	Analgesic, antibacterial, antidiabetic, anti-inflammatory, antimicrobial, antispasmodic, cold, colic, diarrhea, digestive, dysentery, emmenagogue, epilepsy, flu, gastritis, gastrointestinal disorders, hypoglycemic, inflammation, menstrual disorders, sedative, sudorific
Colombia	Tumors
Paraguay	Anthelmintic, antimicrobial, infections, vermifuge
Uruguay	Antiseptic, antispasmodic, digestion, emmenagogue, impotence, inflammation, menstrual disorders, sedative
Venezuela	Diabetes, emmenagogue, impotence

PHYTOCHEMICALS

alnustin, alpha-pinene, alpha-pyrone, auricepyrone,6-o-demethyl-23-methyl, beta-caryophyllene, beta-ocimene, caffeic acid, callerianin, caffeoyl, calleryanin, caryatin, caryophyllene, caryophyllene oxide, caryophyllene-1-10-epoxide, chlorogenic acid, cineol, 1-8-coumarin, delta-cadinene, flavone, 5-8-dihydroxy-3-7-dimethoxy, flavone, 3-5-7-8-tetramethoxy, flavonoids, galangin, galangin-3-methyl ether, germacrene D, gnapahaliin, ISO, gnaphaliin, italidipyrone, lauricepyrone, 6-o-demethyl-23-methy, luteolin, 6-(4'-hydroxy-trans-s, tyryl)-4-methoxy, protocatechuoyl, quercetagetin, quercetin, quercetin-3-methyl ether, scoparol, scoparone, tamarixetin, tamarixetin-7-glucoside

MANACÁ

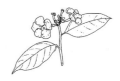

Family: Solanaceae

Genus: *Brunfelsia*

Species: *uniflorus, grandiflora*

Common Names: Manacá, manacán, chiric sanango, chuchuwasha, manaka, vegetable mercury, managá caa, gambá, jeratacaca

Parts Used: Root, bark

Medicinal Properties: Abortifacient, alterative, analgesic, anesthetic, anti-inflammatory, antirheumatic, diaphoretic, diuretic, emmenagogue, hypertensive, hypothermal, laxative, narcotic, purgative

MANACÁ IS A medium-sized, shrubby tree that grows up to 8 m high and is indigenous to the Amazon rainforest. It is often cultivated as an ornamental because it produces pretty, yellowish-white, highly fragrant flowers, from which a perfume is extracted. It can be found in the Amazon regions of Brazil, Bolivia, Peru, Ecuador, Colombia, and Venezuela. In Brazil manacá is known by several botanical names, including *Brunfelsia uniflorus, B. grandiflora*, and *Franciscea uniflora*. In Europe it is known as *B. hopeana*.

Manacá has a long history of indigenous use in the rainforest for both medicine and magic. Its Brazilian common name, manacá, comes from the Tupi Indians in Brazil, who named it after the most beautiful girl in the tribe, Manacán, because of its beautiful flowers. It is a sacred and spiritual plant used by the shamans and *curanderos* in *ayahuasca* (a sacred hallucinogenic), in special initiation ceremonies, and for bad luck. In the Amazon the root of manacá is infused with *aguardiente* (rum) for rheumatism and venereal disease. A decoction of leaves is used externally by indigenous peoples in Peru for arthritis and rheumatism; they also use a decoction of the root for chills. Indigenous tribes in the northwest Amazon consider manacá to be a diaphoretic and diuretic and use it for fever, rheumatism, snakebite, syphilis, and yellow fever. *Curanderos* and herbal healers along the Amazon River and in Ecuador use a root decoction to treat arthritis, rheumatism, colds and flu, uterine pain and cramps, and venereal diseases and to clean the blood, while using a poultice of the leaves as a topical analgesic. One Amazonian *curandero* near Pucallpa, Peru, uses a root tea for adult fevers, arthritis and rheumatism, back pain, common colds and bronchitis, lung disease and tuberculosis, and snakebite and as an enema for kidney disorders and ulcers.

Herbal healers along the Amazon River and in Ecuador use a root decoction of manacá to treat arthritis, rheumatism, colds and flu, uterine pain and cramps, and venereal diseases.

The root of manacá is said to stimulate the lymphatic system, and it has long been used for syphilis, earning the name "vegetable mercury." In herbal medicine manacá is considered to be an abortifacient, alterative, anesthetic, diaphoretic, diuretic, emmenagogue, hypertensive, hypothermal, laxative, and narcotic, and it is employed for arthritis, rheumatism, scrofula, and syphilis. Practitioners and herbalists in the United States use manacá as a diuretic, purgative, and anti-inflammatory to treat arthritis and rheumatism and sexually transmitted diseases and to stimulate the lymphatic system and disperse uric acid. The therapeutic dosage is reported to be 4 to 6 g daily, while the indigenous natural remedy is 1/2 cup of a standard decoction taken 1 to 3 times daily.

The active constituents of manacá include two alkaloids, manaceine and manacine, as well as scopoletin and aesculetin. Manaceine and manacine are thought to be responsible for stimulating the lymphatic system, while aesculetin has demonstrated analgesic, antihepatotoxic, antimutagenic, and anti-inflammatory activities in laboratory tests. Scopoletin is a well-known phytochemical that has demonstrated analgesic, antiasthmatic, anti-inflammatory, antiseptic, antitumor, central nervous system—

stimulant, cancer-preventive, hypoglycemic, hypotensive, myore-laxant, spasmolytic, and uterosedative activity in many different laboratory experiments. Root extracts of manacá have demonstrated marked anti-inflammatory activity in at least two clinical experiments.[1, 2]

WORLDWIDE USES

Region	Uses
Amazonia	Arthritis, colds, fever, flu, lymph, rheumatism, snakebite, syphilis, uterine cramps, uterine disorders, venereal disease, yellow fever
Brazil	Diuretic, purgative, rheumatism
Ecuador	Analgesic, arthritis, cold, flu, lymph, rheumatism, uterine, venereal disease
France	Scrofula
Germany	Rheumatism
Holland	Alterative
Peru	Analgesic, anti-inflammatory, arthritis, back pain, bronchitis, chills, colds, diaphoretic, diuretic, fever, kidney, lung disease, rheumatism, snakebite, syphilis, tuberculosis, ulcers, uterine, venereal disease
Elsewhere	Alterative, diuretic, laxative, rheumatism

PHYTOCHEMICALS

aesculetin, brunfelsene, hopeanine, lactic acid, manaceine, manacine, mandragorine, quinic acid, scopoletin, starch, tartaric acid

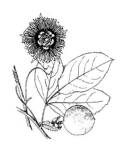

MARACUJA   Passionflower

Family: Passifloraceae

Genus: *Passiflora*

Species: *edulis, incarnata*

Common Names: Maracuja, passionflower, carkifelek, charkhi felek, may-pop, maypop passionflower, saa't gulu, ward assa'ah, zahril aalaam

Parts Used: Vine, leaves, stem

Medicinal Properties: Analgesic, anticonvulsant, antidepressant, anti-inflammatory, antispasmodic, anxiolytic, disinfectant, diuretic, hypnotic, nervine, sedative, spasmolytic, vermifuge

MARACUJA, KNOWN IN Europe and North America as passionflower, is a hardy woody vine that grows up to 10 m long and puts out tendrils, enabling it to climb up and over other plants. It bears striking, large white flowers with pink or purple centers, and and it bears delicious edible fruit. The flowers gave it the name passionflower, or "flower of passion," because Spanish missionaries thought they represented some of the objects associated with the Crucifixion of Christ. Maracuja is indigenous throughout tropical and semitropical zones from South America to North America. There are over 200 species of passionflower; the one most commonly found in the Amazon region is *Passiflora edulis*.

Passionflower was first "discovered" in Peru by a Spanish doctor named Monardes in 1569. He documented the indigenous uses and took it back to the Old World, where it quickly became a favorite herb tea. Spanish conquerors of Mexico and South America also learned its use from the Aztec Indians, and it eventually became widely cultivated in Europe. Since its discovery, maracuja has been widely used as a sedative, antispasmodic, and nerve tonic. Indians throughout the Amazon use the leaf tea as a sedative. When introduced into Europe in the 1500s, it was used as a calming and sedative tea. It was introduced in North American medicine in the mid-1800s as a sedative through native and slave use in the South, where the bruised leaves were also applied topically for headache, bruises, and pain. In many countries in Europe, and in the United States and Canada, the use of passionflower to tranquilize and settle edgy nerves has been documented for over 200 years. Its long-documented history in herbal medicine has included its uses for colic, diarrhea, dysentery, dysmenorrhea, epilepsy, eruptions, insomnia, morphinism, neuralgia, neurosis, ophthalmia, piles, and spasm.

In many countries in Europe, and in the United States and Canada, the use of passionflower to tranquilize and settle edgy nerves has been documented for over 200 years.

Passionflower is widely employed by herbalists and natural health practitioners around the world today. It is mostly employed as a sedative, hypnotic (inducing sleep), nervine, antispasmodic, and pain reliever. In the United States *P. incarnata* is the species most used, to treat insomnia, Parkinson's disease, seizures and convulsions, muscle cramps, hysteria, high blood pressure, tetanus, shingles, neuralgia, dysmenorrhea, menstrual cramps and PMS, and epilepsy and for pain relief. In Europe it is employed for nervous disorders, insomnia, spasms, neuralgia, alcoholism, hyperactivity in children, rapid heartbeat and headaches and as a pain reliever and antispasmodic. In South America *P. edulis* is the species most used, as a sedative, diuretic, antispasmodic, and anthelmintic (expelling intestinal worms) and to treat convulsions, paralysis, alcoholism, headaches, insomnia, colic in infants, diarrhea, grippe, hysteria, neuralgia, menopausal symptoms, and hypertension. In both South and North America, as well as in Europe, maracuja is used topically for skin disorders, inflammation, hemorrhoids, and burns because of its anti-inflammatory and pain-relieving effects.

Passionflower has been the subject of much scientific research. After almost a century of study, its sedative, antispasmodic, and analgesic effects have been firmly established in science; yet these effects have not been correlated to any one chemical or group of chemicals found in the plant. Passionflower contains two major groups of chemicals—glycosides and flavonoids—as well as alkaloids. When these chemicals are isolated and tested individually, they demonstrate reactions opposite to those for which the plant is commonly used; only when the two are combined, as in the whole herb, do researchers observe the plant's sedative effect.[1, 2] The analgesic effects of passionflower were first clinically documented in 1897, while the sedative effects were first recorded in 1904.[1] Antispasmodic, anxiolytic, and hypertensive actions were clinically validated in the early 1980s.[2]

After almost a century of study, passionflower's sedative, antispasmodic, and analgesic effects have been firmly established in science.

The U.S. Food and Drug Administration classifies passionflower as "generally regarded as safe." Passionflower is the subject of various European monographs for medicinal plants and is generally regarded as safe even for children and infants. Herbalists usually recommend 6 g of the herb daily in a standard infusion (tea).

WORLDWIDE USES

Region	Uses
Europe	Alcoholism, antispasmodic, headaches, hyperactivity, hypertension, insomnia, nervine, nervous disorders, neuralgia, pain reliever, sedative, spasms
Iraq	Insomnia, narcotic
Poland	Hysteria, neurasthenia
South America	Alcoholism, analgesic, anthelmintic, antispasmodic, asthma, bronchitis, burn, colic, convulsions, cough, diarrhea, diuretic, grippe, headaches, hemorrhoids, hypertension, hysteria, inflammation, insomnia, menopause, nervine, neuralgia, neurasthenia, paralysis, sedative, skin, spasm, tonic, worms (intestinal)
Turkey	Dysmenorrhea, epilepsy, insomnia, narcotic, neuralgia, neurosis, sedative, soporific, spasm
United States	Antispasmodic, aphrodisiac, burn, convulsions, cyanogenetic, diarrhea, dysmenorrhea, epilepsy, eruption, eye, hemorrhoids, high blood pressure, hysteria, inflammation, insomnia, medicine, menstrual cramps, muscle cramps, nervine, neuralgia, pain reliever, Parkinson's disease, piles, PMS, sedative, seizures, shingles, skin, spasm, tetanus
Elsewhere	Asthma, epilepsy, insomnia, morphinism, narcotic, neuralgia, perfume, spasm

PHYTOCHEMICALS

alkaloids, alpha-alanine, apigenin, D-fructose, D-glucose, flavonoids, gum, gynocardin, harmaline, harmalol, harmine, harmol, homoorientin, isoorientin, isovitexin, kaempferol, lutenin-2, luteolin, maltol, N-nonacosane, orientin, passiflorine, phenylalanine, proline, quercetin, raffinose, rutin, saccharose, saponaretin, saponarine, scopoletin, sitosterol, stigmasterol, sucrose, tyrosine, umbelliferone, valine, vitexin

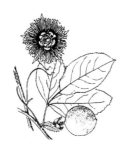

MARACUJA Passion fruit

Family: Passifloraceae

Genus: *Passiflora*

Species: *edulis, incarnata*

Common Names: Maracuja, passionflower, passion fruit, granadilla, purple granadilla, maypop, apricot vine

Part Used: Fruit

Medicinal Properties: Antibacterial, antifungal, nutritive, sedative

ELLOW PASSION FRUIT *(Passiflora edulis)* grows on 3- to 6-meter-long vines, and the fruits are the size of large lemons, wrinkling slightly when ripe. It is the most widely cultivated species in the Amazon and other warm, humid tropics; over 200 species of fruit-bearing *Passiflora* have been cataloged in the Brazilian Amazon alone. Various species of *Passiflora*, climbing vines native to the South American tropics and rainforest, have been domesticated to eat as fresh fruit or to make refreshing and nutritive juices. The yellow, gelatinous pulp is mixed with water and sugar to make drinks, sherbet, ice cream, jam, jellies, and salad dressings.

Passion fruit is catching on as a popular drink in both industrial and developing countries, and a new fruit juice may be hitting the U.S. market in the near future. In a 20-year-old research project, scientists have created a new fruit called "passion pops" by crossbreeding the tropical *P. edulis* with its U.S. relative, *P. incarnata* to produce tennis-ball-sized fruits[1] that range in color from yellow to green, dark maroon, and purple. One of the benefits of the new fruit is that it will grow farther north than the traditional

Medicinal Plants of the Rainforest

U.S. passion fruit and provide an alternative to farmers who have been hurt by winter freezes of citrus crops. Several U.S.-based juice companies have expressed interest in the new fruit, and some new juice products may be on the market in the near future.

Passion fruit has been a food staple for the people and animals of the rainforest for eons. The fruits of many of the *Passiflora* species have been used for centuries by indigenous tribes as a sedative or calming tonic. The fruit of *P. edulis* has been used by the Brazilian tribes as a heart tonic, and passion fruit is still used today in South American traditional medicine. Researcher and author Antonio Bernardes notes: "A cup of maracuja tea [leaves] or 2 glasses of juice will naturally calm down the most hyperactive child, and for this reason it is highly valued by Brazilian mothers." And Daniel B. Mowrey, herbalist and author, notes: "The Brazilians even have a favorite passionflower drink, called *maracuja grande*, that is frequently used to treat asthma, whooping cough, bronchitis, and other tough coughs." In Peruvian traditional medicine today, passion fruit juice is used for urinary infections and as a mild diuretic. Researchers have documented the properties of passion fruit juice in at least four studies showing its antibacterial and antifungal properties as well as its high nutritive value in vitamins, minerals, and amino acids.[2–5]

> Studies of passion fruit juice have shown its antibacterial and antifungal properties as well as its high nutritive value in vitamins, minerals, and amino acids.

WORLDWIDE USES

Region	Uses
Amazonia	Food, heart tonic
Brazil	Asthma, bronchitis, cough, food, sedative, whooping cough
Peru	Diuretic, food, urinary infections

PHYTOCHEMICALS

alkaloids, ascorbic acid, beta-carotene, calcium, carotenoids, catalase, citric acid, EO, ethyl-butyrate, ethyl-caproate, fat, fiber, flavonoids, harman, iron, malic-acid, N-hexyl-butyrate, N-hexyl-caproate, niacin, pectin-methylesterase, phenolase, phosphorus, potassium, protein, riboflavin, sodium, thiamin, water, xanthophylls

We don't have much time. We are talking about an extremely short period during which most of the planet's tropical rainforests may vanish, given current trends. The rainforest is the greatest organic being of this tremendous organic being we call Planet Earth, Gaia, the biosphere, or whatever your name for Mother Earth is. A very central organ of that life support system is threatened with . . . death. And nobody, including the scientists, knows what that means. In reality, we are conducting an extremely perilous experiment on this great organic being that is the Earth, and we have no idea what the full impacts of destroying the forests will be.

—John P. Milton, *Coalitions for the Forest*

MUIRA PUAMA

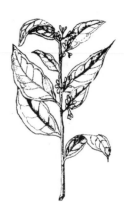

Family: Olacaceae

Genus: *Ptychopetalum*

Species: *olacoides*

Common Names: Muira puama, marapuama, marapama, potency wood, potenzholz

Parts Used: Bark, roots

Medicinal Properties: Antidysenteric, antirheumatic, antistress, aperitif, aphrodisiac, central nervous system stimulant, nervine, neurasthenic, tonic

M UIRA PUAMA, ALSO called "potency wood," is a bush or small tree that grows up to 5 m high and is native to the Brazilian Amazon and other parts of northern Brazil. The small, white flowers have a pungent fragrance similar to jasmine's. Historically, all parts of the plants have been used medicinally, but the bark and roots are the primary parts of the plant utilized.

It has long been used in the Amazon by indigenous peoples for a number of purposes, and the plant found its way into herbal medicine in South America and Europe in the 1920s. Indigenous tribes in Brazil use the roots and bark internally as a tea for treating sexual debility and impotence, neuromuscular problems, rheumatism, grippe, cardiac asthenia, and gastrointestinal asthenia and to prevent baldness. It is also used externally in baths and massages for treating paralysis and beri-beri.

Muira puama has a long history in herbal medicine as an aphrodisiac, a tonic for the nervous system, and an antirheumatic

> **Muira puama has a long history in herbal medicine as an aphrodisiac, a tonic for the nervous system, and an antirheumatic and for gastrointestinal disorders.**

and for gastrointestinal disorders. In 1925 a pharmacological study published on muira puama indicated its effectiveness in treating disorders of the nervous system and sexual impotence, indicating that "permanent effect is produced in locomotor ataxia, neuralgias of long standing, chronic rheumatism, and partial paralysis."[1] In 1930 Meiro Penna wrote about muira puama in his book *Notas Sobre Plantas Brasileriras*. He cited physiological and therapeutic experiments conducted in France by Dr. Rebourgeon that confirmed the efficacy of the plant for "gastrointestinal and circulatory asthenia and impotency of the genital organs."[2]

Two closely related species of *Ptychopetalum, P. olacoides* and *P. uncinatum,* were used interchangeably when the herb became popular in the 1920s and 1930s; a third species, *Liriosma ovata* (which also had a common name of muira puama), was used as well.[3] Early European explorers noted the indigenous uses and the aphrodisiac qualities of muira puama and brought it back to Europe, where it has become part of the herbal medicine of England. Because of the long history of use of muira puama in England, it is still listed in the *British Herbal Pharmacopoeia* (a noted source on herbal medicine from the British Herbal Medicine Association), where it is recommended for the treatment of dysentery and impotence.[4] It has been in the *Brazilian Pharmacopoeia* since the 1950s.[5]

Scientists began searching for the active components in the root and bark of muira puama to determine the reasons for it efficacy in the 1920s.[6-8] Early researchers discovered that the root and bark were rich in free fatty acids, essential oils, plant sterols, and a new alkaloid, which they named muirapuamine.[1] Since it continued to be used successfully throughout the world as an aphrodisiac and treatment for impotence, as well as for hookworms, dysentery, rheumatism, and central nervous system disorders, scientists began researching the plant's constituents and pharmacological properties again in the late 1960s, continuing on until the late 1980s.[9–15] These studies indicated that the active constituents are free long-chain fatty acids, sterols, coumarin, alkaloids, and essential oils. Chemically, muira puama contains 0.05% muira-puamine, 0.4% fat, 0.5% alkaloids, 0.6% pholbaphene, 0.6% alpha-resinic acid, 0.7% beta-resinic acid, 0.5% of a mixture of esters including behenic acid, lupeol and beta-sitosterol, as well as tannin, volatile oils, and fatty acids.

Muira puama is still employed around the world today in herbal medicine. In Brazilian and South American herbal medicine, it is used as a neuromuscular tonic, for asthenia, paralysis, chronic rheumatism, sexual impotence, grippe, ataxia, and central nervous system disorders. In Europe it is used to treat impotence, infertility, neurasthenia, menstrual disturbances, and dysentery. Muira puama has been gaining in popularity in the United States, where herbalists and health care practitioners are using it to treat impotence, menstrual cramps and PMS, neurasthenia, and central nervous system disorders. The benefits of treating impotence with muira puama have recently been studied in two human trials, which proved muira puama to be effective in improving libido and treating erectile dysfunction. In a study conducted in Paris, France, of 262 male patients experiencing lack of sexual desire and the inability to attain or maintain an erection, 62% of the patients with loss of libido reported that the extract of muira puama "had a dynamic effect," and 51% of patients with erectile dysfunctions felt that muira puama was beneficial.[16, 17] The second study, conducted by J. Waynberg in France, evaluated the positive psychological benefits of muira puama in 100 men with male sexual asthenia.[18] The therapeutic dosage used was 1.5 g daily of a muira puama extract.

While so-called aphrodisiacs have come and gone in history, muira puama has risen above this class of products and may well provide the most effective natural therapeutic approach for

> **Muira puama has been gaining in popularity in the United States, where herbalists and health care practitioners are using it to treat impotence, menstrual cramps and PMS, neurasthenia, and central nervous system disorders.**

erectile dysfunctions. Consumers must be aware, however, that to achieve the beneficial effects of the plant, proper preparation methods must be employed. The active constituents thought to be responsible for muira puama's effect are not soluble in water, so taking a bark or root powder in a capsule or tablet will not be very effective. High heat for at least 20 minutes or longer and alcohol are necessary to dissolve and extract the volatile and essential oils, terpenes, gums, and resins found in the bark and root that have been linked to muira puama's beneficial effects.

WORLDWIDE USES

Region	Uses
Amazonia	Asthenia, baldness, beri-beri, cardiac asthenia, gastrointestinal, grippe, impotence, neuromuscular, paralysis, rheumatism, sexual debility
Brazil	Aphrodisiac, asthenia, ataxia, baldness, beri-beri, central nervous system disorders, debility, depression, dysentery, frigidity, gastrointestinal, grippe, heart, impotence, menstrual cramps, neuralgia, neurasthenia, neuromuscular, paralysis, PMS, rheumatism, tonic
Europe	Aphrodisiac, dysentery, impotence, infertility, menstrual disturbances, nervine, neurasthenia, tonic
United States	Aphrodisiac, central nervous system disorders, impotence, menstrual, nervine, neurasthenia, PMS

PHYTOCHEMICALS

alkaloids, alpha-resinic acid, arachidic acid, behenic acid, beta-resinic acid, beta-sitosterol, campesterol, cerotic acid, coumarin, dotriacontanoic acid, EO, heptacosanoic acid, lignoceric acid, lupeol, melissic acid, montanic acid, muirapuamine, nonacosanoic acid, pentacosanoic acid, phlobaphene, trichosanic acid, uncosanic acid

MULATEIRO

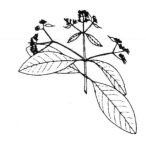

Family: Rubiaceae

Genus: *Calycophyllum*

Species: *spruceanum*

Common Names: Mulateiro, pau mulato, capirona

Part Used: Bark

Medicinal Properties: Anthelmintic, antifungal, emollient, vermifuge,
vulnerary

M ULATEIRO, OR PAU MULATO, is a fascinating tree native to the Amazon region. It grows to a height of about 30 m and has long been used as a source of good, high-density lumber. The tree propagates easily and is found near water, where it can be periodically flooded. Mulateiro is marked by its ability to completely shed and regenerate its bark on a yearly basis, making it a totally renewable resource. The bark, which is very smooth, as if polished,[1] changes colors throughout the year as it matures, going from a green tone to a brownish tone.

Use of mulateiro bark is deeply ingrained in the native culture. It is used as an admixture in the *ayahuasca* (spiritual) rituals, and has many different uses in folkloric medicine. A poultice made from the bark has been used topically in treating cuts, wounds, and burns, due to its antifungal, emollient, and vulnerary qualities.[2] The natives also use a tea made from the bark on their bodies after bathing and then sun-dry themselves. This forms a thin film covering their bodies, believed to help fight the effects of aging.[2] Other

> A poultice made from mulateiro bark has been used topically in treating cuts, wounds, and burns, due to its antifungal, emollient, and vulnerary qualities.

Amazonian tribes have traditionally used the bark of this tree for various skin ailments, as a decoction for fighting skin parasites, and in powder form for fungal infections of the skin. Indigenous peoples of the Amazon boil 1 kg of mulateiro bark in 10 l of water to obtain 4 l of medicine, which is drunk (150 ml per day) for three consecutive months to "cure" diabetes. Peruvian tribes use the bark for mycoses and against *sarna negra*, a nasty little arachnid that lives under the skin and is commonly found in the Amazon Basin area.

There is little research on the active ingredients in the mulateiro bark as of yet, although it is known to have a high content of tannins.

WORLDWIDE USES

Region	Uses
Amazonia	Diabetes, fungal infections, parasites, skin, vulnerary, wounds

MULLACA

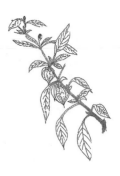

Family: Solanaceae

Genus: *Physalis*

Species: *angulata*

Common Names: Mullaca, camapu, bolsa mullaca, cape gooseberry, wild tomato, winter cherry, juá-de-capote, capulí cimarrón, battre-autour, k'u chih, 'urmoa batoto bita, cecendet, dumadu harachan, hog weed, nvovo, polopa, saca-buche, thongtheng, tino-tino, topatop, wapotok

Parts Used: Whole plant, leaves, roots

Medicinal Properties: Analgesic, antiasthmatic, anticoagulant, antigonorrheal, anti-inflammatory, antileukemic, antimutagenic, antiseptic, antispasmodic, antiviral, cytotoxic, diuretic, expectorant, febrifuge, hypotensive, immunostimulant, trypanocidal

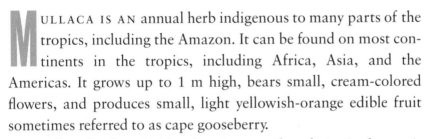

MULLACA IS AN annual herb indigenous to many parts of the tropics, including the Amazon. It can be found on most continents in the tropics, including Africa, Asia, and the Americas. It grows up to 1 m high, bears small, cream-colored flowers, and produces small, light yellowish-orange edible fruit sometimes referred to as cape gooseberry.

Mullaca has long held a place in natural medicine in the tropical countries where it grows. Its use by rainforest Indians in the Amazon is well documented, and its edible sweet-tart fruits are enjoyed by many rainforest inhabitants, animal and human alike. Indigenous tribes in the Amazon use a leaf infusion as a diuretic. Some Colombian tribes believe the fruits and leaves have narcotic properties and decoct them as an anti-inflammatory and disinfectant for skin diseases; others use a leaf tea for asthma. Indigenous peoples in the Peruvian Amazon use the leaf juice internally and externally for worms and the leaves and/or roots for earache, liver problems, malaria, hepatitis, and rheumatism. Indigenous tribes in the Brazilian Amazon use the sap of the plant for earaches and the roots for jaundice.

Mullaca is employed in herbal medicine in both Peru and Brazil. In Peruvian herbal medicine the plant is called mullaca or *bolsa mullaca*. To treat diabetes, the roots of 3 mullaca plants are sliced and macerated in 1/4 l of rum for seven days. Honey is added, and 1/2 glass of this medicine is taken twice daily for 60 days. In addition, an infusion of the leaves is recommended as a good diuretic, and an infusion of the roots is used to treat hepatitis. For asthma and malaria, the dosage is 1 cup of tea made from the aerial parts of the plant. In Brazilian herbal medicine the plant is named *camapu*. There it is employed for chronic rheumatism, for skin diseases and dermatitis, as a sedative and diuretic, for fever and vomiting, and for many types of kidney, liver, and gallbladder problems.

Phytochemical studies on mullaca reveal that it contains flavonoids, alkaloids, and many different types of plant steroids, some of which have never been seen before in science.[1–6] Mullaca has been the subject of recent clinical research that is still ongoing, based on preliminary studies showing that it is an effective immune stimulant, is cytotoxic to numerous types of cancer cells, and has antiviral properties, including against HIV. The new steroids found in mullaca have received the most attention, and many of the documented properties and actions are attributed to these steroids. In several *in vivo* animal tests and *in vitro* lab tests, an extract of the entire plant of mullaca and/or its steroidal fractions demonstrated immune stimulant properties by strongly enhancing blastogenesis, antibody responses, and increased T and B lymphocyte production.[7] Various water, alcohol, and ethanol extracts of mullaca and its plant steroids have shown strong *in vitro* and *in vivo* (in mice) cytotoxic activity against numerous types of cancer cells, including leukemia, lung, colon, cervix, and melanomas.[8–10] Other research groups in Japan have been focusing on mullaca's antiviral actions, and preliminary studies show

> **Preliminary studies of mullaca show that it is an effective immune stimulant, is cytotoxic to numerous types of cancer cells, and has antiviral properties, including against HIV.**

that it is active *in vitro* against polio virus I, as well as HIV I, demonstrating reverse transcriptase inhibitory effects.[11-14] In addition to these actions, mullaca has demonstrated good antibacterial properties *in vitro* against numerous types of bacteria,[15, 16] antispasmodic activities in guinea pigs,[17] hypotensive properties in cats, isotonic muscle contracting properties in toads,[18] and an *in vitro* anticoagulant effect.[19]

Interestingly, much of the clinical research has ignored many of the local and indigenous uses of the plant, thus some of its documented effective uses in herbal medicine remain unexplained. Its tested antibacterial properties could validate its uses as an antiseptic and disinfectant for skin diseases and infections, and to treat gonorrhea. Its antiviral properties could well explain its long history of use for hepatitis, although scientists have not tested it specifically against hepatitis. Possibly the antispasmodic and muscle contractive properties documented for mullaca might explain its widespread use for asthma as well. Yet its use throughout the rainforests for malaria and diabetes is still unexplained by science.

WORLDWIDE USES

Region	Uses
Africa	Sterility, throat
Brazil	Depurative, dermatitis, diuretic, dysuria, earache, fever, gallbladder, jaundice, kidney, liver, rheumatism, sedative, skin disease
Burkina Faso	Analgesic, diarrhea, nausea, sleeping sickness
Central America	Abortion preventative, gonorrhea, malaria
China	Diuretic, expectorant, fever, labor
Colombia	Anti-inflammatory, asthma, disinfectant, narcotic, skin disease

(continues)

WORLDWIDE USES *(continued)*

Region	Uses
Ghana	Fever, stomach, syncope
Haiti	Diuretic, fever, hydropsy
Japan	Antidote, cold, diuretic, fever, swelling, throat
Peru	Anti-inflammatory, asthma, diabetes, disinfectant, earache, hepatitis, liver, malaria, rheumatism, worms
Suriname	Diuretic, gonorrhea, jaundice, malaria, nephritis
Taiwan	Antipyretic, diuretic, hepatitis, liver disease, tumors
Thailand	Boil, rectum
Trinidad	Antiseptic, fever, indigestion, nephritis, rectitis
Elsewhere	Abortion preventative, anti-inflammatory, antiseptic, asthma, childbirth, diabetes, diarrhea, hemorrhage (postpartum), hemostatic, narcotic, ophthalmia, sleeping sickness, tumor (testicle)

PHYTOCHEMICALS

14-alpha-hydroxy ixocarpanolide, ayanin, acetyl choline, beta sitosterol, chlorogenic acid, phygrine, physagulin A, physagulin B, physagulin C, physagulin D, physagulin E, physagulin F, physagulin G, physalin B, physalin D, physalin E, physalin F, physalin G, physalin H, physalin I, physalin J, physalin K, physangulide, vamonolide, withagulatin A, withaminimin, 24-25-epoxy withanolide D, withanolide T, withaphysanolide

MULUNGU

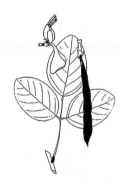

Family: Leguminosae

Genus: *Erythrina*

Species: *mulungu*

Common Names: Mulungu, murungu, muchoco, murungo, totocero, flor-de-coral, árvore-de-coral, pau imortal, mulungu-coral, capa-homem, suiná-suiná

Part Used: Bark

Medicinal Properties: Analgesic, anodyne, anti-inflammatory, hepatotonic, hypnotic, hypotensive, nervine, sedative

MULUNGU IS A medium-sized, well-branched tree that grows up to 8 to 10 m high. It produces a profusion of pretty, reddish-orange flowers at the end of the tree's many branches, and it is sometimes called a coral tree because the flowers are the same color as coral. It produces black seed pods with large red and black seeds inside, which are sometimes used by indigenous peoples to make necklaces and jewelry. It is indigenous to northern Brazil, parts of Peru, and tropical areas in Central America. Mulungu is known by several botanical names, including *Erythrina mulungu*, *E. crista-galli*, and *E. verna*.

There are over 100 species of *Erythrina* in the tropics, several of which are used by indigenous peoples as medicines, insecticides, and fish poisons. Mulungu has long been used in Brazil by indigenous peoples as a natural sedative. In herbal medicine it is considered to be an excellent sedative to calm agitation and nervous coughs and to treat other nervous system problems, including insomnia. It is also widely used for asthma, bronchitis, gingivitis, hepatitis, inflammation in the liver and spleen, intermittent fevers, and insomnia and to clear obstructions in the liver. Herbalists and practitioners in the United States use mulungu to quiet hysteria from trauma or shock, as a mild hypnotic sedative to calm the nervous system, to treat insomnia and promote healthy sleeping patterns by sedating overactive neurotransmitters, to regulate heart palpitations, and to treat hepatitis and liver disorders. Positive regulatory effects on heart palpitations and decreased blood pressure have been reported, and Dr. Donna Schwontkowski, a chiropractor who has used Amazonian plants in her practice, recommends mulungu for hernias, stomachaches, and epilepsy and to help augment milk flow as well. The therapeutic dosage is reported to be 3 to 5 ml of a standard tincture or 1/2 cup 1 to 3 times daily of a standard decoction.

In herbal medicine mulungu is considered to be an excellent sedative to calm agitation and nervous coughs and to treat other nervous system problems, including insomnia.

Mulungu's hypotensive and heart regulatory activity was studied and attributed to a group of alkaloids.[1] Much research has been performed on *Erythrina* alkaloids in the last decade, as they represent a group of very active chemicals with various properties and are almost always present to some degree in all *Erythrina* species of plants.[2] Many of these alkaloids have demonstrated piscicide, anti-inflammatory, cardioactive, narcotic, and hypnotic activities.[2, 3] One novel alkaloid discovered in mulungu is called cristamidine. Its positive effect on the liver was recently demonstrated in a 1995 clinical study with rats.[4] Isoflavones have also been identified in mulungu.[5]

WORLDWIDE USES

Region	Uses
Argentina	Narcotic, pile
Brazil	Asthma, bronchitis, cough, epilepsy, fever, gingivitis, hepatitis, hypnotic, hysteria, inflammation, insomnia, liver, sedative, spleen
United States	Central nervous system disorders, epilepsy, heart, hepatitis, hernia, high blood pressure, hysteria, insomnia, lactagogue, liver, stomachache
Venezuela	Diuretic, piscicide
Elsewhere	Cancer (stomach), cardiotonic, diuretic, narcotic, piscicide, sedative, spasm

PHYTOCHEMICALS

alkaloids, arachidic acid, beta-erythroidine, cristadine, cristamidine, cyanidin-3-glucoside, cyanidin-3-sophoroside, eicosenoic acid, erycristagallin, erysodine, erysonine, erysopine, erysothiopine, erysothiovine, erysovine, erythraline, erythramine, erythratine, erythratinone, hypaphorine, linoleic acid, myristic acid, oleic acid, palmitic acid, pelargonidin-3-glucoside, pelargonidin-3-sophoroside, stearic acid

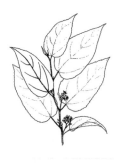

MUTAMBA

Family: Sterculiaceae

Genus: *Guazuma*

Species: *ulmifolia*

Common Names: Mutamba, mutambo, West Indian elm, guazima, guacima, guacimo, guasima de caballo, aquiche, ajya, guasima, cimarrona, guazuma, bolaina, atadijo, ibixuma, cambá-acã, bay cedar, bois d'homme, bois d'orme, bois de hetre, orme d'Amerique

Parts Used: Bark, leaves, root

Medicinal Properties: Antibacterial, antifungal, antimicrobial, antioxidant, antiulcerogenic, astringent, cytotoxic, depurative, diaphoretic, emollient, febrifuge, hepatoprotective, pectoral, refrigerant, stomachic, styptic, sudorific, vulnerary

MUTAMBA IS A medium tree that grows up to 20 m high, with a trunk 30 to 60 cm in diameter. Its oblong leaves are 6 to 12 cm long, and the tree produces small, white to light yellowish flowers. It produces an edible fruit that is covered with rough barbs. It is indigenous to tropical America on both continents and found in the Amazon rainforest.

Mutamba has had a place in herbal medicine in almost every country where it grows. The bark and the leaves are most used medicinally, but sometimes the fresh root is employed. In Belize a small handful of chopped bark is boiled for 10 minutes in 3 cups of water and drunk for dysentery and diarrhea, for prostate problems, and as a uterine stimulant to aid in childbirth. A slightly stronger tea is used externally for skin sores, infections, and rashes. In Brazil a bark tea is considered diaphoretic and used for fevers, coughs, bronchitis, asthma, pneumonia, and liver problems. Mutamba is called *guasima* or *guacima* in Mexico, where it has a very long history of indigenous use. The Huastec Mayans of northeastern Mexico employed the fresh bark boiled in water to aid in childbirth and for gastrointestinal pain, asthma, diarrhea and dysentery, wounds, and fevers.[1] In Peru the dried bark and dried leaves are boiled into tea (standard infusion) and used for kidney disease, liver disease, and dysentery. In other parts of Peru and the Amazon, mutamba is used internally and externally for alopecia, asthma, bronchitis, dermatosis, diarrhea, dysentery, elephantiasis, fever, hepatitis, leprosy, malaria, nephritis, pulmonosis, and syphilis. In Guatemala the dried leaves of the tree are brewed into a tea and drunk for fevers, kidney disease, and skin diseases, as well as used externally for wounds, sores, bruises, dermatitis, skin irruptions and irritations, and erysipelas.[2, 3]

The Huastec Mayans of northeastern Mexico employed fresh mutamba bark boiled in water to aid in childbirth and for gastrointestinal pain, asthma, diarrhea and dysentery, wounds, and fevers.

Its long history of effective uses in herbal medicine propelled researchers to begin studying mutamba's properties and activities in the laboratory beginning in 1968, and it has been the subject of numerous studies since. In the first study published, various water and alcohol mutamba bark extracts demonstrated weak cardiac depressant and cardiotonic activity, as well as hypotensive, smooth muscle–relaxant, and uterine-stimulant activities in animal studies.[4] Various leaf and bark extracts have clinically demonstrated *in vitro* antibacterial and antifungal activity against numerous pathogens in five different studies from 1987 to 1993.[3, 5–8] It also tested to have active properties against gonorrhea *in vitro* in a 1995 study.[9] A weak molluscicidal activity of the bark was documented in a 1974 study.[10]

Of particular note, a Brazilian research group demonstrated that a dried leaf extract was cytotoxic against cancer cells *in vitro*, exhibiting a 97.3% inhibition of cell growth in a 1990 study.[11] Some of the latest research on mutamba has focused on the antioxidants found in the bark and leaves (proanthocyanidins) and their ability to interfere with prostaglandin synthetase, a process by which bacteria and pathogens replicate.[12–14]

WORLDWIDE USES

Region	Uses
Belize	Childbirth, diarrhea, dysentery, prostate, rash, skin, sore
Brazil	Asthma, bronchitis, cough, diaphoretic, dysentery, fever, liver, pneumonia, ulcer
Colombia	Uterine stimulant
Cuba	Astringent, bruise, burn, diuretic, emollient, flu, grippe, hemorrhoids, wounds
Dominican Republic	Diaphoretic, dysentery, fertility (veterinary), lung
Guatemala	Bruise, dermatitis, erysipelas, febrifuge, gonorrhea, kidney disease, skin disease, skin irritation and irruptions, sore, sudorific, ulcers, wounds
Haiti	Antidote (comocladia), astringent, cough, depurative, diarrhea, emollient, fever, flu, fracture, scurvy, skin, stomachic
Jamaica	Elephantiasis, leprosy
Mauritius	Bronchitis, pectoral
Mexico	Asthma, astringent, chest, childbirth, constipation, diarrhea, dysentery, elephantiasis, emollient, fever, gastrointestinal, hemorrhage, kidney, leprosy, malaria, rash, skin, syphilis, uterus, wounds
Peru	Antidysenteric, kidney disease, liver disease
Venezuela	Astringent, emollient, refrigerant, sudorific, syphilis
Elsewhere	Asthma, astringent, chest, elephantiasis, hair, kidney, liver, medicine, obesity, skin, stomach, styptic, sudorific

PHYTOCHEMICALS

alkaloids, beta-sitosterol, caffeine, friedelin-3alpha-acetate, friedelin-3beta-ol, mucilage, tannins, terpenes

NETTLE

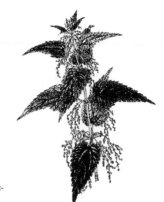

Family: Urticaceae

Genus: *Urtica*

Species: *dioica*

Common Names: Nettle, big string nettle, common nettle, stinging nettle, gerrais, isirgan, kazink, nabat al nar, ortiga, ortiga mayor

Parts Used: Root, leaves

Medicinal Properties: Anodyne, antirheumatic, antiseptic, astringent, bactericide, circulatory stimulant, depurative, diuretic, emmenagogue, galactagogue, hemostatic, hypoglycemic, hypotensive, stomachic, vasodilator, vermifuge

NETTLE, OR STINGING NETTLE, is a perennial plant growing worldwide in wasteland areas. It grows up to 2 m high with pointed leaves and flowers of white to yellowish panicles. Nettle has a reputation for giving a savage sting when skin touches the hairs and bristles on the leaves and stems. The stinging sensation is caused by formic acid and amines (histamine, serotonin, and choline). The tea of the leaves and stems has been used in traditional medicine as a poultice to stop bleeding. An account of this use is recorded by Francis P. Procher, a surgeon and physician in the Southern Confederacy.[1] The nettle leaves were recommended by the plant forager Euell Gibbons as a nutritious food and as a weight loss aid. Many remarkable healing properties have been attributed to nettle, including prevention of baldness, allergic rhinitis, and rheumatic pain.[1, 2] The nettle root is recommended as a diuretic and, relatively recently, for relief of benign prostatic hyperplasia (BPH).[3]

> Many healing properties have been attributed to nettle, including prevention of baldness, allergic rhinitis, and rheumatic pain. The nettle root is recommended as a diuretic and, relatively recently, for relief of benign prostatic hyperplasia.

Nettle root constituents include lignans, scopoletin, sterols (beta-sitosterol and sitosterol-3-o-glucoside), oleannoic acid, and 9-hydroxyl-10-trans-12-cis-octadecanoic acid. Other chemicals are high molecular weight compounds such as five acids and neutral polysaccharides and isolectins.[4]

Several clinical studies document the efficacy of nettle root for BPH. Dr. Varro E. Tyler reported on a paper from the 1995 Congress on Medicinal Plant Research that J. J. Lichius and colleagues showed a reduction in prostatic growth potential in mice with the administration of a high dosage of nettle root extract.[4] Another study using saw palmetto berries and nettle root extracts to treat patients with BPH showed an inhibition of the testosterone metabolites dihydrotestosterone and estrogen, thus proving nettle root to be an effective treatment.[5] Some of the more resent research on BPH and nettles show that nettles can interfere with or block a chemical process in the body that has been linked to prostate disorders. As men age, free-floating testosterone becomes bound to albumin in a process called human sex hormone–binding globulin (SHBG), removing its bioavailability to the body. This chemical process is now believed to be linked to prostate disorders. In several clinical studies, nettle has demonstrated the ability to block this process, which may well explain its documented effectiveness in the treatment of many prostate conditions.[6–9] Since testosterone is a natural aphrodisiac, and nettle may make more testosterone bioavailable for the body's use by blocking SHBG, this may also explain why nettle has recently been regarded as having aphrodisiac properties. The therapeutic dosage of nettle root is reported to be 5 to 6 g daily.

WORLDWIDE USES

Region	Uses
Brazil	Aphrodisiac, depurative, diuretic, dropsy, dyspnea, gout, prostatitis, rheumatism, urticaria
Canada	Ache, alopecia, anodyne, ataxia (locomotor), bruise, chest, counterirritant, parturition, rheumatism
Europe	Alopecia, burn, cholecystitis, cholengitis, constipation, cosmetic, cough, depurative, diuretic, dropsy, dyspnea, epitaxis, gout, hair tonic, hemoptysis, homeopathy, rheumatism, shampoo, tea, urticaria
India	Anodyne, counterirritant, gout, magic, rheumatism, sprain, suppository, swelling
Turkey	Asthma, astringent, blood, bronchitis, depurative, diuretic, emmenagogue, hemostat, purgative, rheumatism, stimulant, tonic, vasoconstrictor, vermifuge
United States	Backache, cancer, epilepsy, fit, insanity, rheumatism, tantrum
Elsewhere	Bactericide, catarrh, dandruff, depurative, diuretic, hematemesis, hematoptysis, hemorrhage, massage, menorrhagia, metrorrhagia, paralysis, shigellosis, sore, stomachic, tumor, vermifuge, wound

PHYTOCHEMICALS

2-methylhepten-(2)-on-(6), 5-hydroxytryptamine, aceticacid, acetophenone, acetylcholine, alpha-tocopherol, beta-carotene, betaine, bromine, butyric acid, caffeic acid, calcium, cellulose, chlorophylls, choline, chromium, ferulic acid, fluorine, folacin, formic acid, glycerol, histamine, koproporphyrin, lecithin, mucilage, P-coumaric acid, protoporphyrin, scopoletin, serotonin, SFA, silicon, sitosterol, sitosterol-glucoside, violaxanthin, xanthophyllepoxide

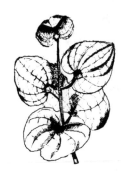

PATA DE VACA

Family: Leguminosae

Genus: *Bauhinia*

Species: *forficata*

Common Names: Pata de vaca, casco de vaca, mororó, pata de boi, unha de boi, unha de vaca, unha de anta

Parts Used: Leaves, bark

Medicinal Properties: Depurative, diuretic, hypoglycemic

PATA DE VACA is a small tree that grows from 5 to 9 m high. It has large, divided leaves resembling a cow's hoof, which are distinctive to the *Bauhinia* genus. It produces large, drooping white flowers and a brown seed pod that looks like the mimosa seed pod. It can be found in the rainforests and tropical parts of Peru and Brazil, as well as in tropical zones of Asia, eastern Paraguay, and northeastern Argentina. It is quite prevalent in Rio de Janeiro and Brazil's Atlantic rainforest in the south.

The indigenous uses of pata de vaca are not well documented, but it has long held a place in Brazilian herbal medicine. It is described as a hypoglycemic, depurative, and diuretic and has been used for over 60 years to balance blood sugar levels in diabetics. It is considered a good blood cleanser, and a leaf decoction is used internally and externally for elephantiasis and snakebite, as well as other skin problems, including those of a syphilitic nature. It is well established in Brazilian herbal medicine and a highly regarded treatment for diabetes, even being called "vegetable insulin." It is widely used in South America by diabetics to help balance blood sugar levels as well as help with other symptoms produced by diabetes, such as polyuria, renal disorders, and other urinary problems. Pata de vaca leaves and tea bags are a common item on pharmacy shelves in South America, and normally a leaf tea (standard infusion) is drunk after each meal to help balance sugar levels.

> **Pata de vaca is widely used in South America by diabetics to help balance blood sugar levels as well as help with other symptoms produced by diabetes, such as polyuria, renal disorders, and other urinary problems.**

Pata de vaca's hypoglycemic activity was first reported in a 1929 clinical study, which was followed by another study in 1931.[1, 2] A study was funded in 1945 to try to determine the active constituents responsible for its activity.[3] However, since a simple leaf tea was shown to help balance sugar levels, it became a popular natural remedy and no other studies were done for many years due to a lack of funding for nonproprietary remedies and drugs. In the mid-1980s, when herbal remedies were again popular, pata de vaca's continued use as a natural insulin substitute was reported once again in two new studies.[4, 5]

Pata de vaca continues to be a popular natural medicine in South America for diabetes. A standard infusion is brewed and drunk after each meal, and pata de vaca is often combined with pedra hume caa for this after-meal tea. North American practitioners and herbalists are now using it for diabetes, hyperglycemia, and polyuria as well.

WORLDWIDE USES

Region	Uses
Brazil	Depurative, diabetes, diuretic, elephantiasis, hypoglycemia, polyuria, renal, snakebite, urinary
Peru	Tonic

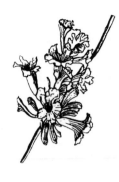

PAU D'ARCO

Family: Bignoniaceae

Genus: *Tabebuia*

Species: *impetiginosa, heptaphylla, avellanedae*

Common Names: Pau d'arco, ipe roxo, lapacho, tahuari, taheebo, tabebuia ipe, tajy

Parts Used: Bark, heartwood

Medicinal Properties: Analgesic, antibacterial, anticarcinomic, antifungal, anti-inflammatory, antileukemic, antimicrobial, antimutagenic, antioxidant, antiparasitic, antirheumatic, antiviral, cytotoxic, immunostimulant, laxative

Pau d'arco is a huge tree of the Amazon rainforest and parts of tropical South America. It grows to 46 m high, and the base of the tree can be 2 to 3 m in diameter. It produces beautiful, large, purple flowers. The *Tabebuia* genus includes many large beautiful flowering trees like pau d'arco, and they are common landscape trees in South American cities because of their beauty. Unfortunately, the tree is also popular with loggers because its high-quality wood is some of the heaviest, most durable wood in the tropics and the rainforest. Pau d'arco wood is widely used in the construction of everything from houses and boats to farm tools.

Pau d'arco has a long and well-documented history of use by the indigenous peoples of the rainforest, who use several species of *Tabebuia*, including *T. heptaphylla, T. impetiginosa, T. rosea,* and *T. serratifolia.* There are even indications that its use may actually antedate the Incas. In fact, throughout South America, tribes living thousands of miles apart have employed it for the same medicinal purposes for hundreds of years. Several Indian tribes of the rainforest have used pau d'arco wood for centuries to make their hunting bows; their common names for the tree mean "bow stick" and "bow stem." The Guarani and Tupi Indians call the tree *tajy*, which means "to have strength and vigor," and use the bark to treat many different conditions. Pau d'arco is recorded to be used by forest inhabitants for malaria, anemia, colitis, respiratory problems, colds, cough, flu, fungal infections, fever, arthritis and rheumatism, snakebite, poor circulation, boils, syphilis, and cancer.[1, 2]

Pau d'arco has also long been used in herbal medicine around the world. In South American herbal medicine, it is considered to be an astringent, anti-inflammatory, antibacterial, antifungal, and laxative and is used to treat ulcers, syphilis, gastrointestinal problems, candidiasis, cancer, diabetes, prostatitis, constipation, and allergies. In herbal medicine in North America, pau d'arco is considered to be an analgesic, antioxidant, antiparasitic, antimicrobial, antifungal, antiviral, antibacterial, anti-inflammatory, and laxative, as well as to have anticancerous properties. It is used externally and internally for fevers, infections, colds, flu, syphilis, cancer, respiratory problems, skin ulcerations, boils, dysentery, gastrointestinal problems of all kinds, arthritis, prostatitis, and circulation disturbances. Pau d'arco is also documented in the United States to be employed to treat lupus, diabetes, ulcers, leukemia, allergies, liver disease, Hodgkin's disease, osteomyelitis, Parkinson's disease, and psoriasis and is a popular remedy for candida and yeast infections. The recorded uses in European herbal medicine reveal that it is used in much the same way as in the United States for the same conditions.

> **In the United States pau d'arco is used to treat lupus, diabetes, ulcers, leukemia, allergies, liver disease, Hodgkin's disease, osteomyelitis, Parkinson's disease, and psoriasis and is a popular remedy for candida and yeast infections.**

The chemical constituents and active ingredients of pau d'arco have been well documented. Its use and reported cures with various types of cancers in the early 1960s fueled much of the early research. Its anticancerous properties were first attributed to a phytochemical found in the bark and wood called lapachol. In a

1968 study lapachol demonstrated highly significant activity against cancerous tumors in rats.[3] Then, in 1974, the NCI reported that Phase I clinical trials failed to produce a therapeutic effect with lapachol without side effects and discontinued further cancer research.[4] Another research group developed a lapachol analog in 1975 that was effective in increasing the life span by over 80% in mice inoculated with leukemic cells.[5] In a small study in 1980 with nine patients with various cancers (liver, kidney, breast, prostate and cervix), pure lapachol demonstrated an ability to shrink tumors and reduce pain caused by tumors and achieved complete remissions in three of the patients.[6]

The Phytochemical Database housed at the U.S. Department of Agriculture has documented lapachol as being antiabscess, anticarcinomic, antiedemic, anti-inflammatory, antimalarial, antiseptic, antitumor, antiviral, bactericide, fungicide, insectifuge, pesticide, protisticide, respiradepressant, schistosomicide, termiticide, and viricide.[7] Besides lapachol, pau d'arco contains at least 20 other active constituents that are attributed to its other actions. It has clearly demonstrated broad clinical applications against a large number of disease-causing microorganisms, which helps explains its wide array of uses in herbal medicine. Its action seems to come from increasing oxygen supply at the local level, destroying bacteria, viruses, fungi, and parasites. Its antimicrobial properties were demonstrated in several clinical trials, in which it exhibited strong activity against various gram-positive bacteria and fungi, including candida, staphylococcus, trichophyton, brucella, tuberculosis, pneumonia, strep, and dysentery.[8–12] Pau d'arco and its constituents have demonstrated antiviral properties against various viruses, including herpes I and II, influenza, polio virus, and vesicular stomatitis virus.[13–15] Its antiparasitic actions against various parasites, including malaria, schistosoma, and trypansoma, have been clinically validated.[13, 16, 17] Bark extracts of pau d'arco have demonstrated anti-inflammatory activity and have been shown to be successful against a wide range of inflammations.[18]

Pau d'arco is an important resource from the rainforest, with many uses and applications in herbal medicine. Unfortunately, its popularity and use have been controversial due to varying results, which are caused by a lack of quality control combined with confusion on which part of the plant to use and how to prepare it. Many species of *Tabebuia*, as well as other completely unrelated tree species exported today from South America as "pau d'arco," have little to none of the active constituents in the true medicinal species studied and used. Even mahogany shavings from the sawmill floors in Brazil are swept up and sold around the world as "pau d'arco" due to the similarity in color and odor of the two woods.[19] In 1987 a chemical analysis of 12 commercially available pau d'arco products showed that only one product contained lapachol in trace amounts.[20] Since lapachol is typically 2% to 7% in true pau d'arco, the study surmised either that the products were not truly pau d'arco, or that processing and transportation damaged the products. Most of the research and studies on pau d'arco have been on the heartwood of the tree, yet most of the commercially available products contain the inner and outer bark of the tree, which is stripped off at sawmills when the heartwood is milled into lumber for construction materials. At least 10 species of *Tabebuia* trees are commercially logged in South America for lumber purposes alone, which explains the varying species of "pau d'arco" bark being sold as natural medicinal products. Finally, many consumers and practitioners are unaware that for the best results when extracting the active constituents (even after obtaining the correct species), the bark and/or wood must be boiled at least 8 to 10 minutes rather than making a simple tea or infusion.

> Many species of *Tabebuia*, as well as other completely unrelated tree species exported today from South America as "pau d'arco," have little to none of the active constituents in the true medicinal species.

With these problems, it is not surprising that consumers and practitioners are experiencing varied results with commercially available pau d'arco products. Yet, with its many effective applications, consumers should take the time to learn about the available products and suppliers and find a reliable source for this important medicinal plant from the rainforest. Relatively new in the marketplace are standardized extracts of pau d'arco that guarantee the amount of lapachol and/or naphthoquinones (a group of phytochemicals that includes lapachol and at least eight others documented in pau d'arco). Although the natural wood and bark are quite effective when the correct species is prepared properly, the new standardized extracts may be the safer purchase (although more expensive) for most laypersons and general consumers.

WORLDWIDE USES

Region	Uses
Brazil	Antifungal, antimutagenic, boils, cancer, candida, colds, colitis, eczema, fever, flu, Hodgkin's disease, leukemia, rheumatism, stomatitis, syphilis, ulcers, warts, wounds
South America	Allergies, anemia, antibacterial, antifungal, anti-inflammatory, arthritis, astringent, cancer, candidiasis, colds, constipation, cough, diabetes, dysentery, fever, flu, gastritis, gastrointestinal, infections, laxative, malaria, prostatitis, respiratory disease, syphilis, ulcers
United States	Allergies, analgesic, antibacterial, antifungal, anti-inflammatory, antimicrobial, antimutagenic, antioxidant, antiparasitic, antiviral, arthritis, boils, cancer, candida, circulation disturbances, cold, diabetes, dysentery, fevers, flu, fungal infections, gastrointestinal, Hodgkin's disease, infections, laxative, leukemia, liver disease, lupus, osteomyelitis, Parkinson's disease, prostatitis, psoriasis, respiratory problems, skin ulcerations, syphilis, ulcers, warts

PHYTOCHEMICALS

aluminum, anthraquinones, ascorbic acid, ash, beta-carotene, beta-sitosterol, calcium, carbohydrates, chromium, chrysophanic acid, cobalt, dehydro-alpha-lapachone, dehydroisolapachone, dehydrotectol, iron, lapachol, magnesium, manganese, naphthoquinones, niacin, phosphorus, potassium, protein, riboflavin, selenium, silicon, sodium, thiamin, tin, zinc

Lesson one in the conservation of tropical rainforests: We are all involved in their destruction and their protection. In our interconnected world of global markets, we are involved in rainforest destruction whether we like it or not. With our wooden picture frames, with the teakwood bowls we place on mahogany coffee tables, we destroy the tropical forest. With our gasoline, our food packaging, our boats and paneled offices, we eradicate the jungle. Living the lives of modern consumers, we eat the tropical forest.

—James D. Nations

PEDRA HUME CAA

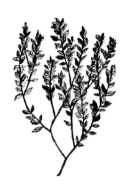

Family: Myrtaceae

Genus: *Myrcia*

Species: *salicifolia, uniflorus*

Common Names: Pedra hume caa, pedra-ume-caa, insulina vegetal

Parts Used: Aerial parts, leaves

Medicinal Properties: Antidysenteric, astringent, hypoglycemic

EDRA HUME CAA is a medium-sized shrub that grows in drier regions of the Amazon and other parts of Brazil. It has small green leaves and large, pretty, orange-red flowers. It is in the Myrtle family, one of more than 150 species of *Myrcia* indigenous to tropical South America and the West Indies.

Pedra hume caa has been used by indigenous tribes in the rainforest for diabetes, diarrhea, and dysentery. The Taiwanos tribe in northwest Amazonia considers the leaves to be astringent and use it for persistent diarrhea. It has had a place in Brazilian traditional medicine for numerous years. Dr. G. L. Cruz, a leading Brazilian practitioner and herbalist, nicknamed it "vegetable insulin" in 1965, noting in his book *Livro Verde das Plantas Medicinais e Industriais do Brasil* that "one uses all parts of the plant in infusions, decoctions or extracts to combat diabetes. Specialists that have made careful study of medicinal plants affirm that the regular use of this plant produces surprising results in the treatment of this ailment, as in a short space of time the sugar disappears from the urine. Hence the name vegetable insulin." Even 30 years later, Dr. Cruz and other Brazilian practitioners are recording the actions and uses of pedra hume caa for diabetes in Brazilian traditional medicine in the same manner. Pedra hume caa remains a very popular natural remedy for diabetes throughout South America; normal treatment is a simple leaf tea with a pleasant, slightly sweet taste. It is also used for diarrhea, hypertension, enteritis, hemorrhages, and mouth ulcers. Practitioners generally recommend 1 to 3 cups daily of a standard infusion taken with meals.

Pedra hume caa's hypoglycemic activity has been studied and validated by Brazilian scientists from 1929 to 1978.[1-4] Two recent clinical studies have demonstrated again its hypoglycemic activity. In a 1990 clinical study with Type II diabetic patients, pedra hume caa demonstrated its ability to lower plasma insulin levels.[5] In a 1993 study with rats, it demonstrated the ability to reduce the hyperglycemia, polyphagia, polydipsia, urine volume, and urinary excretion of glucose and urea in diabetic rats.[6] The study concluded that "aqueous extracts of *Myrcia* have a beneficial effect on the diabetic state, mainly by improving metabolic parameters of glucose homeostasis."

> Taken as a simple leaf tea, pedra hume caa remains a popular natural remedy for diabetes throughout South America.

WORLDWIDE USES

Region	Uses
Brazil	Astringent, diabetes, diarrhea, diuretic, dysentery, enteritis, hemorrhages, hypertension, ulcers (mouth)

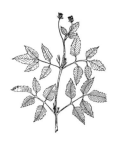

PICAO PRETO

Family: Asteraceae

Genus: *Bidens*

Species: *pilosa*

Common Names: Picao preto (in Brazil), amor seco (in Peru), aceitilla, cadillo, chilca, pacunga, pirco, cuambu, carrapicho, erva-picão, alfiler, clavelito de monte, romerillo, saltillo, yema de huevo, z'aiguille, jarongan, ketul, pau-pau pasir

Parts Used: Aerial parts, whole herb

Medicinal Properties: Antibacterial, antidysenteric, anti-inflammatory, antimicrobial, astringent, diuretic, emmenagogue, emollient, hepatoprotective

PICAO PRETO IS a small, erect annual herb that grows up to 1 m high. It has bright green leaves with serrated, prickly edges and produces small, yellow flowers. It is indigenous to the rainforest and other tropical areas of South America, Africa, the Caribbean, and the Philippines and is considered a weed in many places. It is a Southern cousin to *Bidens tripartita*, the European bur marigold, which has an ancient history in European herbal medicine.

Picao preto has a long history of use by the indigenous people of the Amazon, and virtually all parts of the plant are used. In the Peruvian Amazon picao preto is used for aftosa, angina, diabetes, dysentery, dysmenorrhea, edema, hepatitis, jaundice, laryngitis, and worms. In Piura a decoction of the roots is used for alcoholic hepatitis and worms. The Cuna tribe mixes the crushed leaves with water to treat headaches. Near Pucallpa, Peru, the leaf is balled up and applied to a toothache and the leaves are also used for headaches. In other parts of the Amazon a decoction of the plant is mixed with

> The Cuna tribe mixes crushed picao preto leaves with water to treat headaches. Near Pucallpa, Peru, the leaf is balled up and applied to a toothache.

lemon juice and used to treat angina, sore throat, water retention, hepatitis, and dropsy. The Exuma tribes grind the sun-dried leaves with olive oil to make poultices for sores and lacerations; and in Tonga an infusion of the flowers is used to treat upset stomach in food poisoning. Botanist James Duke reports: "Chewing or gargling may help angina and sores in the mouth; infusions used as emmenagogue, antidysenteric, and to alleviate chills." He also reports that indigenous peoples in Brazil use the plant as a diuretic and to treat jaundice.

In Peruvian herbal medicine today, the plant is called *amor seco* (not to be confused with *Desmodium adscendens,* page 41) or *cadillo*. It is considered diuretic, anti-inflammatory, and hepatoprotective and is commonly used for hepatitis, conjunctivitis, abscesses, mycosis, and urinary infections, as a weight loss aid, and to stimulate childbirth. In Brazilian herbal medicine it is called picao preto or *cuambu* and is considered an emollient, astringent, and diuretic, used for fevers, blennorrhagia, leucorrhea, jaundice, diabetes, sore throat, tonsillitis, obstructions in the liver and other liver disorders, urinary infections, and vaginal infections.[1] The reported therapeutic dosage used is generally 4 to 5 g daily.

> In 1996, a picao preto extract was shown to inhibit prostaglandin-synthesis activity, which is linked to headaches and inflammatory diseases.

Picao preto has been the subject of recent clinical studies that have explained many of its uses in herbal medicine. Its antibacterial activity against gram-positive bacteria was demonstrated in a 1997 study.[2] New bioactive phytochemicals discovered in 1996 showed growing actions against normal and transformed human cell lines.[3] Also in 1996, a picao preto extract was shown to inhibit prostaglandin-synthesis activity.[4] Prostaglandin synthesis is a process linked to headaches and inflammatory diseases. A research group in Taiwan documented its hepatoprotective (liver-protecting) activity, stating that *B. pilosus* can "protect liver injuries from various hepatotoxins and have potential as broad spectrum antihepatic agents."[5] This same research group clinically demonstrated picao preto's significant anti-inflammatory activities one year earlier, in 1995.[6] In 1991 Swiss scientists isolated several known phytochemicals with antimicrobial and anti-inflammatory properties, which led them to believe that the presence of these compounds "may rationalize the use of this plant in traditional medicine in the treatment of wounds, against inflammation and against bacterial infection of the gastrointestinal tract."[7] During the same year, scientists in Egypt were studying and documenting *B. pilosa*'s antimicrobial activity as well.[8] Even as early as 1979 and 1980, scientists demonstrated that specific chemicals found in picao preto were phototoxic to bacteria and fungi.[9, 10]

WORLDWIDE USES

Region	Uses
Amazonia	Aftosa, angina, chills, diabetes, diuretic, dysentery, dysmenorrhea, edema, emmenagogue, headache, hepatitis, jaundice, laryngitis, sore mouth, sore throat, stomachache, toothache, vulnerary, worms, wounds
Bahamas	Cancer, carminative, diuretic, fever, heat-rash itch, sore
Brazil	Astringent, blennorrhagia, diabetes, diuretic, emollient, fever, jaundice, leucorrhea, liver, liver obstructions, sclerosis (glands), sore throat, tonsillitis, urinary infections, vaginal infections
Burkina Faso	Bronchitis, colic, cough, diarrhea, intestine, snakebite
Dominican Republic	Diuretic, emmenagogue, lactogogue, pectoral, sialogogue, toothache
Ghana	Allergy, ear, eye, styptic, urticaria
Haiti	Aftosa, amygdalitis, angina, catarrh, diabetes, lactagogue, stomatitis
Malaya	Antidote, conjunctivitis, cough
Mexico	Diabetes, diuretic, pectoral

(continues)

WORLDWIDE USES *(continued)*

Region	Uses
Peru	Abscess, anti-inflammatory, childbirth, conjunctivitis, diuretic, hepatitis, hepatoprotective, mycosis, obesity, urinary infections, weight loss
Philippines	Boil, intoxicant
Venezuela	Dysentery, vulnerary
Elsewhere	Boil, cold, conjunctivitis, cough, dysentery, eye, food poisoning, inflammation, liver, rheumatism, stomach, styptic, toothache

PHYTOCHEMICALS

acetylenes, B-amyrin, B-sitosterol, beta-D-glucopyranosyloxy-3-hydroxy-6(E)- tetradecen-8, 10,12-triyne, esculetin, flavoniods, friedelin, friedelan-3 beta-ol, limonene, linolic acid, linolenic acid, lupeol, phenylheptatriyne, phytosterin-B, sterols, tannins, tridecapentyn-1-ene, trideca-2,12-diene-4, 6,8,10-tetrayne-1-ol, trideca-3,11-diene-5,7,9-triyne-1,2-diol, trideca-5-ene-7,9,11-triyne-3-ol volatile oil, xanthophylis

SAMAMBAIA

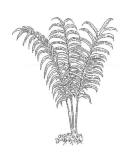

Family: Polypodiaceae

Genus: *Polypodium*

Species: *lepidopteris, decumanum*

Common Names: Samambaia, calaguala, huayhuashi-shupa, cotochupa

Parts Used: Rhizome, aerial parts

Medicinal Properties: Alterative, anti-inflammatory, antirheumatic, diaphoretic, diuretic, expectorant, hypotensive, pectoral, sudorific, tonic

SAMAMBAIA IS A fern that grows in the rainforests of South America. The Polypody family contains three-quarters of all ferns—over 6,000 species of plants, mostly in the tropics of both hemispheres. There are 75 species of plants in the *Polypodium* genus, many of which have been used medicinally for centuries. The name is derived from *poly,* meaning "many," and *podus,* meaning "a foot," because of the many foot-like divisions of the root or rhizomes of polypody ferns.

Samambaia, like most ferns, has a large creeping and dividing root or rhizome system; it is this rhizome, as well as the fronds or leaves, that is most used medicinally. In the Amazon rainforest a maceration of samambaia rhizome is used for fever, while the root is grated fresh or made into a tea for whooping cough and renal indispositions. The Boras indigenous tribe in the Peruvian Amazon prepares the leaves in a drink for coughs. Other Peruvian indigenous tribes use the rhizome for problems of the pancreas. In the rainforest in Guyana, Creole indigenous groups use a decoction of the rhizome in ritual baths for infants. Indigenous groups in Latin

America call the plant *calaguala* and use the rhizome for many different remedies, including for cancer and psoriasis.

Many types of ferns are used in traditional medicine around the world. *Polypodium vulgare* is a common fern indigenous to the forests of Europe, where it has held a place in herbal medicine for centuries. Most ferns, including the European *P. vulgare* and the South American *P. decumanum,* are considered alterative, tonic, pectoral, and expectorant and are used for numerous types of upper respiratory conditions. In Brazilian traditional medicine samambaia is considered alterative, sudorific, antirheumatic, tonic, pectoral, and expectorant; it is widely used for coughs, bronchitis, grippe, and other upper respiratory problems, as well as for rheumatism and skin problems. In Peruvian herbal medicine the rhizome is used for coughs, fevers, and urinary infections, as well as skin problems such as psoriasis, boils, ulcers, and abscesses.

Indigenous groups in Latin America call samambaia *calaguala* and use the rhizome for many different remedies, including for cancer and psoriasis.

There has been a great deal of scientific interest in *Polypodium* plants recently. Numerous potentially biodynamic compounds have been found in this family of plants, including flavonoids, polyphenols, tannins, phloroglucides, tetracyclic triterpenes, and alkaloids.[1] A northern relative of samambaia indigenous to Guatemala, *P. leucotomos*, has been the subject of research in the past three years for its immunomodulating effects and its application in numerous autoimmune diseases.[2, 3] This immunomodulating effect has been attributed to a phytochemical called anapsos, which is also present in samambaia.

Most of the recent research on samambaia has been for its use in treating psoriasis. Psoriasis is a common chronic skin disease that is now believed to be linked to immunological mechanisms.[4] The clinical effect of samambaia has been demonstrated in a number of studies from 1974 to 1987, in which patients with psoriasis and atopic dermatitis were successfully treated using an extract of the aerial parts of *P. decumanum*.[4] Scientists have been searching for the reason samambaia has been successful in treating psoriasis and dermatitis ever since. Scientists have shown that one possibility of its beneficial effects against psoriasis is its immuno-modulating activity with the phytochemical anapsos.[5, 6] Its

immunomodulatory effects were also demonstrated in clinical experiments with healthy volunteers, showing that samambaia extracts increased the number of T-suppressor lymphocytes (T8+) without affecting the number of T-helper (T4+) lymphocytes or B-cells.[4]

In addition, recent findings have indicated that PAF (platelet-activating factor) might be involved in the pathogenesis of psoriasis. In a 1992 clinical study, a phytochemical isolated in samambaia, called adenosine, was shown to significantly inhibit this activity.[7] In 1997 another phytochemical, called sulphoquinovosyl diacylglycerol, was isolated and shown to significantly inhibit this activity as well.[8] Samambaia is also a rich source of essential fatty acids. A number of unsaturated fatty acids have been shown to affect another chemical process in the body, which produces a chemical called leukotriene.[4] Researchers have proven that psoriatic skin has abnormally high quantities of leukotriene, which is believed to be one of the causes of the inflammation in psoriasis. In a 1994 clinical study, the fatty acid components in samambaia were shown to be effective in blocking this process of producing excess leukotriene.[8]

Scientists will probably continue studying samambaia and why it works, while natural health practitioners around the world continue using it effectively for many purposes without knowing which specific chemicals are creating the beneficial effects. In addition to psoriasis, practitioners in the United States are now using samambaia for coughs, bronchitis, chest colds, flu, disorders of the respiratory passages and immune system, rheumatism, gout, and high blood pressure. The reported therapeutic dosage used is generally 3 to 5 g daily.

WORLDWIDE USES

Region	Uses
Amazonia	Cancer, cough, fever, pancreas, psoriasis, renal, whooping cough
Brazil	Alterative, bronchitis, coughs, expectorant, gout, grippe, pectoral, psoriasis, respiratory, rheumatism, skin, sudorific, tonic
Mexico	Cough, fever, pectoral, sudorific
Peru	Abscess, boils, cough, fever, psoriasis, skin, urinary infections, whooping cough
United States	Bronchitis, colds, cough, flu, gout, hypertension, immune disorders, respiratory disorders, rheumatism
Venezuela	Purgative, venereal disease
Elsewhere	Cancer, psoriasis, respiratory disorders, skin, tumor

PHYTOCHEMICALS

(+)-catechin-7-l-arabinoside, 5-beta-20-hydroxyecdysterone, 9(11)-fernen, 17,21-epoxyhopane, 20-hydroxyecdysone, 22-hopene, 24-lophenol-methylene, 26-o-methylpolypodosaponin, 31-norcycloartanol, 31-norcyclolaudenol, anapsos, benzoic acid, beta-sitosterol, butyric acid, caffeic acid, calagualine, caoutchouc, catechins, citric acid, citrostadienol, crusecdysone, cycloartanol, cyclolaudenol, delta-7-cholestanol, ecdysones, ecdysterone, filicin, fucosterol, glucocaffeic acid, glycyrrhizin, hopene-1-oxide, isofucosterol, isovalerianic acid, lauric acid, lophenol, malic acid, methyl-salicylate, methylethylacetic acid, osladin, phloroglucin, phytosterols, pollinastanol, polydine, polypodin-a, polypodaureine, polypodosaponin, resin, rhamnose, salicylic acid, samambain, serratine, starch, stearic acid, sulphoquinovosyl diacylglycerol

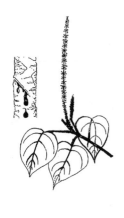

SANGRE DE GRADO

Family: Euphorbiaceae

Genus: *Croton*

Species: *lechleri, salutaris*

Common Names: Sangre de grado, sangre de drago, dragon's blood, drago, sangue de drago, sangue de agua

Parts Used: Bark, resin

Medicinal Properties: Antibacterial, antihemorrhagic, anti-inflammatory, antiseptic, antitumorous, antiviral, cicatrizant, hemostatic, vulnerary

ANGRE DE GRADO is a medium-sized to large tree that grows from 10 to 20 m high. Although tall, the trunk is usually less than 30 cm in diameter and is covered by smooth mottled bark. It has large, heart-shaped, bright green leaves and unique greenish-white flowers on long stalks. *Sangre de grado* means "blood of the dragon" in Spanish. When the trunk of the tree is cut or wounded, a dark red sappy resin oozes out as if the tree is bleeding, earning this local name. It is found throughout the tropics and the Amazon regions of South America. The genus *Croton* is a large one, with 750 species of trees and shrubs distributed in the tropical and subtropical regions of both hemispheres. *Crotons* are rich in active alkaloids, and several species are well-known medicinal plants used as purgatives and tonics.

> When the trunk of the sangre do grado tree is cut or wounded, a dark red sappy resin oozes out as if the tree is bleeding, earning it the name "dragon's blood."

Sangre de grado's red resin, or "blood," along with its bark, has a long history of indigenous use in the rainforest and South America. The earliest written reference dates its use to the 1600s, when Spanish naturalist and explorer P. Bernabé

Cobo found that the curative power of the sap was widely known throughout the indigenous tribes of Mexico, Peru, and Ecuador. For centuries, the sap has been painted on wounds to help stop bleeding, to accelerate healing, and to seal and protect the injury from infection. The sap dries quickly and forms a barrier, like a second skin. It is used internally as well as externally by indigenous tribes and local people in Peru for wounds, leucorrhea, fractures, and piles, as well as for intestinal and stomach ulcers. Other indigenous uses include treating intestinal fevers and pyorrhea, in vaginal baths before childbirth, for hemorrhaging after childbirth, and for skin disorders.

Sangre de grado resin and bark are used in traditional medicine in South America in much the same way as the indigenous uses. In Peruvian herbal medicine it is recommended for hemorrhaging, as an antiseptic vaginal douche, for wounds, and for ulcers in the mouth, throat, and stomach, as well as for skin disorders like eczema. In Brazilian traditional medicine the sap is used for wounds, hemorrhaging, and mouth ulcers and as a general tonic. Although thousands of pounds of bark and resin are imported into the United States, American consumers and practitioners know very little of sangre de grado and its effective uses. Rather, imports of sangre de grado are going to a U.S.-based pharmaceutical company, Shaman Pharmaceuticals, Inc. Shaman has filed patents on two pharmaceutical drugs that are in Phase I and Phase II FDA-approved clinical trials and that contain antiviral constituents they isolated and extracted from the bark and resin of sangre de grado. Their drugs include Provir, an oral product for the treatment of respiratory viral infections, and Virend, a topical antiviral product for the treatment of herpes.

Since much of the research on sangre de grado has been performed in the course of developing proprietary drugs, most of the research has not been published or made available to the public.

> For centuries, the sap has been painted on wounds to help stop bleeding, to accelerate healing, and to seal and protect the injury from infection.

The active constituents in sangre de grado include proanthocyanadins (antioxidants), tannins, a lignan named dimethylcedrusine, and an alkaloid called taspine. The taspine alkaloid from sangre de grado was first documented with anti-inflammatory actions in 1979.[1] In 1985 taspine was documented with anti-inflammatory, antisarcomic, and antiviral actions.[2] Its cicatrizant or wound-healing action was first related to the alkaloid taspine in 1989.[3] Several later studies, in 1991 and 1993, also concentrated on the wound-healing[4] and antitumor properties of taspine.[5] The lignan, dimethylcedrusine, was isolated by scientists in 1993 and was shown to play a central role in sangre de grado's effective wound-healing action as well.[6] This Belgian study revealed that the crude resin stimulated contraction of wounds, helped in the formation of a crust at the wound site, regenerated skin more rapidly, and assisted in the formation of new collagen. While the lignan was found to stimulate collagen formation, the crude resin was found to be four times more effective at wound healing and collagen formation than the lignan or the isolated alkaloid, taspine.[6] The Belgian scientists also determined that taspine was active against herpes; however, according to Shaman Pharmaceuticals, neither taspine nor dimethylcedrusine is the source of their new drugs. In 1994 other phytochemicals were found, including phenolic compounds, proanthocyanadins, and diterpenes, which showed potent antibacterial activity as well as wound-healing properties.[7]

As the research reveals, the indigenous uses of sangre de grado have certainly been validated. It is a wonderful new sustainable rainforest resource that consumers should learn about and take advantage of as it becomes available in the marketplace. Applied directly to the affected area, it is helpful for all types of cuts, scrapes, external wounds, rashes, and skin problems. Internal dosages based on documented indigenous uses and South American herbal medicine practices are generally 20 to 30 drops of resin placed in water and taken 1 to 3 times daily.

WORLDWIDE USES

Region	Uses
Brazil	Astringent, cicatrizant, hemorrhage, hemostat, tonic, tumor, ulcer (mouth), vulnerary, wounds
Dominican Republic	Hemostat, wounds
Mexico	Fever, gum, wounds
Peru	Antiseptic, cicatrizant, eczema, fracture, hemorrhage, hemostat, leucorrhea, piles, skin, throat, ulcers (intestinal, mouth, and stomach), vaginitis, vulnerary, wounds

PHYTOCHEMICALS

alpha-calacorene, alpha-copaene, alpha-pinene, alpha-thujene, beta-caryophyllene, beta-elemene, beta-pinene, betaine, borneol, calamenene, camphene, cuparophenol, D-limonene, dimethylcedrusine, dipentene, EO, eugenol, euparophenol, gamma-terpinene, gamma-terpineol, lignin, linalool, methylthymol, myrcene, p-cymene, pectic acid, proanthocyanadins, resin, tannin, taspine, terpinen-4-ol, vanillin

SARSAPARILLA

Family: Smilacaceae

Genus: *Smilax*

Species: *officinalis*

Common Names: Sarsaparilla, salsaparrilha, khao yen, saparna, smilace, smilax, zarzaparilla

Part Used: Roots

Medicinal Properties: Alterative, antibiotic, anti-inflammatory, antipruritic, antirheumatic, antiseptic, antisyphilitic, aphrodisiac, carminative, depurative, diaphoretic, diuretic, febrifuge, hepatoprotective, hormonal, steroidal, stimulant, stomachic, tonic

SARSAPARILLA IS A large, woody vine that grows up to 50 m long. The root, used for medicinal purposes, is long and tuberous and supports a ground-trailing vine with paired tendrils for climbing. The fragrance of the root is considered pleasant, and it has a spicy sweet taste. It is native to South America, Jamaica, the Caribbean, Mexico, Honduras, and the West Indies. There are many species of *Smilax* around the world that are very similar in appearance, uses, and even chemical structure, including *S. officinalis*, *S. regeli*, *S. aristolochiaefolia*, *S. febrifuga*, *S. sarsaparilla*, and *S. ornata*. Sarsaparilla vine should not be confused with the tree sasparilla, which was once used to flavor rootbeer.

Sarsaparilla has been used for centuries by the indigenous peoples of Central and South America for sexual impotence, rheumatism, and skin ailments and as a tonic for physical weakness. Sarsaparilla root was used as a general tonic by indigenous tribes in South America, where New World traders found it and introduced it into European medicine in the 1400s. European physicians considered it an alterative tonic, blood purifier, diuretic, and diaphoretic.[1] A *Smilax* root from Mexico was introduced into European medicine in 1536, where it developed a strong following as a cure for syphilis and rheumatism.[1] Since this time, the *Smilax* genus has a long history of use for syphilis and other sexually transmitted diseases throughout the world. With its reputation as a blood purifier, it was registered as an official herb in the *U.S. Pharmacopoeia* as a syphilis treatment from 1820 to 1910. From the 1500s to the present, sarsaparilla has been used as a blood purifier and general tonic and has been used all over the world for the same conditions, namely, gout, syphilis, gonorrhea, wounds, arthritis, fevers, coughs, scrofula, hypertension, digestive disorders, psoriasis, skin diseases, and cancer. The therapeutic dosage is reported to be 1 to 3 g daily.

Clinical research on the pharmacological actions of sarsaparilla has been varied over the years. The Chinese have used sarsaparilla in the treatment of syphilis; clinical observations in China demonstrated that sarsaparilla is effective, according to blood tests, in about 90% of acute cases and 50% of chronic cases.[2] In 1942 it was shown clinically to dramatically improve psoriasis, which continued its validation and use as a blood purifying remedy.[3] In the 1950s the antibiotic properties of sarsaparilla were documented.[4, 5] Its effective use as an adjuvant for the treatment of leprosy was documented in a human trial in 1959.[6] Its anti-inflammatory[7] and hepatoprotective[8] effects have been shown in rats, and improvement of appetite and digestion as well as diuretic actions in humans have also been documented.[9] Sarsaparilla's blood-purifying actions were demonstrated when it exhibited the ability to attack and neutralize microbial sub-

According to the Rainforest Action Network, the United States imports about $2.2 billion worth of tropical hardwoods each year, over one-fourth of the $8 billion annual trade in tropical timbers. For every foot of tropical plywood or paneling we buy, much more forest is destroyed in the logging process

—Suzanne Head,
The Consumer Connection

stances in the bloodstream.[10] The majority of sarsaparilla's pharmacological properties and actions have been attributed to a pharmacologically active group of phytochemicals called steroids and saponins. The saponins have been reported to facilitate the body's absorption of other drugs and phytochemicals,[2, 11] which accounts for its history of use in herbal formulas as a bioavailability and herbal enhancement agent.

> **Sarsaparilla's blood-purifying actions were demonstrated when it exhibited the ability to attack and neutralize microbial substances in the bloodstream.**

Sarsaparilla contains the following steroids: sarsasapogenin, smilagenin, sitosterol, stigmasterol, and pollinastanol; and the following saponins: sarsasaponin, smilasaponin, sarsapariloside, and sitosterol glucoside, among others.[2] Saponins and plant steroids found in many species of plants, including sarsaparilla, can be chemically synthesized into human steroids, such as estrogen and testosterone. This chemical synthesization has never been documented to occur in the human body—only in the laboratory. Plant steroids and their actions in the human body are still a subject of much interest, too little research, and, unfortunately, misinformation, mainly for marketing purposes. Sarsaparilla has been erroneously touted to contain testosterone and/or other anecbolic steroids. While it is a rich source of steroids and saponins, it has never been proven to have any anecbolic effects, nor has testosterone been found in sarsaparilla or any other plant source thus far.[2, 12] No known toxicity or side effects have been documented for sarsaparilla; however, ingestion of large dosages of saponins may cause gastrointestinal irritation.[12, 13]

WORLDWIDE USES

Region	Uses
Argentina	Aphrodisiac, diaphoretic, rheumatism
Brazil	Alterative, aphrodisiac, depurative, diaphoretic, diuretic, fever, impotence, psoriasis, purgative, rheumatism, skin, sterility, sudorific, syphilis, urinary
China	Aphrodisiac, rheumatism, stimulant, syphilis
India	Aphrodisiac, spasm
Malaya	Aphrodisiac, rheumatism
Mexico	Burn, depurative, diuretic, inflammation, rash, rheumatism, skin, stimulant
Turkey	Alterative, aphrodisiac, blood, depurative, diuretic, emetic, scrofula, sudorific, tonic
United States	Arthritis, cough, depurative, digestive disorders, fever, gonorrhea, gout, hypertension, psoriasis, scrofula, skin disorders, syphilis, tonic, wounds
Elsewhere	Aperitif, aphrodisiac, cancer, conjunctivitis, impotence, leprosy, rheumatism, sterility, stimulant, syphilis, tonic, toothache, venereal disease

PHYTOCHEMICALS

aluminum, ash, beta-sitosterol, calcium, cetyl-alcohol, chromium, cobalt, EO, epsilon-sitosterol, glucose, iron, magnesium, manganese, parigenin, parillin, phosphorus, pollinastanol, potassium, resin, saponin, sarasaponin, sarsaparilloside, sarsaponin, sarsasapogenin, selenium, silicon, sitosterol-d-glucoside, smilagenin, smilasaponin, stigmasterol, tin, zinc

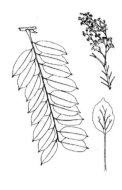

SIMARUBA

Family: Simaroubaceae

Genus: *Simarouba*

Species: *amara, glauca*

Common Names: Simaruba, gavilan, negrito, marubá, marupá, dysentery bark, palo blanco, robleceillo, daguilla, frene, Juan primero, palo amargo, quasia amarga, quassia amer, quinquina d'Europe, bois amer, bois blanc, bois frene, bois negresse

Parts Used: Bark, wood, leaves

Medicinal Properties: Amebicide, analgesic, anthelmintic, antibacterial, antileukemic, antimalarial, antimicrobial, cytotoxic, emmenagogue, febrifuge, stomachic, sudorific, tonic, vermifuge

SIMARUBA IS A medium-sized tree that grows up to 25 m high, with a trunk 50 to 80 cm in diameter. It produces bright green leaves 20 to 50 cm in length and small red fruits. It is indigenous to the Amazon rainforest and other tropical areas in Mexico, Cuba, Haiti, Jamaica, and Central America.

The leaves and bark of simaruba have a long history of use as natural medicine in the tropics. Simaruba was first imported into France from Guyana in 1713 as a remedy for dysentery. When France suffered a dysentery epidemic from 1718 to 1725, simaruba bark was one of the few effective treatments.[1] French explorers "discovered" this effective remedy when they found that the indigenous tribes in the Guyana rainforest used simaruba bark as an effective treatment for malaria and dysentery, much as they still do today. Other indigenous tribes throughout the South American rainforest use simaruba bark for fevers, malaria, and dysentery, as a hemostat to stop bleeding, and as a tonic.

> When France suffered a dysentery epidemic from 1718 to 1725, simaruba bark was one of the few effective treatments.

Simaruba also has a long history in herbal medicine in many other countries. In Cuba, where it is called *gavilan,* an infusion of the leaves or bark is considered an astringent, digestive, anthelmintic, and emmenagogue. It is taken internally for diarrhea, dysentery, malaria, and colitis and used externally for wounds and sores. In Belize the tree is called *negrito* or "dysentery bark"; the bark and sometimes the root are boiled in water to yield a powerful astringent and tonic used to wash skin sores as well as to treat dysentery, diarrhea, stomach and bowel disorders, hemorrhages, and internal bleeding. In Brazil it is employed much the same way against fevers, diarrhea, dysentery, intestinal parasites, and dyspepsia, as well as anemia. In Brazil simaruba bark tea is highly recommended as the best and most effective natural remedy against chronic and acute dysentery.

Simaruba bark's uses for dysentery caused by amebic infections were reported in 1918. A military hospital in England demonstrated that the bark tea had antiamebic activity in humans, reporting the bark tea was an effective treatment for amebic dysentery.[2] Scientists first looked at simaruba's antimalarial properties in 1947, when they determined a water extract of the bark as well as the root demonstrated strong activity against the malaria-causing organism *Plasmodium gallinaceum* in chickens.[3] The study showed that doses of only 1 mg of bark extract to 1 kg of body weight exhibited strong antimalarial activity.[3] In 1962 researchers found that the seeds of simaruba showed active antiamebic activities in humans,[4] and the National Cancer Institute verified that simaruba seed was 91.8% effective against intestinal amoebiasis in humans in a 1976 study.[5] In many of the early studies, the plant constituents found in the bark, root, and leaves of simaruba attributed with the antimalarial and antiamebic properties were a group of quassinoids, similar to those found in quinine bark. In 1978 scientists discovered a new quassinoid in simaruba that significantly inhibited the growth of lymphocytic leukemia *in vitro.*[6] A similar quassinoid, called glaucarubinone, is found in simaruba as well as other plants in the Simaroubaceae family, which has demonstrated antileukemic and cytotoxic activities in other studies.[7]

Scientists began studying simaruba again when new strains of malaria, parasites, and intestinal bacteria began to develop resistance against existing antibacterial and antimalarial drugs.

It wasn't until fairly recently, when new strains of malaria, parasites, and intestinal bacteria began to develop resistance against existing antibacterial and antimalarial drugs, that scientists began studying simaruba again. Two English studies in 1988 demonstrated that simaruba was effective against malaria *in vitro* as well as *in vivo* in rats.[8, 9] A 1990 *in vitro* study showed that simaruba was active against various resistant and nonresistant strains of enterobacteria, which are the common causes of gastrointestinal disorders.[10] Most recently, simaruba was shown to be effective against resistant strains of malaria *in vivo* and *in vitro* in a 1997 clinical study.[11] It is little wonder that the indigenous peoples of the rainforest are still using simaruba as a natural remedy for malaria and dysentery as they have for many years. Traditionally, a standard decoction is made and 1/2 cup drunk 2 to 3 times daily.

WORLDWIDE USES

Region	Uses
Belize	Diarrhea, dysentery, excessive menstruation, hemorrhage, internal bleeding, sores, tonic
Brazil	Diarrhea, dysentery, dyspepsia, febrifuge, hemorrhage, inappetite, intestinal parasites, tonic
Cuba	Emmenagogue
Dominican Republic	Colic, diarrhea, gonorrhea, malaria
Haiti	Ache (body), anemia, anodyne, dysentery, dyspepsia, emetic, emmenagogue, fever, purgative, rheumatism, skin, sudorific
Mexico	Amebicide, dyspepsia, fever, malaria
Salvador	Amebiasis, intoxicant, stomachic
Elsewhere	Cold, diarrhea, dysentery, fevers, malaria, soap

PHYTOCHEMICALS

15-hydroxyailanthone, 15-o-beta-d-glucopyranosylglaucarubol, 15-o-beta-d-glucopyranosylglaucarubolone, arachidic acid, delta-13(18)-glaucarubin, glaucarubin, glaucarubinone, glaucarubolone, linoleic acid, linolenic acid, oleic acid, palmitic acid, palmitoleic acid, stearic acid

STEVIA

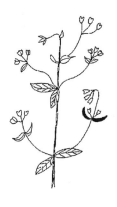

Family: Asteraceae

Genus: *Stevia*

Species: *rebaudiana*

Common Names: Stevia, sweet leaf of Paraguay, caa-he-é, kaa jheé, ca-a-jhei, ca-a-yupi, azucacaa, eira-caa, capim doce, erva doce

Part Used: Leaves

Medicinal Properties: Antifungal, cardiotonic, diuretic, hypoglycemic, hypotensive, tonic, vasodilator

TEVIA IS A perennial shrub that grows up to 1 m tall and has 2- to 3-cm-long leaves. It belongs to the Aster family, which is indigenous to the northern regions of South America, and is still found growing wild in the highlands of the Amambay and Iguacu districts (a border area between Brazil and Paraguay). It is grown commercially in many parts of Brazil, Paraguay, Uruguay, Central America, Israel, Thailand, and China.

For hundreds of years, indigenous peoples in Brazil and Paraguay have used the leaves of stevia as a sweetener. The Guarani Indians of Paraguay call it *kaa jheé* and have used it to sweeten their yerba mate tea for centuries. They have also used stevia to sweeten other medicinal teas and foods and have used it medicinally as a cardiotonic, for obesity, hypertension, and heartburn, and to help lower uric acid levels.

Europeans first learned about stevia in the sixteenth century, when Spanish conquistadores sent word to Spain that the natives of South America had used the plant to sweeten herbal tea since ancient times. Western interest in stevia began around the turn of the nineteeth century, when researchers in Brazil started hearing about a plant with leaves so sweet that just one leaf would sweeten a whole gourd full of bitter mate tea. It was first studied in 1899 by Paraguayan botanist Moises S. Bertoni, who wrote some of the earliest articles on stevia in the early 1900s. The constituents responsible for stevia's sweetness were documented in 1931, when eight novel phytochemicals called glycosides were discovered and named.[1] Of these eight glycosides, one called stevioside is considered the "sweetest" and has been tested to be approximately 300 times sweeter than saccharose.[2] Stevioside, making up 6% to 18% of the constituents of stevia leaves, is also the most prevalent glycoside present in the leaves.[2] Stevioside is considered 300 times sweeter than sucrose at 0.4% sucrose concentration, 150 times sweeter at 4% sucrose, and 100 times sweeter at 10% sucrose concentration.[2, 3] Because of the great interest in stevia as a natural sweetener, there have been many studies on it, including toxicological studies. Stevioside has been found to be nontoxic in acute toxicity studies with rats, rabbits, guinea pigs, and fowl, showing that it is excreted without structural modification.[3] It has also been shown not to be mutagenic or genotoxic, nor did it produce effects on fertility.[3]

> **For hundreds of years, indigenous peoples in Brazil and Paraguay have used the leaves of stevia as a sweetener**

For nearly 20 years, millions of consumers in Japan and Brazil, where stevia is approved as a food additive, have been using stevia extracts as safe, natural, noncaloric sweeteners. Japan is the largest consumer of stevia leaves and extracts in the world, and there it is used to sweeten everything from soy sauce to pickles, confections, and soft drinks. Even multinational giants like Coca Cola and Beatrice Foods use stevia extracts to sweeten foods (as a replacement for NutraSweet and saccharin) for sale in Japan, Brazil, and other countries where it is approved as a food additive. Not so in the United States, however, where stevia is specifically prohibited from use as a sweetener or as a food additive.

Why? Many people believe that the national noncaloric sweetener giants have been successful in preventing this all-natural, inexpensive, and nonpatentable sweetener from being used to replace their patented, synthetic, more expensive sweetener products. Today, stevia products and steviosol extracts may only be sold in the United States as foods and food supplements, not as food additives. In fact, in 1991 the Food and Drug Administration (FDA) even banned all imports of stevia into the country.[4] This political move was viewed by many to have monetary ties to the sweetener industry, such as NutraSweet and others, which stood to lose a lot, and it created a huge public outcry in the natural products industry. The import ban was lifted in 1995, after much lobbying led by the American Herbal Products Association. This allowed stevia to be sold as a dietary supplement under new legislation called the Dietary Supplement Health and Education Act of 1994. The FDA, in one of its more politically incorrect debacles of this century, has ruled that stevia is presumed safe as a dietary supplement but is considered unsafe as a food additive today. This ruling seemingly continues to protect the profit margins of the sweetener giants. In the words of Rob McCaleb, president of the Herb Research Foundation and a newly appointed member of the President's Commission on Dietary Supplements, "The FDA may have painted itself into a corner on this one. Its policy simply makes no sense."[5]

In addition to being a sweetener, stevia is considered by Brazilian herbal medicine to be hypoglycemic, hypotensive, diuretic, and tonic. It is used as a cardiotonic as well as for treating diabetes and high blood pressure. American practitioners are using stevia in much the same manner. Several clinical studies validate these uses. A crude extract of stevia demonstrated hypotensive activity in a 1996 clinical study with rats, showing that "at dosages higher than used for sweetening purposes, [stevia extract] is a vasodilator agent in normo- and hy-

> In Brazilian herbal medicine stevia is used as a cardiotonic as well as for treating diabetes and high blood pressure.

pertensive animals."[6] Several earlier studies on both stevia extracts as well as isolated glycosides demonstrated this hypotensive action as well as a diuretic action.[7, 8] The same Brazilian scientist recorded stevioside's ability to lower systemic blood pressure in rats in 1991.[9] Another Brazilian research group demonstrated that water extracts of stevia leaves had a hypoglycemic effect and increased glucose tolerance in humans, reporting that it "significantly decreased plasma glucose levels during the test and after overnight fasting in all volunteers."[10] Another team of scientists tested the hypoglycemic effects of the individual glycosides in stevia and attributed the effect on glucose production to the glycosides steviol, isosteviol, and glucosilsteviol.[11] The main sweetening glycoside, stevioside, did not produce this effect.[11] Its effects and uses as a cardiotonic to normalize blood pressure levels, to regulate heartbeat, and for other cardiopulmonary indications were first reported in rat studies in 1978.[12, 13]

WORLDWIDE USES

Region	Uses
Brazil	Cardiotonic, diabetes, diuretic, hypertension, hypoglycemic, hypotensive, sweetener, tonic, vasodilator
Paraguay	Contraceptive, diabetes, sweetener
South America	Diabetes, sweetener

PHYTOCHEMICALS

aluminum, ascorbic acid, ash, austroinulin, beta-carotene, calcium, chromium, cobalt, dulcosides, iron, magnesium, manganese, niacin, phosphorus, potassium, protein, rebaudiosides, riboflavin, selenium, silicon, sodium, steviol, stevioside, thiamin, tin, zinc

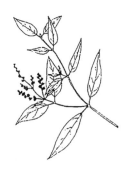

SUMA

Family: Amaranthaceae

Genus: *Pfaffia*

Species: *paniculata*

Common Names: Suma, Brazilian ginseng, pfaffia, para toda, corango-acu

Part Used: Root

Medicinal Properties: Anabolic, analgesic, anti-inflammatory, antimutagenic, aphrodisiac, estrogenic, hypocholesterolemic, immunostimulant, nutritive, sedative, steroidal, tonic

UMA IS A large, rambling, shrubby ground vine with an intricate and deep root system. It is indigenous to the Amazon Basin area and other tropical parts of Brazil, Ecuador, Panama, Paraguay, Peru, and Venezuela. Since its first botanical recording in 1826, it has been referred to by several botanical names, including *Pfaffia paniculata*, *Hebanthe paniculata*, and *Gomphrena paniculata*.[1] The genus *Pfaffia* is well known in Central and South America, with over 50 species growing in the warmer tropical regions of the area.

In South America suma is known as *para toda* (which means "for all things") and as Brazilian ginseng, since it is widely used as an adaptogen for many things, much like regular ginseng. The indigenous peoples of the Amazon region who named it *para toda* have used suma root for generations for a wide variety of health purposes, including as a general tonic, as an energy and rejuvenating tonic, and as a general cure-all for many types of illnesses.[2] Suma has been used as a tonic, an aphrodisiac, and a calming agent and to treat ulcers for at least 300 years and is an important herbal remedy in the folk medicine of several indigenous Indian tribes today.[3]

In herbal medicine throughout the world today, suma is considered an adaptogen. The word *adaptogen* was coined in 1947 by a Russian scientist named N. V. Lazarev. His definition of the word was a medicinal substance fulfilling three criteria: (1) It must cause only minimal disorders in the body's physiological functions; (2) it must increase the body's resistance to adverse influences not by specific action, but by a wide range of physical, chemical, and biochemical factors; and (3) it must have an overall normalizing effect, improving all kinds of conditions and aggravating none. Suma, with its wide range of documented uses, certainly meets these criteria. In herbal medicine in Ecuador today, suma is considered a tonic for the cardiovascular system, the central nervous system, the reproductive system, and the digestive system, and it is used to treat hormonal disorders, sexual dysfunction and sterility, arteriosclerosis, diabetes, circulatory and digestive disorders, rheumatism, and bronchitis.[4] Thomas Bartram, in *Encyclopedia of Herbal Medicine,* reports that suma is used in Europe to restore nerve and glandular functions, to balance the endocrine system, to strengthen the immune system, for infertility, for menopausal and menstrual symptoms, to minimize the side effects of birth control medications, for high cholesterol, to neutralize toxins, and as a general restorative tonic after illness. In North and South American herbal medicine, suma root is used as an adaptogenic and regenerative tonic regulating many systems of the body, as an immunostimulant, and to treat exhaustion resulting from Epstein-Barr disease and chronic fatigue syndrome, hypoglycemia, impotence, arthritis, anemia, diabetes, cancer, tumors, mononucleosis, high blood pressure, PMS, menopause and hormonal disorders, and many types of stress. The reported therapeutic dosage generally used is 4 to 5 g daily.

The indigenous peoples of the Amazon region have used suma root for a wide variety of health purposes, including as a general tonic, as an energy and rejuvenating tonic, and as a general cure-all for many types of illnesses.

Suma has also been called "the Russian secret" because it is taken by Russian Olympic athletes to increase muscle-building and endurance without the side effects associated with steroids. This action is attributed to the anabolic-type agent beta-ecdysterone, as well as to three novel ecdysteroid glycosides that are found in high amounts in suma.[5, 6] Suma is such a rich source of beta-ecdysterone that it is the subject of a Japanese patent for the extraction methods employed to obtain it from this root.[7] Two other plant hormones are found in suma, sitosterol and stigmasterol, and some practitioners believe they help to encourage estrogen production. For this reason some practitioners employ suma for menopausal symptoms.

Russian Olympic athletes have taken suma to increase muscle-building and endurance without the side effects associated with steroids.

Nutritionally, suma root contains 19 different amino acids, a large number of electrolytes, and trace minerals, including iron, magnesium, cobalt, silica, zinc, and vitamins A, B1, B2, E, K, and pantothenic acid.[6] The high content of germanium accounts for its properties as an oxygenator at the cellular level. The root of suma is composed of up to 11% saponins.[8] These saponins include a group of novel chemicals called pfaffosides, as well as pfaffic acids, glycosides, and nortriterpenes. These saponins have clinically demonstrated the ability to inhibit cultured tumor cell melanomas and help to regulate blood sugar levels.[9–11] The pfaffosides and pfaffic acid derivatives in suma have been patented as antitumor compounds in two Japanese patents.[12, 13]

WORLDWIDE USES

Region	Uses
Brazil	Anemia, arthritis, asthma, cancer, chronic fatigue syndrome, diabetes, Epstein-Barr, hypertension, hypoglycemia, immunostimulant, impotence, leukemia, mononucleosis, tonic, tumors
Ecuador	Arteriosclerosis, bronchitis, circulatory, diabetes, digestive, hormonal, rheumatism, sexual dysfunction, sterility, tonic
Europe	Endocrine, fertility, high cholesterol, immunostimulant, menopause, menstrual disorders, nerve, nervine, tonic
Japan	Cancer, steroidal, tumor
Russia	Muscle growth, tonic
United States	Chronic fatigue syndrome, diabetes, Epstein-Barr, hormonal disorders, hypertension, impotence, menopause, mononucleosis, nervine, PMS

PHYTOCHEMICALS

beta-ecdysone; cobalt; germanium; iron; magnesium; nortriterpenoids; pantothenic acid; pfaffic acids; saponins; silica; sitosterol; stigmasterol; vitamins A, B1, B2, E, K; zinc

TAYUYA

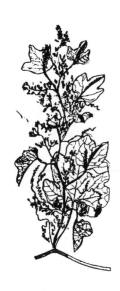

Family: Cucurbitaceae

Genus: *Cayaponia*

Species: *tayuya*

Common Names: Tayuya, taiuia, taioia, abobrinha-do-mato, cabeca-de-negro, tomba

Part Used: Root

Medicinal Properties: Analgesic, antibacterial, antifungal, anti-inflammatory, antimicrobial, antioxidant, antirheumatic, antisyphilitic, choleretic, depurative, digestive, diuretic, laxative, metabolic regulator, purgative, stomachic, tonic

AYUYA IS A woody vine found throughout Brazil and in many parts of the Amazon rainforest. This important Amazon plant belongs to the gourd family. There are many plants in the Cucurbitaceae family, most of which are characterized by long, tuberous roots. Tayuya is known by several botanical names, including *Cayaponia tayuya, Trianosperma tayuya, Bryonia tayuya,* and *Cayaponia ficcifolia;* however, all of these scientific names refer to the same plant.

Indians have been using tayuya since prehistoric times, and the value of this herb is undisputed. It has traditionally been used as a tonic and blood cleanser, usually combined with a bit of honey or stevia to tone down the strong, bitter taste. In the Amazon rainforest, Indians have used the root of tayuya for snakebite and rheumatism for centuries.[1] Indians in Colombia use a derivative of the plant for sore eyes; indigenous tribes of Peru use it for skin problems.

Tayuya has a long history in Brazilian herbal medicine. Botanist J. Monteiro da Silva states, "Tayuya is used . . . for treatment of all types of pain . . . It has a calming action on pain . . .

It is recommended as an anti-syphilitic agent."[2] Monteiro also believes that tayuya helps regulate the metabolism. In Brazil today, tayuya is used as an analgesic, anti-inflammatory, tonic, and blood purifier and detoxifier, as a diuretic to treat diarrhea, and for epilepsy, metabolism regulation, backache, sciatic pain, headaches, gout, neuralgia, constipation, anemia, cholera, dyspepsia, stomach problems, fatigue and debility, skin disorders, arthritis and rheumatism, syphilis, tumors (especially in the joints), and as a general analgesic for many conditions.

Tayuya is currently employed in North and South America because of its pain-reducing properties, as well as other properties. Natural health practitioners in the United States today are using tayuya to treat irritable bowel syndrome, dyspepsia and sluggish digestion, neuralgia, sciatica, gout, headaches, and rheumatism and as a metabolic regulator. Because of its reported effectiveness as a blood purifier and detoxifier, it is also being used to treat water retention, wounds, splotchiness on the face, eczema, herpes, severe acne, and other skin problems. It is also being used in athletic training and recovery to help remove lactic acid accumulation and to reduce swelling, and to relieve emotional fatigue and depression. The reported therapeutic dosage generally used is 3 to 4 g daily.

> Tayuya's analgesic and anti-inflammatory properties were scientifically validated in a 1991 study that supported many of its indigenous and folkloric uses.

Tayuya's analgesic and anti-inflammatory properties were scientifically validated in a 1991 study that supported many of its indigenous and folkloric uses.[1] Cucurbitacins, glucosides, and phytochemicals with antioxidant, anti-inflammatory, and analgesic properties have been isolated in tayuya.[3-5] Saponins, sterols, and phenolics are also known to occur in other plants of the same family. According to another study, entitled "Superoxide scavenging properties of flavonoids in a non-enzymic system," some phytochemicals in tayuya act as potent scavengers of free radicals, providing an antioxidant effect.[6] Another recent study, conducted by T. Konoshima, et. al., suggests that phytochemicals in tayuya have significant inhibitory effects on Epstein-Barr virus as well as antitumor effects on mouse skin.[7]

WORLDWIDE USES

Region	Uses
Brazil	Analgesic, arthritis, backache, cholera, depurative, diarrhea, digestive disorders, diuretic, dyspepsia, epilepsy, fatigue, gout, headache, metabolism, neuralgia, purgative, rheumatism, sciatica, syphilis, tonic, tumor (joint)
Colombia	Eye (sore)
Peru	Rheumatism, skin disorders, snakebite
United States	Acne, arthritis, depression, digestion disorders, dyspepsia, eczema, edema, gout, headache, herpes, irritable bowel syndrome, metabolism, nervine, neuralgia, rheumatism, sciatica, skin disorders

PHYTOCHEMICALS

29-nor-cucurbitacin glucosides, alkaloids, amentoflavone, cayaponosides, cucurbitacins, cucurbitane triterpenoids, datiscetin, eriodictyol, flavonoids, isoorientin, leucocyanidol, malic acid, orientin, resins, robinetin, saponins, sterols

VASSOURINHA

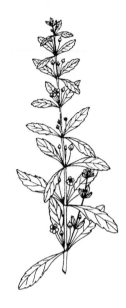

Family: Scrophulariaceae

Genus: *Scoparia*

Species: *dulcis*

Common Names: Vassourinha, escobilla, piqu pichana, ñuñco pichana, cancharagua, mastuerzo, amarga, anisillo, balai doux, balye du, bitterbroom, boroemia, broomweed, brum sirpi, brum tahplira, du-jhanga, escoba lisa, balai doux, bunyiga, guekan, haraspata, hierba de dolor, hafai-duanha, mat mat, nuc-nuc pichana, osim-miseng, pottipooli, rice weed, salle jhar, sirsaika, sisibi wiwiri, sweet broom, teeth bush, typycha kuratu, cha padang, ginje jepun, ginje menir, pokok delis, pokok kelambu, the makao, wild rice

Parts Used: Entire plant, roots

Medicinal Properties: Analgesic, antibacterial, antidiabetic, antifungal, antiherpetic, anti-inflammatory, antiseptic, antispasmodic, antiviral, emmenagogue, emollient, expectorant, febrifuge, hypocholesterolemic, hypotensive, pectoral, refrigerant

VASSOURINHA IS AN erect annual herb that grows up to 1/2 m high and produces serrated leaves and many small white flowers. It is widely distributed in many tropical countries in the world and is found in abundance in South America and the Amazon rainforest. Vassourinha has long held a place in herbal medicine in every tropical country where it grows, and its use by indigenous Indian tribes is well documented.

Indigenous tribes in Ecuador brew a tea of the entire plant to reduce swellings, aches, and pains. The Tikunas make a decoction for washing wounds, and women drink the same decoction for three days each month during menstruation as a contraceptive and/or an abortifacient. In the rainforests of Guyana, indigenous tribes use a leaf decoction as an antiseptic wash for wounds, as an antiemetic for infants, as a soothing bath for fevers, and in poultices for migraine headaches. Indigenous peoples in Brazil use the leaf juice to wash infected wounds and place it in the eyes for eye problems, and they make an infusion of the entire plant for an expectorant and emollient. Indigenous tribes in Nicaragua use a hot water infusion and/or decoction of vassourinha leaves or the whole plant for stomach pain, for menstrual disorders, as an aid in childbirth, to clean the blood, for insect bites, fevers, heart problems, liver and stomach disorders, malaria, and venereal disease, and for a general tonic.

Vassourinha is still employed in herbal medicine throughout the tropics. In Peru a decoction of the entire plant is recommended for upper respiratory problems, menstrual disorders, and fever, while the leaf juice is still employed externally for wounds and hemorrhoids. In Brazilian herbal medicine the plant is considered an emollient, febrifuge, hypoglycemic, emmenagogue, hypotensive, pectoral, and expectorant; it is used for upper respiratory disorders, bronchitis, coughs, menstrual disorders, diabetes, and hypertension, just to name a few of its many roles.

> Indigenous peoples in Brazil use the leaf juice to wash infected wounds and place it in the eyes for eye problems.

Some of vassourinha's many uses in herbal medicine have been validated by research. In laboratory tests, vassourinha showed active properties against gram-positive bacteria (but not gram-negative) and strong antifungal actions as well.[1, 2] Phytochemical screening of vassourinha has shown that it is a source of novel flavonoids and terpene plant chemicals, some of which have not been seen in science before.[3, 4] Many of vassourinha's tested biological activities are attributed to these phytochemicals, the main ones being scopadulcic acids A and B, scopadiol, scopadulciol, scopadulin, and scoparic acids A, B, and C.[5–12] Vassourinha's hypoglycemic actions in two diabetic patients were reported in 1985.[13] In animal studies between 1993 and 1996, researchers showed that different extracts of vassourinha demonstrated anti-inflammatory activity in rats, antispasmodic activity in guinea pigs and rats, analgesic actions in mice, and hypertensive properties in rats and dogs.[14, 15] In these animal studies they reported no toxicity in amounts of up to 2 grams per kilogram of body weight. The antitumorous activity of scopadulcic acid B, one of vassourinha's main active constituents, was demonstrated in a 1993 study.[16] This same phytochemical and another called scopadulin demonstrated antiviral properties in two prior studies, including against herpes simplex I *in vivo* in hamsters.[17, 18] An ethanol extract of the whole plant of vassourinha demonstrated an ability to inhibit receptor binding to both dopamine and serotonin receptors in another recent study.[19]

Scientists have been trying since the mid-1990s to synthesize several phytochemicals found in vassourinha, including scopadulcic acid B, for their use in the pharmaceutical industry. Herbalists and natural health practitioners have used and will continue to use the natural plant as an effective natural remedy for upper respiratory problems and viruses, for menstrual problems. and as a natural hypotensive, analgesic, and antispasmodic agent when needed. The reported therapeutic dosage generally used is 2 to 3 g daily or 1 to 2 cups daily of a standard decoction in 1/2-cup dosages.

This is the land of our forefathers, and their forefathers before them. If we don't do something to protect the little that is left, there will be nothing for our children. Our forests are mowed down, the hills leveled, the sacred graves of our ancestors have been desecrated, our water and streams are contaminated, our plant life is destroyed, and the forest animals are killed or have run away. What else can we do now but make our protests heard, so that something can be done to help us?

Avek matai ame maneu mapat. (Until we die we will block this road.)

—The Penan, Melabit, and Kayan indigenous tribal protesters in Sarawak, Indonesia

WORLDWIDE USES

Region	Uses
Africa	Conjunctivitis, cough, diuretic, earache
Amazonia	Abortifacient, aches, antiemetic, bronchitis, contraceptive, cough, diarrhea, erysipelas, eye, fever, hemorrhoids, kidney disease, pains, sores (gonorrheal), swelling, wounds
Brazil	Analgesic, bronchitis, cardiopulmonary disorders, cough, diabetes, earache, emollient, expectorant, fever, gastric disorders, hemorrhoids, hypertension, insect bite, insecticide, menstrual disorders, pectoral, respiratory disorders, skin, vermifuge, wounds
Central America	Bruise, diarrhea, emmenagogue, fever, gonorrhea, gravel, grippe, hepatosis, insecticide, kidney, menstrual disorders, purgative, sore throat, stomach disease, stomach pain, wound
Dominican Republic	Astringent, diabetes, sore throat
Haiti	Amygdalosis, antiseptic, astringent, blennorrhagia, cough, diabetes, diuretic, dysmenorrhea, earache, emetic, gonorrhea, headache, inflammation, menorrhagia, nerve, piles, sore, sore throat, spasm, toothache, tumor
India	Antivenin, blennorrhagia, dysentery, earache, fever, headache, stomach, toothache
Malaya	Childbirth, cough, expectorant, labor, opium substitute, stomachache, syphilis
Nicaragua	Anemia, childbirth, depurative, diarrhea, fever, heart, insect bite, itch, liver, malaria, menstrual disorders, snakebite, stomach disorders, tonic, venereal disease
Nigeria	Analgesic, antidiabetic, antipyretic, diuretic, expectorant
Peru	Astringent, colic, febrifuge, hallucinogen, hemorrhoids, mucolytic, respiratory disorders, wounds
Surinam	Bronchitis, coughs, diabetes, febrifuge, jaundice, rash

WORLDWIDE USES (*continued*)

Region	Uses
Trinidad	Antidote, depurative, diabetes, dysmenorrhea, eczema, evil eye, jaundice, mange, marasmus, ophthalmia, rash, sore
Venezuela	Astringent, blennorrhagia, diarrhea, menorrhagia, metroxenia
West Indies	Diabetes, diarrhea, dysmenorrhea
Elsewhere	Albuminuria, anemia, aphrodisiac, bronchitis, childbirth, cicatrizant, cough, diabetes, diarrhea, diuretic, dysentery, emetic, fever, gravel, hyperglycemia, hypertension, ketonuria, kidney, leprosy, menstrual disorders, purgative, refrigerant, retinitis, snakebite, toothache, venereal disease, vermifuge

PHYTOCHEMICALS

3'-4'-5-5'-7-8-hexahydroxy flavone, 6-methoxy benzoxazolin-2-one, 6-methoxy benzoxazolinone, 7-o-methyl scutellarein, 7-o-beta-d-glucuronide, acacetin, alpha amyrin, apigenin, benzoxazolinone, beta sitosterol, betulinic acid, cynaroside, D mannitol, dulcinol, dulcioic acid, gentisic acid, glut-5(6)-en-3-beta-ol, glutinol, hymenoxin, ifflaionic acid, iso vitexin, linarin, luteolin, para coumaric acid, scopadiol, scopadulcic acid A, scopadulcic acid B, scopadulciol, scopadulin, scoparic acid A, scoparic acid B, scoparic acid C, scoparinol, scutellarein, scutellarein-7-o-beta-d-glucuronide, scutellarin, scutellarin methyl ester, vicenin 2, vitexin

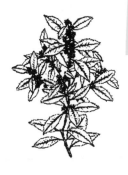

YERBA MATE

Family: Aquifoliaceae

Genus: *Ilex*

Species: *paraguariensis, paraguayiensis*

Common Names: Yerba mate, mate, erva mate, Paraguay cayi, Paraguay tea, South American holly

Part Used: Leaves

Medicinal Properties: Alterative, analeptic, antioxidant, aperient, astringent, depurative, diuretic, glycogenolytic, immunostimulant, lipolytic, purgative, stimulant, stomachic, sudorific, tonic

ERBA MATE IS a widely cultivated, medium-sized evergreen tree that grows 4 to 8 m high. It is in the holly family, with holly-like leaves that are somewhat leathery. In the wild, yerba mate grows near streams. The white flowers produce small red, black, or yellow berries, but it is *Ilex*'s leaves that are used medicinally and as a natural refreshing tea beverage throughout South America. It is indigenous to Paraguay, Brazil, and other South American countries.

Yerba mate is a wild plant that has a distinct aroma and taste that has never been surpassed through plantation cultivation, although it is widely cultivated now to keep up with demand. In South America yerba mate is considered a "national drink," and in Europe it is called "the green gold of the Indios." In Brazil and Paraguay, the leading exporting nations, some production still comes from wild stands, most of which are found in the humid depressions of the foothills. It is not unusual for one wild tree to yield 30 to 40 kg of dried leaves annually. In harvesting, mate gatherers, called *tarrafeiros* or *yebateros,* travel through the jungle searching for a stand of trees called a *mancha.* Harvesting is done between May and October, when the tree is in full leaf, and leaves are picked from the same tree only every third year, thus protecting the tree for the ensuing crop.

Yerba mate is the subject of a German monograph that lists its uses for mental and physical fatigue and describes it as having "analeptic, diuretic, positively inotropic, positively chronotropic, glyco-genolytic and lipolytic effects." Yerba mate has been used medicinally as a diuretic, tonic, and central nervous system stimulant. Another traditional use has been as a depurative (to promote cleansing and excretion of waste).[1] Herbalist Daniel Mowrey reports that yerba mate is a "whole body tonic, even in large amounts" and "promotes balances in many body systems without overstimulating any system." He believes that yerba mate's tonic effect on the body helps to regulate sleep cycles and reduce fatigue. Around the world, yerba mate is used to reduce appetite, invigorate the body, and reduce fatigue.

Around the world, yerba mate is used to reduce appetite, invigorate the body, and reduce fatigue.

In Europe yerba mate is used for weight loss, "as the ideal slimming remedy which facilitates losing weight in a natural way and stills the distressing feelings of hunger and thirst."[2] Dr. James Balch, M.D., recommends yerba mate for arthritis, headache, hemorrhoids, fluid retention, obesity, fatigue, stress, constipation, allergies, and hay fever, stating that it "cleanses the blood, tones the nervous system, retards aging, stimulates the mind, controls the appetite, stimulates the production of cortisone, and is believed to enhance the healing powers of other herbs." Generally, 2 to 3 cups of a standard infusion (leaf tea) is taken daily with meals. Powdered leaves and leaf extracts with standardized caffeine content are being used in capsules and formulas in herbal products as well.

Research on the active constituents of yerba mate was reported in the mid-1970s through mid-1980s.[3, 4] The primary active chemical constituency of yerba mate is made up of 0.3%

to 2.0% caffeine, theobromine, theophylline, saponins, and 10% chlorogenic acid. Sterols resembling ergosterol and cholesterol are also present in Yerba Mate. In addition, yerba mate is a rich source of minerals, and 15 amino acids are present in the leaves.[5] In a study by Swantson-Flatt with the closely related *Ilex* species guayusa, the mate extract "retarded the development of hyperglycaemia" in streptozotocin diabetic mice and "reduced the hyperphagia, polydipsia, body weight loss, and glycated haemoglobin."[6] This study suggests the presence of potentially useful antidiabetic agents in mate. The antioxidant properties demonstrated by yerba mate were reported in two clinical studies showing its high antioxidant values linked to rapid absorption of known antioxidant phytochemicals found in mate leaves.[7, 8] Of most recent clinical interest is a group of known and novel saponins that researchers have isolated in mate leaves. Saponins are a group of phytochemicals with known pharmacological activities, including, as the latest research shows on yerba mate, stimulating the immune system.[9–11]

WORLDWIDE USES

Region	Uses
Brazil	Digestion, diuretic, heart, obesity, stimulant, stomachic, tea, tonic, urinary
Mexico	Coffee
Paraguay	Tea
South America	Aperient, astringent, coffee, rheumatism
Turkey	Diuretic, purgative, scurvy, stimulant, sudorific, tea
United States	Allergies, arthritis, cardiotonic, constipation, depurative, diuretic, fatigue, hayfever, headache, hemorrhoids, obesity, stress
Elsewhere	Cardiotonic, diuretic, fatigue, stimulant, tonic

PHYTOCHEMICALS

2,5-xylenol, 4-oxolauric-acid, 5-o-caffeoylquinic-acid, alpha-amyrin, ash, beta-amyrin, butyric acid, caffeine, caffetannin, chlorogenic acid, chlorophyll, choline, EO, fiber, inositol, isobutyric acid, isocapronic acid, isovaleric acid, neochlorogenic acid, nicotinic acid, nitrogen, pantothenic acid, protein, pyridoxine, resin, resinic acid, riboflavin, rutin, stearic acid, tannin, theobromine, theophylline, trigonelline, ursolic acid, vanillin

Part Three

Rainforest Resources

Rainforest Remedy Recipes

~~~~~~

THE FOLLOWING RECIPES are commonly used by rainforest shamans and healers, natural health practitioners in North and South America, and others using rainforest herbs to positively impact their health. The recipes are a general guide as to how these rainforest plants are being used. No health claims are made for these plants or recipes and they are not intended to treat, cure, or mitigate any disease nor replace proper health care. The definitions and standard methods of preparing infusions, decoctions, and tinctures like those described below can be found starting on page 237.

Allergy Remedy

Combine 2 parts nettle root and one part each of yerba mate, jatoba, gervão, picao preto, and carqueja. Take 1 gram of this herbal mixture 2 to 3 times daily as needed for allergy symptoms. This remedy can also be made into a standard infusion or standard tincture. Try 1/2 to 1 cup of the tea/infusion or 1 teaspoon of the tincture 2 to 3 times daily.

Arthritis Relief Remedy

Combine equal parts of amor seco, cat's claw, chuchuhuasi, tayuya, iporuru, mullaca, and sarsaparilla. Put in capsules and try

1 gram 2 to 3 times daily as needed. This remedy can also be prepared as a standard tincture and teaspoon used 2 to 3 times daily as needed.

Calming Tea Remedy

When dealing with stress, try this calming blend of herbs as a natural tea. Steep 1 tablespoon of these mixed herbs in a cup of boiling water: 2 parts each passion flower and chamomile, and 1 part each damiana, fedegoso, and muira puama.

Cold and Flu Remedy

Combine equal parts picao preto, fedegosa, Brazilian peppertree, amor seco, mullaca, samambaia, gervão, and cat's claw. For colds and flu, try 1 gram 2 to 3 times daily. This combination can also be made into a standard infusion and 1 cup of tea drunk 3 times daily, but most people find the taste unpleasant.

Digestion Support Remedy

Combine 2 parts each of jurubeba, carqueja, and espinheira santa, and 1 part each of boldo and gervão. This herbal mixture (1 to 2 grams) can be taken in capsules with meals, or take 1 teaspoon of a standard tincture just before meals to help aid digestion. It is also a very good natural antacid remedy.

Energy Tonic

Combine equal parts of jatoba bark, guarana seed, and yerba mate leaf. Stuff in capsules and/or take the equivalent of 1 to 2 grams when needed for added energy. This can also be prepared as an infusion by placing a heaping teaspoon of the herb mixture in a cup of boiling water, letting it steep, and drinking it as a refreshing energy tea.

Fungal/Yeast Remedy

Combine 2 parts jatoba with one part each fedegosa, Brazilian peppertree, and pau d'arco. This can be taken for internal candida, 2 grams twice daily for at least 15 days and up to 30 days. This can also be prepared as a strong decoction, boiling it for at least 10 to 15 minutes until the water is reduced to half. Add at least 1 teaspoon of lemon juice per 2 cups of water or to taste when boiling. The remedy can be taken warm or cold in 1/2-cup dosages daily (refrigerate the remainder). This decoction can also be used on topical fungal problems such as athlete's foot and nail fungus; apply it liberally to the affected area. For a natural douche remedy for yeast infections, use 1 cup of this decoction (you can replace lemon juice with cider vinegar) to douche with daily.

Heart Tonic

Prepare a standard tincture or decoction with 2 parts cat's claw to 1 part each erva tostão, fedegosa, graviola, guarana, and yerba mate. To nutritionally support heart functions, try 1/2 to 1 cup of a standard decoction or 1 tablespoon of a standard tincture 1 to 2 times a week. This amount can be taken daily if needed.

Immune-Building Tonic

Use in capsules, prepare a standard decoction, or make a standard tincture with 2 parts cat's claw, 1 part mullaca, 1 part macela, 1 part suma, and 1 part chuchuhuasi. To nutritionally support general immune functions, try 2 grams in capsules, 1/2 cup of the decoction, or 1 tablespoon of the tincture once or twice weekly. For weakened immune systems or during periods of special need, these amounts can be taken daily.

Kidney Tonic

Combine 3 parts chanca piedra and 1 part each erva tostão, ja-toba, espinheira santa, sarsaparilla, and Brazilian peppertree. This remedy can be prepared in capsules, as a standard infusion, or as a tincture. To nutritionally support healthy kidney and uri-nary tract functions, try 1 cup of a standard infusion, 1 teaspoon of a standard tincture, or 1 to 2 grams in capsules 1 to 2 times a week. These amounts can be taken once or twice daily during times of special need.

Liver Tonic

Combine 2 parts each carqueja, artichoke, chanca piedra, and jurubeba to 1 part each picao preto, erva tostão, boldo, and gervão. This herbal combination can be prepared as an infusion or tincture or placed in capsules. To nutritionally support healthy liver functions, try 1 cup of a standard infusion, 1 tablespoon of a standard tincture, or 1 to 2 grams in capsules once or twice a week. In times of special need, these amounts can be taken once or twice daily.

Menstrual Pain Relief

For menstrual pain and difficulties, try combining 2 parts each abuta, tayuya, and iporuru and 1 part each vassourinha and gervão. These herbs have a strong taste, and this remedy is normally placed in capsules because of the objectionable taste of a tea or tincture. Try 1 gram 2 to 3 times daily as needed for menstrual cramps and pain.

Parasite Remedy

Combine equal parts macela, graviola, carqueja, fedegosa, boldo, gervão, simaruba, and epazote (Chenopodium ambrosioides), and try 1 gram twice daily for 15 to 30 days. This herbal formula can also be made into a standard tincture with 1 teaspoon taken twice daily for the same period of time.

Prostate Tonic

Combine 3 parts jatoba and 1 part each mutamba, Brazilian peppertree, chanca piedra, and sarsaparilla. This remedy can be placed in capsules or prepared as a decoction or tincture. To nutritionally support healthy prostate functions, try 3/4 cup of a standard decoction, 1 teaspoon of a standard tincture, or 1 to 2 grams in capsules once or twice a week. These amounts can be taken once or twice daily during times of special need.

METHODS OF PREPARING HERBAL REMEDIES

Medicinal plants are used and prepared in various ways, and different parts of the plant may be used for different purposes. For example, the leaves of a plant may be drunk as a hot tea (infusion) for one type of illness, while the bark of the same plant is extracted in alcohol (tincture) to help a completely different type of illness. Below some common methods of preparing herbal remedies are defined.

Decoction

A standard method of preparing a plant by boiling it in water for approximately 1 hour. A standard decoction calls for boiling 30 g dried herb or 60 g fresh herb in approximately 750 ml of water until it is reduced to approximately 500 ml (approximately 2 oz fresh or 1 oz dried herb to 3 cups of water, reduced to 2 cups). Normal dosage for a decoction is generally 1/2 cup.

Infusion

A standard method of preparing a plant, much like making a tea. A standard infusion generally calls for 30 g dried or 60 g fresh herb to 500 ml of just boiling water (approximately 1 oz dried or 2 oz fresh herb to 2 cups water). The boiling water is poured on top of the herb, then the pot is covered tightly and left to steep/infuse for 10 minutes. The infusion can be drunk warm or cold. A normal dosage for an infusion is generally 1/2 cup.

Maceration

A standard method of preparing a plant; also called a cold infusion. A standard maceration calls for pouring 500 ml of cold water over 25 g dried or 50 g fresh herb (2 cups of water over 3/4 ounce dried or 1-1/2 ounce fresh herb). It is normally allowed to soak/macerate for 12 to 24 hours and is then strained. Standard dosage is 1/2 cup.

Tincture

A standard method of preparing a plant with alcohol. A standard 1:5 tincture calls for 1 part plant material to 5 parts alcohol/water (by volume or weight). Depending on the plant, 25% to 80% alcohol will be used, and the remaining percentage made up of water. Normally, the tincture is left to macerate/soak with the plant material in it for approximately 2 weeks, shaken occasionally, and then strained to remove the plant.

Rainforest Plant Tables

~~~~~~

THE INFORMATION IN Table 1, Documented Properties and Actions of Rainforest Plants, and Table 2, Documented Worldwide Ethnic Uses of Rainforest Plants, was compiled from over 500 published sources of documentation referenced in the Notes section of this book. The information on the following pages is for education and information purposes only and is not intended to be used to diagnose, prescribe, or replace proper medical care.

Table 1
DOCUMENTED PROPERTIES AND ACTIONS OF RAINFOREST PLANTS

Plant/Scientific Name	Properties and Actions
Abuta *Cissampelos pareira*	analgesic, anticarcinomic, anti-inflammatory, antileukemic, antiseptic, antispasmodic, aperient, diuretic, emmenagogue, expectorant, febrifuge, hepatoprotective, hypotensive, piscicide, purgative, stimulant, stomachic, tonic
Acerola *Malpighia glabra*	antioxidant, astringent, nutritive
Alcachofra (artichoke) *Cynara scolymus*	cholagogue, choleretic, choliokinetic, depurative, detoxifer, diuretic, hepatoprotective, hypocholesterolemic, hypotensive, stimulant, tonic
Amor seco *Desmodium adscendens*	antianaphylactic, antiasthmatic, antihistamine, anti-inflammatory, antispasmodic, bronchodilator, depurative, diuretic, laxative, vulnerary
Andiroba *Carapa guianensis*	analgesic, anti-inflammatory, antiparasitic, antiseptic, cicatrizant, emollient, febrifuge, insecticide, vermifuge
Annatto *Bixa orellana*	antibacterial, antidysenteric, antigonorrheal, anti-inflammatory, antioxidant, antiseptic, antitussive, astringent, cicatrizant, depurative, diuretic, emollient, expectorant, febrifuge, hepatoprotective, hypoglycemic, hypotensive, nutritive, parasiticide, purgative, stomachic
Balsam of Tolu, Peru *Myroxylon balsamum, pereirae*	antibacterial, antifungal, anti-inflammatory, antiparasitic, antiseptic, antitussive, cicatrizant, expectorant, respiratory, vulnerary
Boldo *Peumus boldus*	anodyne, anthelmintic, antiseptic, cholagogue, choleretic, demulcent, depurative, detoxifier, diuretic, hepatic, hepatotonic, sedative, stimulant, stomachic, tonic, vermifuge
Brazilian peppertree *Schinus molle*	analgesic, antibacterial, antidepressant, antifungal, antimicrobial, antispasmodic, antiviral, astringent, balsamic, cytotoxic, diuretic, expectorant, hypotensive, purgative, stomachic, tonic, uterine stimulant, vulnerary
Brazil nut *Bertholletia excelsa*	antioxidant, emollient, insecticide, nutritive

Plant/Scientific Name	Properties and Actions
Cajueiro (cashew) *Anacardium occidentale*	antidysenteric, anti-inflammatory, antitussive, aphrodisiac, astringent, diuretic, febrifuge, hypoglycemic, hypotensive, purgative, refrigerant, stomachic, tonic
Camu-camu *Myrciaria dubia*	anti-inflammatory, antioxidant, astringent, emollient, nutritive
Carqueja *Baccharis genistelloides*	analgesic, antacid, anthelmintic, antihepatotoxic, anti-inflammatory, antirheumatic, antiulcerogenic, aperient, depurative, digestive, diuretic, febrifuge, gastrotonic, hepatic, hepatoprotective, hepatotonic, hypoglycemic, laxative, refrigerant, stomachic, tonic, vermifuge
Cat's claw (uña de gato) *Uncaria tomentosa*	antibacterial, anti-inflammatory, antimutagenic, antioxidant, antitumorous, antiviral, cytostatic, depurative, diuretic, hypotensive, immunostimulant, vermifuge
Catuaba *Erythroxylum catuaba*	antibacterial, antiviral, aphrodisiac, central nervous system stimulant, tonic
Chanca piedra *Phyllanthus niruri*	anodyne, antibacterial, antihepatotoxic, anti-inflammatory, antispasmodic, antiviral, aperitif, carminative, choleretic, digestive, diuretic, emmenagogue, febrifuge, hepatotonic, hypoglycemic, hypotensive, immunostimulant, laxative, stomachic, tonic, vermifuge
Chuchuhuasi *Maytenus krukovit*	adrenal supportive, analgesic, anodyne, antiarthritic, antidiarrheic, anti-inflammatory, antirheumatic, antitumor, aphrodisiac, immunostimulant, muscle relaxant, stimulant, stomachic, tonic
Copaiba *Copaifera officinalis*	antibacterial, anti-inflammatory, antimicrobial, astringent, cicatrizant, disinfectant, diuretic, emollient, expectorant, laxative, stimulant, vulnerary
Damiana *Turnera aphrodisiaca*	aphrodisiac, astringent, diuretic, emmenagogue, laxative, nervine, stimulant, stomachic, tonic
Erva tostão *Boerhaavia diffusa*	anthelmintic, antiamebic, antibacterial, anticonvulsant, antifibrinolytic, anti-inflammatory, antispasmodic, antiviral, choleretic, depurative, diuretic, hemostatic, hepatoprotective, hepatotonic, hypotensive, lactagogue, laxative, vermifuge
Espinheira santa *Maytenus ilicifolia*	analgesic, antacid, antiasthmatic, antibiotic, antileukemic, antiseptic, antitumorous, antiulcerogenic, cicatrizant, detoxifier, disinfectant, diuretic, laxative, stomachic, tonic

(continues)

Plant/Scientific Name	Properties and Actions
Fedegoso *Cassia occidentalis*	analgesic, antibacterial, antifungal, antihepatotoxic, anti-inflammatory, antiparasitic, antiseptic, antispasmodic, antiviral, carminative, diaphoretic, emmenagogue, febrifuge, hepatoprotective, hepatotonic, insecticidal, laxative, parasiticide, purgative, stomachic, sudorific, vermifuge
Gervão *Stachytarpheta jamaicensis*	analgesic, antacid, anthelmintic, diuretic, emmenagogue, febrifuge, hypotensive, lactagogue, laxative, purgative, sedative, spasmogenic, stomachic, sudorific, tonic, vasodilator, vermifuge, vulnerary
Graviola *Annona muricata*	antibacterial, antiparasitic, antispasmodic, astringent, cytotoxic, febrifuge, hypotensive, insecticide, nervine, pectoral, piscicide, sedative, stomachic, vasodilator, vermifuge
Guarana *Paullinia cupana*	analgesic, antibacterial, aphrodisiac, astringent, cardiotonic, diuretic, febrifuge, nervine, purgative, stimulant, tonic, vasodilator
Guava *Psidium guajava*	antibacterial, antimicrobial, antispasmodic, astringent, cicatrizant, emmenagogue, hypoglycemic, laxative, nutritive
Iporuru *Alchornea castaneifolia*	analgesic, anodyne, antiarthritic, antibacterial, anti-inflammatory, antimicrobial, aphrodisiac, laxative
Jaborandi *Pilocarpus jaborandi*	anti-inflammatory, diaphoretic, diuretic, emetic, febrifuge, lactagogue
Jatoba *Hymenaea courbaril*	antibacterial, antifatigue, antifungal, anti-inflammatory, antioxidant, antispasmodic, astringent, decongestant, diuretic, expectorant, hemostatic, hepatoprotective, hypoglycemic, laxative, stimulant, stomachic, tonic, vermifuge
Jurubeba *Solanum paniculatum*	anti-inflammatory, carminative, cholagogue, decongestive, digestive, diuretic, emmenagogue, febrifuge, gastrotonic, hepatotonic, hypotensive, stomachic, tonic
Maca *Lepidium meyenii*	antifatigue, aphrodisiac, immunostimulant, nutritive, steroidal, tonic
Macela *Achyrocline satureoides*	analgesic, anti-inflammatory, antimutagenic, antiseptic, antispasmodic, antitumorus, antiviral, cytotoxic, digestive, emmenagogue, genotoxic, hypoglycemic, immunostimulant, insecticidal, muscle relaxant, sudorific, vermifuge
Manacá *Brunfelsia uniflorus*	abortifacient, alterative, analgesic, anesthetic, anti-inflammatory, antirheumatic, diaphoretic, diuretic, emmenagogue, hypertensive, hypothermal, laxative, narcotic, purgative

Plant/Scientific Name	Properties and Actions
Maracuja (passionflower) *Passiflora incarnata*	analgesic, anticonvulsant, antidepressant, anti-inflammatory, antispasmodic, anxiolytic, disinfectant, diuretic, hypnotic, nervine, sedative, spasmolytic, vermifuge
Maracuja (passion fruit) *Passiflora edulis*	antibacterial, antifungal, nutritive, sedative
Muira puama *Ptychopetalum olacoides*	antidysenteric, antirheumatic, antistress, aperitif, aphrodisiac, central nervous system stimulant, nervine, neurasthenic, tonic
Mulateiro *Calycophyllum spruceanum*	anthelmintic, antifungal, emollient, vermifuge, vulnerary
Mullaca *Physalis angulata*	analgesic, antiasthmatic, anticoagulant, antigonorrheal, anti-inflammatory, antileukemic, antimutagenic, antiseptic, antispasmodic, antiviral, cytotoxic, diuretic, expectorant, febrifuge, hypotensive, immunostimulant, trypanocidal
Mulungu *Erythrina mulungu*	analgesic, anodyne, anti-inflammatory, hepatotonic, hypnotic, hypotensive, nervine, sedative
Mutamba *Guazuma ulmifolia*	antibacterial, antifungal, antimicrobial, antioxidant, antiulcerogenic, astringent, cytotoxic, depurative, diaphoretic, emollient, febrifuge, hepatoprotective, pectoral, refrigerant, stomachic, styptic, sudorific, vulnerary
Nettle *Urtica dioica*	anodyne, antirheumatic, antiseptic, astringent, bactericide, circulatory stimulant, depurative, diuretic, emmenagogue, galactagogue, hemostatic, hypoglycemic, hypotensive, stomachic, vasodilator, vermifuge
Pata de vaca *Bauhinia forficata*	depurative, diuretic, hypoglycemic
Pau d'arco *Tabebuia impetiginosa*	analgesic, antibacterial, anticarcinomic, antifungal, anti-inflammatory, antileukemic, antimicrobial, antimutagenic, antioxidant, antiparasitic, antirheumatic, antiviral, cytotoxic, immunostimulant, laxative
Pedra hume caa *Myrcia salicifolia*	antidysenteric, astringent, hypoglycemic
Picao preto *Bidens pilosa*	antibacterial, antidysenteric, anti-inflammatory, antimicrobial, astringent, diuretic, emmenagogue, emollient, hepatoprotective

(continues)

Plant/Scientific Name	Properties and Actions
Samambaia *Polypodium lepidopteris*	alterative, anti-inflammatory, antirheumatic, diaphoretic, diuretic, expectorant, hypotensive, pectoral, sudorific, tonic
Sangre de grado *Croton lechleri*	antibacterial, antihemorrhagic, anti-inflammatory, antiseptic, antitumorous, antiviral, cicatrizant, hemostatic, vulnerary
Sarsaparilla *Smilax officinalis*	alterative, antibiotic, anti-inflammatory, antipruritic, antirheumatic, antiseptic, antisyphilitic, aphrodisiac, carminative, depurative, diaphoretic, diuretic, febrifuge, hepatoprotective, hormonal, steroidal, stimulant, stomachic, tonic
Simaruba *Simarouba amara*	amebicide, analgesic, anthelmintic, antibacterial, antileukemic, antimalarial, antimicrobial, cytotoxic, emmenagogue, febrifuge, stomachic, sudorific, tonic, vermifuge
Stevia *Stevia rebaudiana*	antifungal, cardiotonic, diuretic, hypoglycemic, hypotensive, tonic, vasodilator
Suma *Pfaffia paniculata*	anabolic, analgesic, anti-inflammatory, antimutagenic, aphrodisiac, estrogenic, hypocholesterolemic, immunostimulant, nutritive, sedative, steroidal, tonic
Tayuya *Cayaponia tayuya*	analgesic, antibacterial, antifungal, anti-inflammatory, antimicrobial, antioxidant, antirheumatic, antisyphilitic, choleretic, depurative, digestive, diuretic, laxative, metabolic regulator, purgative, stomachic, tonic
Vassourinha *Scoparia dulcis*	analgesic, antibacterial, antidiabetic, antifungal, antiherpetic, anti-inflammatory, antiseptic, antispasmodic, antiviral, emmenagogue, emollient, expectorant, febrifuge, hypocholesterolemic, hypotensive, pectoral, refrigerant
Yerba mate *Ilex paraguariensis*	alterative, analeptic, antioxidant, aperient, astringent, depurative, diuretic, glycogenolytic, immunostimulant, lipolytic, purgative, stimulant, stomachic, sudorific, tonic

Table 2

DOCUMENTED WORLDWIDE ETHNIC USES OF RAINFOREST PLANTS

Plant/Scientific Name	Ethnic Uses
Abuta *Cissampelos pareira*	anabolic, antidote, antiecbolic, aphrodisiac, asthma, bladder, blennorrhagia, boil, bronchitis, burn, calculus, chill, cholera, cold, constipation, convulsion, cough, cystitis, delirium, diabetes, diarrhea, digestion, diuretic, dog bite, dropsy, dysentery, dyspepsia, emmenagogue, epilepsy, erysipelas, expectorant, eye, febrifuge, gonorrhea, gravel, hematuria, hemorrhage, hydropsy, hypertension, itch, jaundice, kidney, leucorrhea, lithontriptic, malaria, menorrhagia, nephritis, palpitation, parturition, pimples, piscicide, poultice, purgative, rabies, rheumatism, snakebite, sore, stimulant, stomachache, styptic, testiculitis, tonic, urinary infection, urogenital, uterine disorders, uterine hemorrhage, venereal
Acerola *Malpighia glabra*	astringent, breast, diarrhea, dysentery, fever, hepatitis, liqueur, tenesmus
Alcachofra *Cynara scolymus*	albuminuria, anemia, arteriosclerosis, calculus, cancer, cholagogue, cystitis, diabetes, diuretic, dropsy, dyspepsia, gallbladder, gallstones, high cholesterol, hydropsy, hyperglycemia, hypertension, kidney, liver, rheumatism, snakebite, tonic, uremia
Amor seco *Desmodium adscendens*	ache (back, body, joint, muscle), anthelmintic, aphrodisiac, asthma, blennorrhagia, blood, bronchitis, cataplasm, colic, constipation, contraceptive, convulsion, cough, depurative, detoxifier, diarrhea, digestive, dysentery, fracture, galactagogue, headache, hemorrhage, inflammation, kidney disorders, laxative, leucorrhea, magic, malaria, marasmus, nervousness, oliguria, ovary, oxytoxic, ringworms, sore, urinary, vaginal infections, vaginitis, venereal disease, wounds
Andiroba *Carapa guianensis*	analgesic, arthritis, bruise, cancer, cold, cough, feet, fever, flu, herpes, insect insectifuge, insect bite, insecticide, insectifuge, insect repellent, itch, leprosy, malaria, muscle pain, parasiticide, pediculicide, psoriasis, rash (skin), skin, skin disease, soap, tetanus, ulcers (skin), vermifuge, wounds
Annatto *Bixa orellana*	antidote, antiseptic, aphrodisiac, astringent, burn, cancer, cholesterolemia, cicatrizant, coloring, conjunctivitis, cordial, cosmetic, cystitis, depurative, diabetes, diuretic, douche, dye, dysentery, epilepsy, erysipelas, excitant, fainting, fever, flu,

(continues)

Plant/Scientific Name	Ethnic Uses
Annatto *cont.*	gonorrhea, hair oil, headache, heartburn, hepatitis, hyperglycemia, hypertension, inflammation, insect repellent, jaundice, kidney, liver, malaria, obesity, oliguria, parasiticide, prostate, purgative, refrigerant, renal, skin disorders, stomachache, stomachic, stomatitis, styptic, throat, tumor, unguent, urinary, urogenital, vaginitis, venereal
Balsam of Tolu, Peru *Myroxylon balsamum, pereirae*	abscess, amenorrhea, antiseptic, asthma, bactericide, bronchitis, cancer, catarrh, chilblains, cold, colic, cough, deodorant, diuretic, dysmenorrhea, expectorant, freckle, fumigant, fungicide, gout, headache, itch, osteomyelitis, parasiticide, pectoral, pediculosis, perfume, rash (skin), rheumatism, ringworms, scabies, sclerosis, skin, sore, spasm, sprain, stimulant, stomachache, stomachic, swelling, tonic, tuberculosis, tumor, ulcers (skin), umbilicus, venereal, vermifuge, wound
Boldo *Peumus boldus*	anodyne, anthelmintic, antiseptic, choleretic, cold, digestion, diuretic, dyspepsia, earache, gallbladder, gallstones, gastrointestinal, gonorrhea, gout, hepatosis, hepatotonic, jaundice, laxative, liver, rheumatism, sedative, stimulant, stomach, stomachic, syphilis, tonic, urogenital, vermifuge, worms
Brazilian peppertree *Schinus molle*	amenorrhea, antidepressant, antiseptic, aposteme, arrhythmia, asthma, astringent, balsamic, blennorrhagia, bronchitis, cataract, cicatrizant, colds, colic, collyrium, conjunctivitis, cough, cystitis, diarrhea, digestive disorders, diuretic, dysmenorrhea, edema, emmenagogue, expectorant, eye, fever, foot, fractures, gingivitis, gonorrhea, gout, grippe, gum, hemoptysis, hypertension, inflammation, liqueur, masticatory, menstrual disorders, mouth, piscicide, poison, preventative, purgative, respiratory tract disorders, respiratory tract infections, rheumatism, sore, spice, stimulant, stomachache, stomachic, swelling, tea, tonic, toothache, tuberculosis, tumor, ulcer, urethritis, urinary tract disorders, urinary tract infections, urogenital, venereal, viricide, vulnerary, wart, wound
Brazil nut *Bertholletia excelsa*	emollient, food, insect repellent, liver, soap
Cajueiro (cashew) *Anacardium occidentale*	analgesic, antiseptic, aphrodisiac, asthenia, asthma, astringent, bronchitis, callosity, catarrh, caustic, cold, colic, congestion, constipation, corn, cough, debility, dermatosis, diabetes,

Plant/Scientific Name	Ethnic Uses
Cajueiro cont.	diarrhea, diuretic, douche, dysentery, dyspepsia, eczema, fever, flu, freckle, gargle, genital, impotence, infection, infections (skin), intestinal colic, leishmaniasis, leprosy, liqueur, mouthwash, muscular debility, nausea, piscicide, poison, psoriasis, purgative, scrofula, scurvy, skin, sore throat, stimulant, stomach-ache, swelling, syphilis, throat, thrush, tonsillitis, tumor, ulcers (mouth, skin, stomach), urinary, vaginitis, venereal, vesicant, wart, wounds
Camu-camu *Myrciaria dubia*	cold, flu, food
Carqueja *Baccharis genistelloides*	allergies, anemia, angina, antacid, anthelmintic, bitter, bloating, calculus, circulation, constipation, depurative, diabetes, diarrhea, digestive, dyspepsia, febrifuge, gallbladder, gallstones, gastritis, gastroenteritis, gout, grippe, hydropsy, impotence, indigestion, intestinal gas, intestines, kidney, leprosy, liver, malaria, nausea, sore throat, sterility, stomach, stomachic, tonic, tonsillitis, ulcers, urinary, venereal disease, vermifuge
Cat's claw (uña de gato) *Uncaria tomentosa*	abscesses, anti-inflammatory, arthritis, asthma, blood disorders, bowel, cancer, cardiotonic, chronic fatigue syndrome, cirrhosis (liver), colds, colitis, contraceptive, Crohn's disease, cytostatic, depression, detoxifier, diabetes, diverticulitis, dysentery, fever, flu, gastritis, gonorrhea, hemorrhages, hemorrhoids, herpes, hypertension, immune disorders, immunostimulant, inflammation, intestinal disorders, irritable bowel syndrome, kidney, leukemia, liver, lupus, menstrual, parasites, psoriasis, rheumatism, shingles, skin, tonic, tumor, ulcer (gastric), urinary, urinary tract disorders, wounds
Catuaba *Erythroxylum catuaba*	aphrodisiac, cancer (skin), central nervous system stimulant, fatigue, impotence, insomnia, intestines, liver, neurasthenia, stomach, tonic
Chanca piedra *Phyllanthus niruri*	aperitif, asthma, bladder, blennorrhagia, bronchitis, calculus, cancer, carminative, cirrhosis, cold, colic, constipation, cough, dermatosis, diabetes, diarrhea, digestive, diuretic, dropsy, dysentery, dyspepsia, emmenagogue, fever, flu, gallbladder, gallstones, gonorrhea, hepatitis, hydropsy, hyperglycemia, inflammation, itch, jaundice, kidney, kidney stones, malaria, medicine, miscarriage, piscicide, poultice, rectitis, renal, renosis, stomachache, stomachic, syphilis, tenesmus, tonic, tumor (abdomen), typhoid, urinary infection, uterine relaxant, vaginitis, vertigo

(continues)

Plant/Scientific Name	Ethnic Uses
Chuchuhuasi *Maytenus krukovit*	ache (menstrual, muscle), analgesic, anodyne, aphrodisiac, arthritis, backache, bronchitis, cancer (skin), diarrhea, fatigue, fever, hemorrhoids, impotence, insect repellent, menstrual irregularities, osteoarthritis, rheumatism, sterility, stomachache, stomachic, tonic, tumors (skin), virility
Copaiba *Copaifera officinalis*	bronchitis, catarrh, cicatrizant, cystitis, dermatitis, diarrhea, gonorrhea, hemorrhoids, herpes, incontinence, inflammation, psoriasis, skin disorders, sores (skin), syphilis, tumor (prostate), ulcers (stomach)
Damiana *Turnera aphrodisiaca*	amaurosis, antidepressant, aphrodisiac, astringent, catarrh, cold, diabetes, diuretic, dysentery, dysmenorrhea, dyspepsia, enuresis, expectorant, headache, intestine, laxative, liqueur, malaria, nerve, nervine, panacea, paralysis, renitis, stimulant, stomachache, syphilis, tonic, urinary, venereal
Erva tostão *Boerhaavia diffusa*	abdomen, abdominal pain, abortifacient, abscess, albuminuria, anemia, anthelmintic, anticonvulsant, antiflatulent, anti-inflammatory, aphrodisiac, appetite stimulant, ascites, asthma, beri-beri, blennorrhagia, blood purifier, boil, calculi, cancer (abdominal), cataract, childbirth, cholagogue, cholera, convulsions, cough, cystitis, debility, diuretic, dropsy, dysmenorrhagia, dyspepsia, edema, emetic, epilepsy, erysipelas, expectorant, eye, febrifuge, fever, food, gallbladder, gonorrhea, guinea worms, heart ailments, heart disease, hemorrhages (childbirth, thoracic), hemorrhoids, hepatitis, hepatoprotective, hepatotonic, hydropsy, inflammation (internal), jaundice, joint pain, kidney disorders, lactagogue, laxative, liver, lumbago, menstrual, nephritis, ophthalmic, renal, rheumatism, sclerosis (liver), snakebite, spleen (enlarged), sterility, stomachic, tonic, urinary, urinary disorders, urticaria, weakness, yaws
Espinheira santa *Maytenus ilicifolia*	acne, adrenal, analgesic, anemia, antacid, antifertility, aperitif, aphrodisiac, astringent, cancer, cicatrizant, colic, constipation, contraceptive, detoxifier, dyspepsia, gastritis, indigestion, intestine, kidney, laxative, leukemia, liver disorders, stomach, stomachic, tea, tonic, ulcers (gastric, stomach),
Fedegoso *Cassia occidentalis*	abdominal pain, abortifacient, abscess, acne, anemia, anodyne, anthelmintic, antifertility, antifungal, anti-inflammatory, antiseptic, antispasmodic, asthma, astringent, athlete's foot, bilious, bite (scorpion), bronchitis, burn, carminative, cataract, chancre, childbirth, chill, cholagogue, coffee, cold, colic, collyrium, constipation, contraceptive, dermatosis, diabetes, diaphoretic, diarrhea, diuretic, dropsy, dysentery, dysmenorrhea, dyspepsia, earache, eczema, emmenagogue, energy, erysipelas, eye,

Plant/Scientific Name	Ethnic Uses
Fedegoso, *cont.*	febrifuge, fever, fungal disease (skin), furuncle, gonorrhea, guinea worms, headache, heart, heart attack, hematuria, hemorrhage, herpes, hypertension, inflammation, insecticide, itch, jaundice, kidney, leprosy, liver, liver tonic, malaria, menstrual pain, nausea, ophthalmia, pain, palpitation, parasiticide, poultice, puerperium, purgative, rash, respiratory infections, rheumatism, ringworms, scabies, skin, skin diseases, snakebite, sore throat, spasm, stomach, stomachache, stomachic, sudorific, swelling, syncope, tetanus, tonic, toothache, tuberculosis, tumor, typhoid, ulcer, urinary disorders, uterine pain, venereal, vermifuge, womb, wounds, yellow fever
Gervão *Stachytarpheta jamaicensis*	abortifacient, alopecia, amenorrhea, anodyne, anthelmintic, antifertility, asthma, boil, bronchitis, bruise, cardiac, cataract, cathartic, chest cold, childbirth, colds, cough, depurative, diarrhea, dropsy, dysentery, dysmenorrhea, eczema, emetic, emmenagogue, erysipelas, fever, flu, gonorrhea, headache, heart, inflammation, intestinal worms, itch, lactagogue, liver, liver disease, malaria, nausea, nerve, nervousness, neuralgia, parasites, poison, puerperium, purgative, rash, rectitis, rheumatism, rhinitis, rhinosis, sedative, skin, sore, sprain, stomach, stomachache, stomachic, sudorific, syphilis, tea, tumor, ulcers (skin), venereal, vermifuge, vitiligo, worms, yellow fever
Graviola *Annona muricata*	analgesic, anthelmintic, antiphlogistic, antispasmodic, arthritis, asthenia, asthma, astringent, bilious, boil, cataplasm, childbirth, chill, cicatrizant, cough, cyanogenetic, depurative, dermatosis, diarrhea, diuretic, dysentery, dyspepsia, emetic, fainting, febrifuge, fever, flu, galactagogue, gallbladder, grippe, hypertension, insecticide, insomnia, internulcer, kidney, lactagogue, liqueur, malaria, nervousness, neuralgia, palpitation, parasites, parturition, pectoral, pediculicide, pellagra, piscicide, rash, rheumatism, ringworm, scurvy, sedative, skin disease, soporific, sore, spasm, stomach, stomachic, tea, tranquilizer, ulcer (stomach), vermifuge, worms
Guarana *Paullinia cupana*	arteriosclerosis, astringent, cardiotonic, coffee, detoxifier, diarrhea, fatigue, fevers, flatulence, headache, heart, intoxicant, migraine, nervine, neuralgia, obesity, stimulant
Guava *Psidium guajava*	antiseptic, astringent, bactericide, bowel, bronchitis, cachexia, catarrh, cholera, chorea, cicatrizant, cold, colic, convulsion, cough, deafness, dentifrice, depurgative, dermatosis, diarrhea, dysentery, dyspepsia, emmenagogue, epilepsy, fattening, fever, gingivitis, hemostat, hysteria, itch, jaundice, laxative, menstrual, nausea, nephritis, pile, respiratory, rheumatism, scabies, skin, sore, sore throat, spasm, stomachache, swelling, tonic, toothache, ulcer, vermifuge, vertigo, vulnerary, wound

(continues)

Iporuru
Alchornea castaneifolia

ache (muscle), analgesic, aphrodisiac, arthritis, cough, diabetes, diarrhea, fertility, headache, laxative, osteoarthritis, pain, rheumatism, wound

Jaborandi
Pilocarpus jaborandi

antidote (atropine, belladonna), baldness, Bright's disease, bronchitis, diaphoretic, diuretic, dropsy, emetic, enterocolitis, fever, flu, glaucoma, lactagogue, laryngitis, neurosis, pneumonia, prurigo, psoriasis, renal, renitis, rheumatism, stomatitis

Jatoba
Hymenaea coubaril

antiseptic, antispasmodic, arthritis, asthma, beri-beri, bexiga, bladder, blennorrhagia, bronchitis, bruise, bursitis, candida, cardiopulmonary, catarrh, constipation, cough, cystitis, decongestant, diarrhea, dysentery, dyspepsia, emphysema, energy, expectorant, fatigue, fracture, fungal infections, fungicide, headache, hematuria, hemorrhages, hemorrhoids, indigestion, intestine, kidney, laryngitis, laxative, liqueur, lung, prostatitis, purgative, respiratory, rheumatism, sedative, sore, spasm, stomach, stomachic, tonic, ulcer, venereal, vermifuge

Jurubeba
Solanum paniculatum

abscess (internal), anemia, bladder, boil, bowel, catarrh, Crohn's disease, decongestant, digestive disorders, diuretic, dyspepsia, erysipelas, fever, gastritis, hangover, hepatitis, hepatotonic, high blood pressure, hydropsy, inappetence, indigestion, irritable bowel syndrome, liver, skin, spleen, stomachic, tonic, tumor (uterine), urinary disorders

Maca
Lepidium meyenii

anemia, aphrodisiac, energy, fertility, impotence, memory, menopause, menstrual tonic, tuberculosis

Macela
Achyrocline satureoides

analgesic, anthelmintic, antibacterial, antidiabetic, anti-inflammatory, antimicrobial, antiseptic, antispasmodic, asthma, carminative, cold, colic, diabetes, diarrhea, digestion, digestive, dysentery, emmenagogue, epilepsy, flu, gastritis, gastrointestinal disorders, hypoglycemic, impotence, infections, inflammation, menstrual disorders, menstrual regulation, sedative, sudorific, tumors, vermifuge

Manacá
Brunfelsia uniflorus

abortifacient, alterative, analgesic, anesthetic, anti-inflammatory, arthritis, back pain, bronchitis, chills, cold, diaphoretic, diuretic, fever, flu, kidney, laxative, lung disease, lymph, purgative, respiratory, rheumatism, scrofula, snakebite, syphilis, tuberculosis, ulcers, uterine, uterine cramps, venereal, yellow fever

Maracuja (passionflower)
Passiflora edulis, incarnata

analgesic, antispasmodic, aphrodisiac, asthma, bronchitis, burn, convulsions, cough, cyanogenetic, diarrhea, diuretic, dysmenorrhea, epilepsy, eruption, eye, hemorrhoid, high blood pressure, hysteria, inflammation, insomnia, medicine, menopause, menstrual cramps, morphinism, muscle cramps, narcotic, nervine, neuralgia, neurasthenia, neurosis, pain reliever, paralysis, Parkinson's disease, perfume, piles, PMS, sedative, seizures, shingles, skin, soporific, spasm, tetanus, tonic, worms (intestinal)

Plant/Scientific Name	Ethnic Uses
Maracuja (passion fruit) *Passiflora edulis, incarnata*	asthma, bronchitis, cough, diuretic, food, heart tonic, sedative, urinary infections, whooping cough
Muira puama *Ptychopetalum olacoides*	aphrodisiac, asthenia, baldness, beri-beri, cardiac asthenia, cramps (menstrual), depression, frigidity, gastrointestinal, grippe, impotence, medicine, nervine, neuralgia, neurasthenia, neuro-muscular, paralysis, PMS, rheumatism, sexual debility, tonic
Mulateiro *Calycophyllum spruceanum*	diabetes, fungal infections, fungicide, parasites, skin, vulnerary, wounds
Mullaca *Physalis angulata*	abortion preventative, analgesic, antidote, anti-inflammatory, antiseptic, asthma, boil, childbirth, cold, depurative, dermatitis, diabetes, diarrhea, disinfectant, diuretic, dysuria, earache, expectorant, fever, gallbladder, gonorrhea, hemorrhage (post-partum), hemostatic, hepatitis, hydropsy, indigestion, jaundice, kidney, labor, liver, liver disease, malaria, narcotic, nausea, nephritis, ophthalmia, rectitis, rectum, rheumatism, sedative, skin disease, sleeping sickness, sterility, stomach, swelling, syncope, throat, tumor (testicle), tumors, worms
Mulungu *Erythrina mulungu*	asthma, bronchitis, cancer (stomach), cardiotonic, central nervous system disorders, cough, diuretic, epilepsy, fever, gingivitis, heart, hepatitis, hernia, high blood pressure, hypnotic, hysteria, inflammation, insomnia, lactagogue, liver, narcotic, pile, piscicide, sedative, spasm, spleen, stomachache
Mutamba *Guazuma ulmifolia*	antidote (comocladia), antidysenteric, asthma, astringent, bronchitis, bruise, burn, chest, childbirth, constipation, cough, depurative, dermatitis, diaphoretic, diarrhea, diuretic, dysentery, elephantiasis, emollient, erysipelas, febrifuge, fertility (veterinary), fever, flu, fracture, gastrointestinal, gonorrhea, grippe, hair, hemorrhage, hemorrhoids, irruptions, kidney, kidney disease, leprosy, liver, liver disease, lung, malaria, medicine, obesity, pectoral, pneumonia, prostate, rash, refrigerant, scurvy, skin, skin disease, skin irritation, sore, stomach, stomachic, styptic, sudorific, syphilis, ulcers, uterine stimulant, uterus, wounds
Nettle *Urtica dioica*	ache, alopecia, anodyne, asthma, astringent, ataxia (locomotor), backache, blood, bronchitis, bruise, burn, cancer, catarrh, chest, cholecystitis, cholengitis, constipation, cough, counter-irritant, dandruff, depurative, diuretic, dropsy, dyspnea, emmenagogue, epilepsy, epitaxis, evil eye, fit, gout, hair tonic, hematemesis, hemoptysis, hemorrhage, hemostat, homeopathy, insanity, massage, menorrhagia, paralysis, parturition, prostate, purgative, rheumatism, shampoo, shigellosis, sore, sprain, stimulant, stomachic, suppository, swelling, tea, tonic, tumor, urticaria, vasoconstrictor, vermifuge, wound

(continues)

Pata de vaca
Bauhinia forficata

depurative, diabetes, diuretic, elephantiasis, hypoglycemia, polyuria, renal, snakebite, tonic, urinary

Pau d'arco
Tabebuia impetiginosa

allergies, analgesic, anemia, antibacterial, antifungal, anti-inflammatory, antimicrobial, antimutagenic, antioxidant, anti-parasitic, antiviral, arthritis, astringent, boils, cancer, candida, circulation, cold, colitis, constipation, cough, diabetes, dysentery, eczema, fever, flu, fungal infections, fungicide, gastritis, gastrointestinal, Hodgkin's disease, infections, laxative, leukemia, liver disorders, lupus, malaria, osteomyelitis, Parkinson's disease, prostatitis, psoriasis, respiratory disorders, rheumatism, stomatitis, syphilis, ulcers (skin, stomach), warts, wounds

Pedra hume caa
Myrcia salicifolia

astringent, diabetes, diarrhea, dysentery, enteritis, hemorrhages, hypertension, ulcers (mouth)

Picao preto
Bidens pilosa

abscess, aftosa, allergy, amygdalitis, angina, antidote, anti-inflammatory, astringent, blennorrhagia, boil, bronchitis, cancer, carminative, catarrh, childbirth, chills, cold, colic, conjunctivitis, cough, diabetes, diarrhea, diuretic, dysentery, dysmenorrhea, ear, edema, emmenagogue, emollient, eye, fever, food poisoning, headache, heat rash, hepatitis, hepatoprotective, inflammation, intestine, intoxicant, itch, jaundice, lactagogue, laryngitis, leucorrhea, liver, mycosis, obesity, pectoral, rheumatism, sclerosis (glands), sialogogue, snakebite, sore, sore (mouth, throat), stomach, stomachache, stomatitis, styptic, tonsillitis, toothache, urinary infections, urticaria, vaginitis, vulnerary, weight loss, worms, wounds

Samambaia
Polypodium lepidopteris

abscess, alterative, boil, bronchitis, cancer, cold, cough, expectorant, fever, flu, gout, grippe, high blood pressure, immune disorders, immunostimulant, pancreas, pectoral, psoriasis, purgative, renal, respiratory, rheumatism, skin disorders, sudorific, tonic, tumor, urinary infections, venereal, whooping cough

Sangre de grado
Croton lechleri

antibacterial, antifungal, antimicrobial, antiseptic, astringent, cicatrizant, eczema, fever, flu, fracture, gum, hemorrhage, hemostat, herpes, leucorrhea, piles, respiratory, skin, throat, tonic, tumor, ulcer (intestinal, mouth, stomach), vaginitis, vulnerary, wounds

Sarsaparilla
Smilax officinalis

alterative, aperitif, aphrodisiac, arthritis, blood, burn, cancer, conjunctivitis, cough, depurative, diaphoretic, digestive disorders, diuretic, emetic, fever, gonorrhea, gout, hypertension, impotence, inflammation, leprosy, psoriasis, purgative, rash, rheumatism, scrofula, skin, spasm, sterility, stimulant, sudorific, syphilis, tonic, toothache, urinary, venereal, wounds

Simaruba
Simarouba amara

ache (body), amebiasis, amebicide, anemia, anodyne, cold, colic, diarrhea, dysentery, dyspepsia, emetic, emmenagogue, excessive menstruation, febrifuge, gonorrhea, hemorrhage, inappetence, internal bleeding, intestinal parasites, intoxicant,

Simaruba *cont.*

malaria, purgative, rheumatism, skin, soap, sores, stomachic, sudorific, tonic

Stevia
Stevia rebaudiana

cardiotonic, contraceptive, diabetes, diuretic, high blood pressure, hyperglycemia, hypertension, sweetener, tonic, vasodilator

Suma
Pfaffia paniculata

anemia, aphrodisiac, arteriosclerosis, arthritis, asthma, bronchitis, cancer, chronic fatigue syndrome, circulatory disorders, diabetes, digestive, endocrine, Epstein-Barr, high blood pressure, high cholesterol, hormonal disorders, hypoglycemia, immunostimulant, impotence, infertility, leukemia, menopause, menstrual disorders, mononucleosis, muscle growth, nerve, nervine, PMS, rheumatism, sterility, tonic, tumor

Tayuya
Cayaponia tayuya

ache (back), acne, analgesic, arthritis, blennorrhagia, bowel, cholera, constipation, debility, depression, depurative, detoxifier, diarrhea, digestion, digestive disorders, diuretic, dyspepsia, eczema, edema, epilepsy, erysclepia, eye (sore), fatigue, fever, gout, headache, herpes, hydropsy, irritable bowel syndrome, liver, metabolism, nerve, nervine, neuralgia, purgative, rheumatism, sciatica, skin, snakebite, spleen, syphilis, tonic, tumor (joint), ulcer, wound

Vassourinha
Scoparia dulcis

abortifacient, aches, albuminuria, amygdalosis, analgesic, anemia, antidiabetic, antidote, antiemetic, antiseptic, antivenin, aphrodisiac, astringent, bite (insect), blennorrhagia, bronchitis, bruise, cardiopulmonary disorders, childbirth, cicatrizant, colic, conjunctivitis, contraceptive, cough, depurative, diabetes, diarrhea, diuretic, dysentery, dysmenorrhea, earache, eczema, emetic, emmenagogue, emollient, erysipelas, evil eye, expectorant, eye, fever, gastric disorders, gonorrhea, gravel, grippe, hallucinogen, headache, heart, hemorrhoids, hepatosis, hyperglycemia, hypertension, inflammation, insecticide, itch, jaundice, ketonuria, kidney, kidney disease, labor, leprosy, liver, malaria, mange, marasmus, menorrhagia, menstrual (excessive bleeding), menstrual disorders, metroxenia, mucolytic, nerve, ophthalmia, opium substitute, pains, pectoral, pile, purgative, rash, refrigerant, respiratory disorders, retinitis, skin, snakebite, sore, sores (gonorrheal), sore throat, spasm, stomachache, stomach, stomach disorders, swelling, syphilis, tonic, toothache, tumor, venereal disease, vermifuge, wounds

Yerba mate
Ilex paraguaiensis

allergies, aperient, arthritis, astringent, cardiotonic, coffee, constipation, depurative, digestion, diuretic, fatigue, hayfever, headache, heart, hemorrhoids, nervine, obesity, purgative, rheumatism, scurvy, stimulant, stomachic, stress, sudorific, tea, tonic, urinary

Sustainable Rainforest Products

~~~~~~

THE GROWTH AND health of our economy today is defined by the intensive exploitation of natural resources. Our present economic model ignores environmental degradation when assessing profits. If we are to survive, principles of sustainability must become integrated into our system. Sustainability means that the functions and processes of an ecosystem can be maintained (or sustained) and the needs of the present can be met: all without compromising the needs of future generations. Please be a responsible consumer and buy sustainable rainforest products.

Many factors must be taken into consideration, but two are key. The first step is to support the land and resource rights and economies of indigenous peoples: Preserving indigenous cultures is key to saving the rainforest. These knowledgeable people and their ancestors have inhabited rainforests for millennia without destroying them. We need them to teach us how to use the forests without damaging them. Medicines, foods, and other unknown treasures can be harvested without jeopardizing the future. People from developed countries have much to learn from indigenous peoples in terms of our relationship with the Earth. By respecting and allowing them to lead the way toward a true, stable utilization of this bountiful resource, if they choose to utilize it in any commercial way at all, we have the potential of achieving true sustainability.

The second step is to be a responsible consumer—and that's hard work. How can you tell if a product has been sustainably harvested? Ask questions. Where do purchases really come from? Where are your dollars really going? Who is benefiting from the profit? Is any of the profit returned to the people who are supplying rainforest products or raw materials? How much? Who receives the funds there? As a consumer, you are directly affecting the economy and ecology of the globe.

As we promote products like those listed below, we must also be aware that only a limited amount can be consumed. The concept of sustainability transcends the traditional rules of "supply and demand," as each ecosystem determines the ceiling of its productivity. Overconsumption is a driving force behind deforestation. The primary question for us must not be, "Which herbal supplement, ice cream, or candy should I buy?" but, "Do I need to buy this?"

Blue Planet Trading Co.
717 Simundson Drive, #111
Point Roberts, WA 98281
(604) 251-4277

Rainforest Riches Chocolates. A great variety of chocolate products with cashews and Brazil nuts.

Cultural Survival Inc.
53A Church Street
Cambridge, MA 02138
(617) 495-2562

All natural and preservative-free Rainforest Crunch Cashew and Brazil Nut Brittle and Rainforest Crunch Cookies (chocolate and Brazil nut). Retail and wholesale cashew fruit. Cashew fruit is eaten fresh, made into fruit drinks, jams, or butters. It is also dried to a date-like consistency. This is a nonprofit organization that supports indigenous cultures.

From the Rainforest
270 Lafayette Street
New York, NY 10002
(800) EAR-TH96

All natural, preservative-free nut and fruit mixes, including mango, papaya, pineapple, banana chips, cashews, Brazil nuts, and coconut.

Life Plus, Inc.

268 W. Main
Batesville, AK 72501
(800) 572-8446
Internet: http://lifeplus.com
Rainforest herbal supplements ecologically harvested by the indigenous tribes of the rainforest, sold through a network marketing plan. A portion of profits is returned to the rainforest.

Moonshine Trading Co.

PO Box 896
Winters, CA 95694
(916) 753-0601
Gourmet nut butters, spreads, honey.

Rainforest Action Network

450 Sansome Street, Suite 700
San Francisco, CA 94111
(415) 398-4404
Rainforest Essentials soap, shampoo, conditioner, and other body care products. All natural, vegetable-based products made with copaiba oil harvested by rubber tappers in the rainforests.

The Rainforest Company

701 North 15th Street, Suite 500
Saint Louis, MO 63103
(314) 621-1330
Internet: http://www.the-rainforest-co.com
Produces and distributes a range of natural food and personal care products that includes Rainforest Crunch, candy and confections, trail mixes, sauces and condiments, shampoo, and body wash, all with sustainably harvested rainforest ingredients.

The Rainforest Market

1601 W. Koenig Lane
Austin, TX 78756
(800) 780-5902
Internet: http://www.rain-tree.com/rfm_web
E-mail: rain2@bga.com
Rainforest herbs, supplements, and indigenous arts and crafts from the Amazon rainforest are featured at this unique retail store. Also offers mail order.

Rainforest Products, Inc.

PO Box 250
Mill Valley, CA 94942
(415) 383-8111

Natural granola cereal with cashews, Brazil nuts, and other edible snacks.

Raintree Marketing, Inc.
Raintree Nutrition, Inc.
1601 W. Koenig Lane
Austin, TX 78756
(800) 780-5902
Internet: http://www.rain-tree.com
E-mail: raintree@bga.com

Rainforest medicinal botanicals ecologically harvested by the indigenous peoples of the rainforest. Sold in bulk, in proprietary formulas, and as labeled supplements. A portion of all profits are returned to nonprofit rainforest organizations.

Toucan Chocolates
31 Wyman Street
Waban, MA 02168
(617) 964-8696

Boxed chocolates containing Brazil nuts and cashews. Colorful packaging is environmentally sensitive.

Walnut Acres
Penns Creek, PA 17862
(800) 433-3998

Two varieties of honey mixed together. The honey is gathered from wild beehives by rural cooperatives in Zambia and Tanzania. Available in bulk wholesale or retail.

Ward's Pond Farm
RFD 3, Box 1380
Morrisville, VT 05661
(802) 888-3001

Quality fancy Brazilian cashew pieces prepared with maple syrup and sea salt. Smoked or roasted.

Nonprofit Rainforest Organizations

Amazon Center for Environmental Education and Research (ACEER)
Ten Environs Park
Helena, AL 35080
(800) 255-8206
A nonprofit organization committed to rainforest conservation through education and research.

APECA
12 South Main Street, Suite 302
West Hartford, CT 06107
(860) 232-6971
Internet: http://www.apeca.org
APECA (Association Promoting Education and Conservation of the Amazon) is a nonprofit organization dedicated to the conservation of the Peruvian Amazon rainforest, its native peoples, and their cultures. Founded in 1993, APECA began as a floating health clinic, delivering medical services to the remote Amazon River villages of Loreto, Peru. Since then, APECA has established programs in health education, nutrition, natural medicine, and sanitation.

Center for World Indigenous Studies
PO Box 2574
Olympia, WA 98507-2574
Fax: (360) 956-1087
Internet: http://www.halcyon.com/FWDP/cwisinfo.html
An independent, nonprofit research and education organization dedicated to wider understanding and appreciation of the ideas and knowledge of indigenous peoples. The center fosters better understanding between peoples through the publication and distribution of literature written and voiced by leading contributors from fourth-world nations. The center gathers and stores information and makes it internationally accessible through a computerized "Fourth World Documentation Project" on the Internet.

Conservation International
1015 18th Street, NW
Suite 1000
Washington, DC 20036
(202) 429-5660
Internet: http://www.conservation.org/ciap.htm

A nonprofit organization using science, economics, policy, and community involvement to promote biodiversity conservation in rainforests and other endangered ecosystems worldwide.

The Rainforest Action Network
301 Broadway, Suite A
San Francisco, CA 94133
Internet: http://www.ran.org

A nonprofit organization working to protect the Earth's rainforests and support the rights of their inhabitants through education, grassroots organizing, and nonviolent direct action.

Rainforest Conservation Fund
2038 Borth Carl, Suite 233
Chicago, IL 60614
(312) 975-7571

Nonprofit organization with various projects in the Amazon region supporting indigenous tribes and providing education and funds to help tribes harvest, market, and provide new tribal income by sustainably harvesting rainforest plants, fruits, and nuts.

Rainforest Preservation Foundation
PO Box 820308
Ft. Worth, TX 76182
(817) 222-1155

Nonprofit foundation that buys endangered rainforest land in Brazil and places it in a trust. Provides land deed certificates to those donating funds showing the amount of land purchased with their donation.

Notes

PART 1

1. The World Wide Fund for Nature, September 1997.
2. Astor, Michael. "Brazil quiet as evidence of Amazon's demise mounts." Associated Press (December 15, 1997).
3. "1997 was the year the world caught fire, says WWF." Agence France-Presse (December 16, 1997).
4. "Deforestation rates in tropical forests and their climatic implications." World Wide Fund for Nature, 1997 Annual Report.

ABUTA

1. Bruneton, Jean. *Pharmaognosy, Phytochemistry, Medicinal Plants.* Andover, England: Intercept Limited, 1995.
2. Werbach, Melvyn R., M.D., and Michael T. Murray, N.D. *Botanical Influences on Illness—A Sourcebook of Clinical Research.* Tarzana, CA: Third Line Press, 1994.
3. Blumenthal, Mark. "Plant medicines from the New World." *Whole Foods Magazine* (April 1997).
4. Kametani, T., M. Ihara, and T. Honda. *Heterocycles* 4 (1976): 483.
5. Guinaudeau, H., M. Leboeuf, and A. Cave. *Lloydia* 38 (1975): 275.
6. Marini-Bettolo, G. B. Acad. *Geneeskund.* Belg. 43 (1981): 185 (C.A. 96:129624t).
7. Anwer, F., et al. "Studies in medicinal plants 3. Protoberberine alkaloids from the roots of *Cissampelos pareira Linn.*" Experientia (October 15, 1968).
8. Bhatnagar, A. K., et al. "Chemical examination of the roots of *Cissampelos pareira Linn.* V. Structure and stereochemistry of hayatidin." *Experientia* (April 15, 1967).
9. Bhatnagar, A.K., et al. "Chemical examination of the roots of *Cissampelos pareira Linn.* IV. Structure and stereochemistry of hayatin." *J. Org. Chem.* (March 1967).
10. Kupchan, S. M., et al. "Tumor inhibitors. VI. Cissampareine, new cytotoxic alkaloid from *Cissampelos pareira.* Cytotoxicity of bisbenzylisoquinoline alkaloids." *J. Pharm. Sci.* (April 1965).
11. Basu, D. K. "Studies on curariform activity of hayatinin methochloride, an alkaloid of *Cissampelos pareira.*" *Jpn. J. Pharmacol.* (June 1970).
12. Kondo, Y., et al. "Inhibitory effect of bisbenzylisoquinoline alkaloids on nitric oxide production in activated macrophages." *Biochem. Pharmacol.* 46 (1993): 1887–92.

261

13. Morita, H., et al. "Conformation of tropolone ring in antileukemic tropoloiso-quinoline." *Chem. Pharm. Bull.* (Tokyo) 41, 8 (August 1993): 1478–80.

14. Morita, H., et al. "Structures and solid state tautomeric forms of two novel an-tileukemic tropoloisoquinoline alkaloids, pareirubrines A and B, from *Cissampelos pareira*." *Chem. Pharm. Bull.* (Tokyo) 41, 8 (August 1993): 418–22.

ACEROLA

1. Berry, R. E., et al. *Food. Prod. Dev.* 14 (1977): 109.

2. Nakasobem, H. Y., et al. *Proc. Am. Soc. Hort. Sci.* 89 (1966): 161.

3. Leme, J. Jr., et al. "Variation of ascorbic acid and beta-carotene content in lyophilized cherry from the West Indies (*Malpighia punicifolia* L.)." *Arch. Latinoam. Nutr.* (June 1973).

4. Medeiros, R. B. de. "Proportion of ascorbic, dehydroascorbic and diketogulonic acids in green or ripe acerola (*Malpighia punicifolia*)." *Rev. Bras. Med.* (July 1969).

5. Caceres, A. "Plants used in Guatemala for the treatment of dermatophytic infec-tions 2. Evaluation of antifungal activity of seven American plants." *J. Ethno-pharmacol.* 40 (1993): 3.

ALCACHOFRA

1. Monograph: Artichoke. *The Lawrence Review of Natural Products* (November 1992). St. Louis, MO: Facts and Comparisons, Inc.

2. Hammouda, R. M., et al. "HPLC evaluation of the active constituents in the newly introduced Romanian strain of *Cynara scolymus* culivate in Egypt." *Planta Medica* 57, suppl. 2 (1991): A119.

3. Puigmacia, M., et al. "Spectroscopic study of caffeolyquinic acid derivatives of *Cynara colymus*." *Planta Medica* 52 (1986): 529.

4. Dranik, L. I. "Quantitative analysis of cynarin in the leaves of the artichoke (*Cynara scolymus* L.)." *Farm. Zh.* (1965).

5. Nichiforesco, E., et al. "On the determination of o-dihydrophenols of caffeic acid type present in artichoke leaves (*Cynara scolymus* L.)." *Ann. Pharm. Fr.* (June 1965).

6. Stary, Frantisek. *The Natural Guide to Medicinal Herbs and Plants.* New York: Dorset Press, 1992.

7. Bianchini, F. *Health Plants of the World.* Milan: Arnoldo Mondadori Editore, 1975.

8. Mowrey, Daniel. *Herbal Tonic Therapies.* USA: Keats Publishing, 1993.

9. Hammouda, F. M., et al. "Flavonoids of *Cynara scolymus* L. cultivated in Egypt." *Plant Foods Hum. Nutr.* (1993).

10. Bartram, Thomas. *Encyclopedia of Herbal Medicine.* Dorset, England: 1995.

11. Sayed, M.D. "Traditional medicine in health care." *J. Ethnopharmacol.* (March 1980).

12. Ruppelt, B. M., et al. "Pharmacological screening of plants recommended by folk medicine as anti-snake venom—I. Analgesic and anti-inflammatory activities." *Mem. Inst. Oswaldo Cruz* (1991).

13. Khalkova, Zh., et al. "An experimental study of the effect of an artichoke prepara-tion on the activity of the sympathetic-adrenal system in carbon disulfide expo-sure." *Probl. Khig.* (1995).

14. Adzet, T., et al. "Hepatoprotective activity of polyphenolic compounds from *Cynara scolymus* against CCl4 toxicity in isolated rat hepatocytes." *J. Nat. Prod.* (July–August 1987).

15. Hinou, J., et al. "Polyphenolic substances of *Cynara scolymus* L. leaves." *Ann. Pharm. Fr.* (1989).

16. Bogaert, J. P., et al. "Organic acids, principally acid-alcohols, in *Cynara scolymus* L. (Compositae)." *Ann. Pharm. Fr.* (June 1972).

17. Maros, T., et al. "Effects of *Cynara scolymus* extracts on the regeneration of rat liver. 2." *Arzneimittel Forschung* (July 1968); T. Maros, et al. "Effects of *Cynara scolymus* extracts on the regeneration of rat liver. 1." *Arzneimittel Forschung* (February 1966).

18. Nichiforesco, E. "Considerations on the stability of o-dihydroxyphenolic derivatives of artichoke leaves (*Cynara scolymus* L.)." *Ann. Pharm. Fr.* (April 1967).

AMOR SECO

1. Brandao, M., et al. "Survey of medicinal plants used as antimalarials in the Amazon." *J. Ethnopharmacol.* 36, 2 (1992): 175–82.

2. Coee, F., et al. "Ethnobotany of the Garifuna of eastern Nicaragua." *Econ. Bot.* 50, 1 (1996): 1–107.

3. Boye, G. and O. Ampopo. "Plants and traditional medicine in Ghana." *Economic and Medicinal Plant Research* 4 (1990): 33–34. Devon, England: Academic Press Ltd., 1990.

4. Ampopo, O. "Plants that heal." *World Health 1977* (1977): 26–30.

5. Addy, M. E., et al. "Effects of the extracts of *Desmodium adscendens* on anaphylaxis." *J. Ethnopharmacol.* 11, 3 (1984): 283–92.

6. Addy, M. E., et al. "Effect of *Desmodium adscendens* fraction F1 (DAFL) on tone and agonist-induced contractions of guinea pig airway smooth muscle." *Phytother Res* 3, 3 (1989): 85–90.

7. Addy, M. E., et al. "Effect of *Desmodium adscendens* fractions on antigen- and arachidonic acid-induced contractions of guinea pig airways." *Can. J. Physiol. Pharmacol.* 66, 6 (1987): 820–25.

8. Addy, M. E., et al. "Dose-response effect of one subfraction of Desmodium adscendens aqueous extract on antigen- and arachidonic acid-induced contractions of guinea pig airways." *Phytother. Res.* 1, 4 (1987): 180–86.

9. Addy, M. E., et al. "Effect of *Desmodium adscendens* fraction 3 on contractions of respiratory smooth muscle." *J. Ethnopharmacol.* 29, 3 (1990): 325–35.

10. Addy, M. E., et al. "Dose-response effects of *Desmodium adscendens* aqueous extract on histamine response, content and anaphylactic reactions in the guinea pig." *J. Ethnopharmacol.* 18, 1 (1996): 13–20.

11. Addy, M. E., et al. "Several chromatographically distinct fractions of Desmodium adscendens inhibit smooth muscle contractions." *Int. J. Crude Drug Res.* 27, 2 (1989): 81–91.

12. Addy, M. E., et al. "An extract of *Desmodium adscendens* activates cyclooxygenase and increases prostaglandin synthesis by ram seminal vesicle microsomes." *Phytother. Res.* 9, 4 (1995): 287–93.

13. Addy, M. E., et al. "Some secondary plant metabolites in *Desmodium adscendens* and their effects on arachidonic acid metabolism." *Prostaglandins Leukotrienes Essent. Fatty Acids* 47, 1 (1992): 85–91.

ANDIROBA

1. Pereira Pinto, G. "O oleo de andiroba." In *Boletin Tecnico* (Instituto Agronomico Norte) 31 (1956): 119.

2. Soukup, J. *Vocabulary of the Common Names of the Peruvian Flora and Catalog of the Genera.* Lima: Editorial Salesiano, 1970, 436.

3. Hammer, M. L., et al. "Tapping an Amazonian plethora: four medicinal plants of Marajó Island, Pará (Brazil)." *J. Ethnopharmacol.* (September 1993).

4. Ollis, W., et al. In *Tetrahedron* 26 (1970): 1637.

5. Lavie, D., et al. In *Bioorganic Chemistry* 2 (1972): 59.
6. Marcelle, G. B., et al. In *Phytochemistry* 14 (1975): 2717.
7. Correa, Pio. *Dicionario de Plantas Uteis do Brasil e Exoticas Cultivadas,* vols. 1–6. Brasilia: IBDF, 1984.
8. Morton, J. F. *Atlas of Medicinal Plants of Middle America, Bahamas to Yucatan.* Springfield, IL: C. Thomas, 1981.

ANNATTO

1. Heinerman, John. *Heinerman's Encyclopedia of Healing Herbs & Spices.* New York: Parber Publishing Co., 1996.
2. Ohasi, E. Y., et al. *Urucu. Uma opcao para o Estado do Para.* Belem: Secretaria de Estado de Agricultura, Boletim informative, No. 6, 1982, 25 pages.
3. Matos, F. J. *Cienc. E Cult.* 39 (7) Supl. (1987): 533.
4. Bressani, R., et al. "Chemical composition, amino acid content and nutritive value of the protein of the annatto seed (*Bixa orellana,* L.)." *Arch. Latinoam Nutr.* 33 (2) (June 1983): 356–76.
5. Angelucci, E., et al. *Ital. Capinas* 11 (1980): 89–96.
6. Morrison, E. Y., et al. "Extraction of an hyperglycaemic principle from the annatto (*Bixa orellana*), a medicinal plant in the West Indies." *Trop. Geogr. Med.* (January–April 1991).
7. Morrison, E. Y., et al. "Toxicity of the hyperglycaemic-inducing extract of the annatto (*Bixa orellana*) in the dog." *West Indian Med. J.* (June 1987).
8. Morrison, E. Y., et al. "The effect of *Bixa orellana* (annatto) on blood sugar levels in the anaesthetized dog." *West Indian Med. J.* (March 1985).
9. Lawrence, B. M. and J. W. Hogg. *Phytochemistry* 12 (1973): 2295.
10. Scita, G. "Retinoic acid and beta-carotene inhibit fibronectin synthesis and release by fibroblasts; antagonism to phorbol ester." *Carcinogenesis* 15 (1994): 1043–48.
11. Zhang, L. X. "Carotenoids up-regulate connexin43 gene expression independent of their provitanin A or antioxidant properties." *Cancer Res.* 52 (1992): 5707–12.
12. Di Mascio, P. "Carotenoids, tocopherols and thiols as biological singlet molecular oxygen quenchers." *Biochem. Soc. Trans.* 18 (1990): 1054–6.
13. Hirose, S. "Energized state of mitochondria as revealed by the spectral change of bound bixin." *Arch. Biochem. Biophys.* 152 (1972): 36–43.
14. Inada, Y. "Spectral changes of bixin upon interaction with respiring rat liver mitochondria." *Arch. Biochem. Biophys.* 146 (1971): 366–7.
15. Campelo, C. R. "Contribuicao ao estudo das plantas medicinais no estado de alagoas III, VII." Simposio de Plantas Medicinais do Brasil, 1–3 de Setembro, 1982, Belo Horizonte-MG, 85m.
16. Terashima S., et al. "Studies on aldose reductase inhibitors from natural products. IV. Constituents and aldose reductase inhibitory effect of *Chrysanthemum morifolium, Bixa orellana and Ipomoea batatas.*" *Chem. Pharm. Bull.* (Tokyo) (December 1991).
17. Cáceres A., et al. "Antigonorrhoeal activity of plants used in Guatemala for the treatment of sexually transmitted diseases." *J. Ethnopharmacol.* (October 1995).

BALSAM OF TOLU, BALSAM OF PERU

1. Blumenthal, Mark. "Plant medicines from the New World." *Whole Foods* (March 1997), 114.
2. Lloyd, J. U. *Origin and History of all the Pharmacopeial Vegetable Drugs.* Cincinnati: Caxton Press, 1929.

3. Morton, J. F. *Major Medicinal Plants: Botany, Culture and Uses.* Springfield, IL: Charles C. Thomas, 1997.

4. Monograph: Balsamum peruvianum. *Bundesanzeiger* 173 (September 18, 1986).

BOLDO

1. Schindler, H. Arzneim. *Forsch.* 7 (1957): 747.

2. Bombardelli, E., et al. *Fitoterapia* 47 (1976): 3.

3. Monograph: Boldo folium. *Bundesanzeiger* 76 (April 23, 1987).

4. Monograph: Boldo. *The Lawrence Review of Natural Products* (May 1991). St Louis, MO: Facts and Comparisons, Inc.

5. Rueggett, A. *Helv. Chim. Acta.* 42 (1959): 754.

6. Hansel, R. *Phytopharmaka*, 2d ed. Berlin: Springer-Verlag, 1991, 186–91.

7. Hughes, D. W., et al. "Alkaloids of *Peumus boldus.* Isolation of (+) reticuline and isoboldine." *J. Pharm. Sci.* 57 (June 1968): 1023.

8. Hughes, D. W., et al. "Alkaloids of *Peumus boldus.* Isolation of laurotetanine and laurolitsine." *J. Pharm. Sci.* (September 1968).

9. Vanhaelen, M. 1973. "Spectrophotometric microdetermination of alkaloids in *Peumus boldus.*" *J. Pharm. Belg.* (May–June 1973).

10. Lanhers, M. C., et al. "Hepatoprotective and anti-inflammatory effects of a traditional medicinal plant of Chile, *Peumus boldus.*" *Planta Med.* (April 1991).

11. Lévy-Appert-Collin, M. C., et al. "Galenic preparations from *Peumus boldus* leaves (Monimiacea)." *J. Pharm. Belg.* (January–February 1977).

12. Backhouse N., et al. "Anti-inflammatory and antipyretic effects of boldine." *Agents Actions* (October 1994).

13. Krug, H., et al. "New flavonol glycosides from the leaves of *Peumus boldus* Molina." *Pharmazie* (Novemeber 1965).

14. Speisky, H, et al. "Boldo and boldine: an emerging case of natural drug development." *Pharmacol. Res.* (January–February, 1994).

15. Tavares, D. C., et al. "Evaluation of the genotoxic potential of the alkaloid boldine in mammalian cell systems in vitro and in vivo." *Mutat. Res.* (May 1994).

16. Hirosue, T., et al. *Chem. Abstr.* 109 229018d (1988).

17. Gotteland, M., et al. "Effect of a dry boldo extract on oro-cecal intestinal transit in healthy volunteers." *Rev. Med. Chil.* 123: 955–60 (1995).

BRAZILIAN PEPPERTREE

1. Kramer, F. L. "The pepper tree *Schinus molle.*" *Econ. Bot.* 11 (1957): 322–26.

2. Yelasco-Negueruela, A. "Medicinal plants from Pampallakta: an Andean community in Cuzco (Peru)." *Fitoterapia* 66, 5 (1995): 447–62.

3. Bhat, R. B., et al.. "Traditional herbal medicine in Transkei." *J. Ethnopharmacol.* 48 1(1995): 7–12 .

4. Burkill, I. H. *Dictionary of the Economic Products of the Malay Peninsula*, vol. 2. Ministry of Agriculture and Cooperatives, Kuala Lumpur, Malaysia, 1966.

5. Elisabetsky, E., et al. "Traditional Amazonian nerve tonics as antidepressant agents: chaunochiton kappleri: a case study." *J. Herbs Spices Med Plants* 1 1/2 (1992): 125–62.

6. Gonzalez, F., et al. "A survey of plants with antifertility properties described in the South American folk medicine." *Abstr. Princess Congress* I, Bangkok, Thailand, December 10–13, 1987, 20 pages.

7. Perez, C., et al. "Inhibition of pseudomonas aerguinosa by argentinean medicinal plants." *Fitoterapia* 65, 2 (1994): 169–72.

8. Terhune, S., et al. "B-spathulene: a new sesquiterpene in *Schinus molle* oil." *Phytochemistry* 13 (1973): 865.

9. Dominguez, X., et al. "A chemical survey of seventeen medicinal Mexican plants." *Planta Med.* 18 (1970): 51.

10. Pozzo-Balbi, T., et al. "The triterpenoid acids of *Schinus molle*." *Phytochemistry* 17 (1978): 2107–10.

11. Dikshit, A. "*Schinus molle:* a new source of natural fungitoxicant." *Appl. Environ. Microbiol.* 51, 5 (1986): 1085–88.

12. L-Keltawi, N. et al. "Antimicrobial activity of some Egyptian aromatic plants." *Herba Pol.* 26, 4 (1980): 245–50.

13. Gundidza, M., et al. "Antimicrobial activity of essential oil from *Schinus molle* Linn." *Central African J. Med.* 39, 11 (1993): 231–34.

14. Ross, S., et al. "Antimicrobial activity of some Egyptian aromatic plants." *Fitoterapia* 51 (1980): 201–5.

15. Simons, J., et al. "Succulent-type as sources of plant virus inhibitors." *Phytopathology* 53 (1963): 677–83.

16. Bhakuni, D., et al. "Screening of Chilean plants for anticancer activity. I." *Lloydia* 39, 4 (1976): 225–43.

17. Bello, R. et al. "Effects on arterial blood pressure of the methanol and dichloromethanol extracts from *Schinus molle* L. in rats." *Phytother. Res.* 10, 7 (1996): 634–35.

18. Zaidi, S. et al. "Some preliminary studies of the pharmacological activities of *Schinus molle*." *Pak. J. Sci. Ind. Res.* 13 (1970): 53.

19. Moreno, M. "Action of several popular medicaments on the isolated uterus." *C R Seances Soc. Biol. Ses. Fil.* 87 (1922): 563–64.

20. Barrachina, M. "Analgesic and central depressor effects of the dichloromethanol extract from *Schinus molle* L." *Phytother. Res.* 11, 4 (1997): 317–19.

21. Bello, R., et al. "Effects on arterial blood pressure of the methanol and dichloromethanol extracts from *Schimus molle* L. in rats." *Phytother. Res.* 10, 7 (1996): 634–35.

22. Wimalaratne, P., et al. "Isolation and identification of house fly, *Musca domestica* L., repellents from pepper tree, *Schinus molle* L." *J. Chem. Ecol.* 22, 1 (1996): 49–59.

BRAZIL NUT

1. Schultes, R. E. "Gifts of the Amazon flora to the world." *Arnoldia* 50, 2 (1990): 21–34.

2. Smith, Nigel, J. Williams, Donald Plucknett, and Jennifer Talbot. *Tropical Forests and Their Crops.* New York: Comstock Publishing, 1992.

3. Chang, J. C., et al. "Selenium content of Brazil nuts from two geographic locations in Brazil." *Chemosphere* (February 1995).

4. Duke, J. A. *Handbook of Northeastern Indian Medicinal Plants.* Boston: Quarterman Publications, 1986.

5. Ip, C., et al. "Bioactivity of selenium from Brazil nut for cancer prevention and selenoenzyme maintenance." *Nutr. Cancer* (1994).

6. Ampe, C., et al. "The amino-acid sequence of the 2S sulfur-rich proteins from seeds of Brazil nut (*Bertholletia excelsa* H.B.K.)." *Eur. J. Biochem.* 159 (1986): 597–604.

7. Sun, S. S., et al. "Properties, biosynthesis and processing of a sulfur-rich protein in Brazil nut (*Bertholletia excelsa* H.B.K.)." *Eur. J. Biochem.* 162 (1987): 477–83.

8. Thorn, J., et al. 1978. "Trace nutrients. Selenium in British food." *Br. J. Nutr.* (March 1978).

CAJUEIRO

1. Mota, M. L., et al. "Anti-inflammatory actions of tannins isolated from the bark of *Anacardium occidentale* L." *J. Ethnopharmacol.* (July 1985).

2. Jurberg, P., et al. "Effect of Niclosamide (Bayluscide WP 70), *Anacardium occidentale* hexane extract and *Euphorbia splendens* latex on behavior of *Biomphalaria glabrata* (Say, 1818), under laboratory conditions." *Mem. Inst. Oswaldo Cruz* (March–April 1995).

3. Laurens, A., et al. "Molluscacidal activity of *Anacardium occidentale* L. (Anacardiaceae)." Ann. Pharm. Fr. (1987).

4. Mendes, N. M., et al. "Molluscacide activity of a mixture of 6-n-alkyl salicylic acids (anacardic acid) and 2 of its complexes with copper (II) and lead (II)." *Rev. Soc. Bras. Med. Trop.* (October–December 1990).

5. de Souza, C. P., et al. "The use of the shell of the cashew nut, *Anacardium occidentale,* as an alternative molluscacide." *Rev. Inst. Med. Trop.,* Sao Paulo, Brazil (September–October 1992).

6. Kubo, et al. "Tyrosinase inhibitors from *Anacardium occidentale* fruits." J. Nat. Prod. 57, 4 (April 1994): 545–51.

7. Laurens, A., et al. "Study of antimicrobial activity of *Anacardium occidentale* L." *Ann. Pharm. Fr.* (July 1982).

8. França, F., et al. "An evaluation of the effect of a bark extract from the cashew (*Anacardium occidentale* L.) on infection by Leishmania (Viannia) braziliensis." *Rev. Soc. Bras. Med. Trop.* (July–September 1993).

9. França. F., et al. "Plants used in the treatment of leishmanial ulcers due to Leishmania (Viannia) braziliensis in an endemic area of Bahia, Brazil." *Rev. Soc. Bras. Med.* Trop. 29, 3 (1996): 229–32.

CAMU-CAMU

1. Beckstrom-Sternberg, S., and J. A. Duke. *Ethnobotany and Phytochemical Databases,* U.S. Dept. of Agriculture, Agricultural Research Service, USDA.

CARQUEJA

1. Pavanm, A. G. "*Baccharis timera* (Carqueja amarga) uma planta da medicino popular brasileira." *Anais. Fac. Farm.* 10 (1952): 205.

2. Soicke, H., et al. "Characterisation of flavonoids from Bacchais trimera and their antihepatotoxic properties." *Planta Medica, Journal of Medicinal Plant Research* 1 (1986): 37–39.

3. Camargo, M. T. L. de A. *Medicina Popular.* Sao Paulo, Brazil: Almed Editora de Livaria, 1985.

4. Costa, A. F. *Farmacognosia,* vol. 2, 2d ed. Lisbon: Fundacai Calouste Gulbenkian, 1978, 1011–12.

5. Gamberini, M. T., et al. "Inhibition of gastric secretion by a water extract from *Baccharis triptera.*" Mart. Mem. Inst. Oswaldo Cruz 86, Suppl 2 (1991): 137–39.

6. Xavier, A. A., et al. "Effect of an extract of *Baccharis genistelloides* on the glucose level of the blood." *C R Seances Soc. Biol. Fil.* 161, 4 (1967): 972–74.

7. Herz, W., et al. "New ent-clerodane-type diterpenoids from *Baccharis trimera.*" *J. Org. Chem.* 42, 24 (November 25, 1977): 3913–17.

8. Sosa, M. E., et al. 1994. "Insect antifeedant activity of clerodane diterpenoids." *J. Nat. Prod.* 57, 9 (September 1994): 1262–65.

9. Fullas, F., *et al.* "Cytotoxic constituents of *Baccharis gaudichaudiana.*" *J. Nat. Prod.* 57, 6 (1994): 8017.

10. Gene, R. M., et al. "Anti-inflammatory and analgesic activity of *Baccharis trimera:* identification of its active constituents." *Planta Med.* 62, 3 (June 1996): 232–35.

CAT'S CLAW

1. Ocampo, T. Palmiro, ed. *Uncaria tomentosa, Aspectos Ethnomedicos, Medicos, Farmacologicos, Botanicos, Agronomicos, Comerciales, Legales, Anthropologicos, Sociales y Politicos.* Lima: Instituto de Desarrollo Rural Peruano (IDDERP), 1994, 74.

2. ACPC. "Uña de Gato Asháninka." Lima: Association for the Conservation of the Patimony of Cutivireni, undated, 4 pages.

3. Jones, Kenneth. *Cat's Claw: Healing Vine of Peru.* Seattle: Sylvan Press, 1995, 180.

4. Cabieses, Fernando. *The Saga of the Cat's Claw.* Lima: Via Lactera Editores, 1994.

5. Krallendorn®, *Uncaria tomentosa* (Willd.) DC Root Extract. Information for *Physicians, and Dispensing Chemists,* 3d rev. ed. Volders, Austria: Immodal Pharmaka GmbH, September 1995, 20 pages.

6. Keplinger, U. M. "Einfluss von Krallendorn extract auf Retrovirale Infektioned," *Zurcher AIDS Kongress.* Zurich, Switzerland, October 16 and 17, 1992, program and abstracts.

7. Keplinger, U. M., "Therapy of HIV-infected individuals in the pathological categories CDC Al and CDC B2 with a preparation containing IMM-207," IV. *Osterreicbiicher AIDS-Kongress,* Vienna, Austria, September 17 and 18, 1993, abstracts: 45.

8. Keplinger, H., et al. "Oxindole Alkaloids Having Properties Stimulating the Immunologic System and Preparation Containing Same." United States Patent 5,302,611, April 12, 1994.

9. Keplinger, H., et al. "Oxindole Alkaloids Having Properties Stimulating the Immunologic System and Preparation Containing the Same." United States Patent 4,940,725, July 10, 1990.

10. Keplinger, H., et al. "Oxindole Alkaloids Having Properties Stimulating the Immunologic System and Preparation Containing the Same." United States Patent 4,844,901, July 4, 1989.

11. Urbina, Humberto Ruiz. "Usos medicinales de la planta peruana 'uña de gato.'" Report presented at the Uña de Gato First International Congress, Geneva, Switzerland, May 30–31, 1994, 9 pages.

12. Montenegro De Matta, S., et al. "Alkaloids and procyanidins of an *Uncaria* sp. from Peru." *Il Farmaco. Ed. Sc.* 31 (1976): 527–35.

13. Ozaki, Y., et al. "Pharmacological studies on *Uncaria* and *Amsonia* alkaloids." *Japanese Journal of Pharmacology* (suppl.) 30 (1980): 137P.

14. Kreutzkamp, B. *Niedermolekulare Inhalstoffe mit Immunstimulierenden Eigenschaften aus Uncaria tomentosa, Okoubaka aubrevillei und anderen Drogen.* Dissertation of the faculty of chemistry and pharmacy of Ludwig Maximilians University, Munich, May 1984.

15. Stuppner, H., et al. "HPLC analysis of the main oxindole alkaloids from *Uncaria tomentosa.*" *Chromatographia* 34, 11/12 (1992): 597–600.

16. Wagner, H., et al. "Die Alkaloide von *Uncaria tomentosa* und ihre Phagozytosesteigernde Wirkung." *Planta Medica* 51 (1985): 419–23.

17. Keplinger, H. "Oxindole Alkaloids Having Properties Stimulating the Immunologic System and Preparation Containing Same," United States Patent 5,302,611, April 12, 1994.

18. Laus, G. and D. Keplinger. "Separation of sterioisomeric oxindole alkaloids from *Uncaria tomentosa* by high performance liquid chromatography." *Journal of Chromatography* A 662 (1994): 243–49.

19. Lavault, M., et al. "Alcaloides de l'*Uncaria guianensis.*" *Planta Medica* 47 (1983): 244–45.

20. Hemingway, S. R. and J. D. Phillipson. "Alkaloids from South American species of *Uncaria* (Rubiaceae)." *Journal of Pharmacy and Pharmacology* 26, suppl. (1974): 113P.

21. Raymond-Hamet, M. "Sur l'alcaloide principal d'une rubiacee des regions tropicales de l'Amerique de Sud: *l'Orouparia guianensis* Aubelt." *Comptes Rendus Hebdomadaires des Seances de l'Academie des Sciences* 235 (1952): 547–50.

22. Gotuzzo, E., et al. "En marcha seria investigacion: Uña de gato y pacientes con el VIH." *De Ciencia y Tecnologia* 34 (October 1993).

23. Inchaustegui and Gonzales, R. "Estudio preliminar sobre. CAS y SIDA." *Utilizando Plantas Medicinales, Anos 1989-1994, Hospital IPSS, Iquitos, Peru.* Iquitos, Peru: Hospital del Instituto Peruano de Seguridad Social Iquitos Comite ETS-SIDA, February 1993, 24 pages.

24. Stuppner, H., et al. "A differential sensitivity of oxindole alkaloids to normal and leukemic cell lines." *Planta Medica* 59, suppl. (1993): A583.

25. Peluso, G., et al. "Effetto antiproliferativo su cellule tumorali di estrattie metaboliti da *Uncaria tomentosa*. Studi in vitro sulla loro azione DNA polimerasi." 11 Congreso Italo-Peruano de Etnomedicina Andina, Lima, Peru, October 27–30, 1993, 21–2.

26. Rizzi, R., et al. "Mutagenic and antimutagenic activities of *Uncaria tomentosa* and its extracts." Première Colloque Européan d'Ethnopharmacologie, Metz, France, March 22–24, 1990.

27. Rizzi, R., et al. "Bacterial cytotoxicity, mutagenicity and antimutagenicity of *Uncaria tomentosa* and its extracts. Antimutagenic activity of *Uncaria tomentosa* in humans." Première Colloque Européan D'Ethnopharmacologie, Metz, France, March 22–24, 1990.

28. Rizzi, R., et al. "Mutagenic and antimutagenic activities of *Uncaria tomentosa* and its extracts." *Journal of Ethnopharmacology* 38 (1993): 63–77.

29. Yepez, A. M., et al. "Quinovic acid glycosides from *Uncaria guianensis*." *Phytochemisty* 30 (1991): 1635–37.

30. Aquino, R., et al. "Plant metabolites. New compounds and anti-inflammatory activity of *Uncaria tomentosa*." *Journal of Natural Products* 54 (1991): 453–59.

31. Aquino R., et al. "New polyhydroxylated triterpenes from *Uncaria tomentosa*." *Journal of Natural Products* (1990): 559–64.

32. Cerri, R., et al. "New quinovic acid glycosides from *Uncaria tomentosa*." *Journal of Natural Products* 51 (1988): 257–61.

33. Yasukawa, K., et al. "Effect of chemical constituents from plants on 12-0-tetradecanoylphorbol-13-acetate-induced inflammation in mice." *Chemical and Pharmaceutical Bulletin* 37 (1989): 1071–73.

34. Recio, M. C., et al. "Structural requirements for the anti--inflammatory activity of natural triterpenoids." *Planta Medica* 61, no. 2 (1995): 182–85.

35. De Simone, F., et al. "New quinovic acid glycosides from *Uncaria tomentosa*." *Journal of Natural Products* 51, no. 2 (March–April 1988): 257–61.

36. Senatore, A., et al. "Ricerche fitochimiche e biologiche sull *Uncaria tomentosa*." *Bollettino Societa di Biologia Sperimentale* 65 (1989): 517–20.

37. Fazzi, Marco A. Costa. *Evaluation de l'Uncaria tomentosa (Uña de Gato) en lan Prevencion de Ulceras Gastricas de Stress Producidas Experimentalmente en Rats.* Dissertation of the faculty of medicine, University Peruana Cayetano Heredia, Lima, Peru, 1989.

38. Aquino, R., et al. "Plant metabolites. Structure and *in vitro* antiviral activity of quinovic acid glycosides from *Uncaria tomentosa* and *Guettarda platypoda*." *Journal of Natural Products* 4, 52 (1989): 679–85.

Notes

39. Yano, S., et al. "Ca2, channel-blocking effects of hirsutine, an indole alkaloid from *Uncaria* genus, in the isolated rat aorta." *Planta Medica* 57 (1991): 403–5.

40. Chan-Xun, C., et al. "Inhibitory effect of rhynchophylline on platelet aggregation and thrombosis." *Acta Pharmacologica Sinica* 13,2 (1992): 126–30.

41. Jin, R. M., et al. "Effect of rhynchophylline on platelet aggregation and experimental thrombosis." *Acta Pharmacologica Sinica* 25 (1991): 246–49.

42. Monograph: Cat's Claw. *Lawrence Review of Natural Products* (April 1996).St. Louis, MO: Facts and Comparisons Inc.

43. Davis, Brent W. "A 'new' world-class herb for A.K. practice: *Uncaria tomentosa*—a.k.a. uña de gato (UDG)." Collected Papers of the International College of Applied Kinesiology (Summer 1992).

44. Whitaker, Julian. "Uña de Gato." *Health & Healing, Tomorrow's Medicine Today* 5, no. 5 (May 1995).

45. Steinberg, Phillip, 1994. "*Uncaria tomentosa* (cat's claw). A wondrous herb form the Peruvian rain forest." *Townsend Letter for Doctors* (May 1994): 442–43.

46. Jones, Kenneth. 1994. "The herb report: uña de gato, life-giving vine of Peru." *Am. Herb Assoc.* 10, 3 (1994): 4.

47. Urbina, Humberto Ruiz. *Experiencias con el Empleor de la Plantas* Uncaria tomentosa *o Uña de Gato en Clinica Veterinaria de Perros y Gatos*. Lima (May 1994), 11 pages.

CATUABA

1. Chian Sing. *Cura com Yoga e Plantas Medicinais*. Rio de Janeiro: Freitas Bastos, 1979.

2. Van Straten, Michael. *Guarana: The Energy Seeds and Herbs of the Amazon Rainforest*. U.S.: C. W. Daniel Company, Ltd. 1994.

3. Altman, R. F. A. "Presenca de ioimbina na catuaba, INPA." *Ser. Quim. Publ.* 1 (1958).

4. Maia, J. G., et al. *Estudos Integrados de Plantas da Amazonia*. V Simposio de Plantas Medicinais do Brasil, Sao Paulo, Brazil (September 6, 1978): 7.

5. Manabe, H., et al. "Effects of catuaba extracts on microbial and HIV infection." *In Vivo* 6, 2 (March–Apri 1992): 161–5.

CHANCA PIEDRA

1. Robineau, L., ed. *Towards a Caribbean Pharmacopoeia*. TRAMIL-4 Workshop, UNAH, Enda Caribe, Santo Domingo, 1991.

2. Jones, Kenneth. *Pau d'Arco: Immune Power from the Rain Forest*. Rochester, VT: Healing Arts Press, 1995, 54–8.

3. L. R., et al. *Tetrahedron* 22 (1966): 2899–2908.

4. Calixto J. B. "Antispasmodic effects of an alkaloid extracted from *Phyllanthus sellowianus:* a comparative study with papaverine." *Braz. J. Med. Biol Res.* 17, 3–4 (1984): 313–21.

5. Syamasundar, K. V. "Antihepatotoxic principles of *Phyllanthus niruri* herbs." *J. Ethnopharmacol.* 14, 1 (1985): 41–44.

6. Shimizu, M. "Studies on aldose reductase inhibitors from natural products. II. Active components of a Paraguayan crude drug, 'paraparai mi,' *Phyllanthus niruri*." *Chem. Pharm. Bull.* (Tokyo) 37, 9 (1989): 2531–32.

7. Ueno, H. "Chemical and pharmaceutical studies on medicinal plants in Paraguay. Geraniin, an angiotensin-converting enzyme inhibitor from 'paraparai mi,' *Phyllanthus niruri*." *J. Nat. Prod.* 51, 2 (1988): 357–59.

8. Santos, A. R. "Analgesic effects of callus culture extracts from selected species of *Phyllanthus* in mice." *J. Pharm. Pharmacol.* 46, 9 (1994): 755–59.

9. Santos, A. R. "Analysis of the mechanisms underlying the antinociceptive effect of the extracts of plants from the genus *Phyllanthus*." *Gen. Pharmacol.* 26, 7 (1995): 1499–1506.

10. Srividya, N. "Diuretic, hypotensive and hypoglycaemic effect of *Phyllanthus amarus*." *Indian J. Exp. Biol.* 33, 11(1995): 861–64.

11. Dixit, S. P. and M. P. Achar. *J. Natl. Integ. Med. Assoc.* 25, 8: 269 (1983).

12. Thyagarajan, S.P. "In vitro inactivation of HBsAg by *Eclipta alba* Hassk and *Phyllanthus niruri* Linn." *Indian J. Med. Res* 76 (1982): 124–30.

13. "Effects of an extract from *Phyllanthus niruri* on hepatitis B and woodchuck hepatitis viruses: in vitro and in vivo studies." *Proc. Natl. Acad. Sci.* USA 84, 1 (1987): 274–78.

14. Wang, M., et al. "Herbs of the genus *Phyllanthus* in the treatment of chronic hepatitis B: observations with three preparations from different geographic sites." *J. Lab. Clin. Med.* 126, (1995): 350–52.

15. Wang, M. X., et al. "Efficacy of *Phyllanthus* spp. in treating patients with chronic hepatitis B." *Chung Kuo Chung Yao Tsa Chih* 19, 12 (1994): 750–51.

16. Yeh, S. F., et al. "Effect of an extract from *Phyllanthus amarus* on hepatitis B surface antigen gene expression in human hepatoma cells." *Antiviral Research* 20 (1993): 185–92.

17. Mehrotra, R. "In vitro studies on the effect of certain natural products against hepatitis B virus." *Indian J. Med. Res* 92 (1990): 133–38.

18. Ogata, T. "HIV-1 reverse transcriptase inhibitor from *Phyllanthus niruri*." *AIDS Res Hum Retroviruses* 8, 11 (1992): 1937–44.

19. Qian-Cutrone, J. "Niruriside, a new HIV REV/RRE binding inhibitor from *Phyllanthus niruri*." *J. Nat. Prod.* 59, 2 (1996): 196–99.

CHUCHUHUASI

1. Kenneth Jones. *Cat's Claw: Healing Vine of Peru.* Toronto: Sylvan Press, 1995.

2. DiCarlo, F. J., et al. "Reticuloendothelial system stimulants of botanical origin." *Journal of the Reticuloendothelial Society* (1964): 224–32.

3. Martinod, P., et al. "Isolation of tingenone and pristimerin from *Maytenus chuchuhuasha*." *Phytochemistry* 15 (1976): 562–63.

4. Gonzalez Gonzalez, J., et al. "Chuchuhuasha--a drug used in folk medicine in the Amazonian and Andean areas. A chemical study of *Maytenus laevis*." *Journal of Ethnopharmacology* 5 (1982): 73–77.

5. Itokawa, H., et al. "Oligo-nicotinated sesquiterpene polyesters from *Maytenus ilicifolia*." *Journal of Natural Products* 56 (1993): 1479–85.

6. Sekar, Kumara V. S., et al. "Mayteine and 6-benzoyl-6-deacetyl-mayteine from *Maytenus krukovii*." *Planta Medica* 61 (1995): 390.

7. Bradshaw, D., et al. "Therapeutic potential of protein kinase C inhibitors." *Agents and Actions* 38 (1993): 135–47.

COPAIBA

1. Lueng, Albert and Steven Foster. *Encyclopedia of Common Natural Ingredients.* New York: Wiley and Sons, 1996.

2. Opdyke, D. L. *Food Cosmet. Toxicol.* 14 (Suppl.) (1976): 687.

3. Marussella, J. C. and N.A. Sicurella. *J. Am. Pharm. Assoc.* 49 (1960): 692.

4. Basile, A. C., et al. "Anti-inflammatory activity of oleoresin from Brazilian Copaifera." *J. Ethnopharmacol.* 22, 1 (January 1988): 101–9.

5. Opdyke, D. L. *Food Cosmet. Toxicol.* 11 (1973):1075.

6. Polhill, R. M. and R. H. Raven. *Proceedings of the International Legume Conference,* vol.2 , Kew, July 24–29, 1978, Royal Botanic Gardens, Kew, England (1981).

7. Monache, G. D., et al. *Tetrahedron Lett.* 8, 659 (1971).

8. Ferrari, M., et al. *Phytochemistry,* 10, 905 (1971).

9. Monache, F. D., et al. *Ann. Chim.* (Rome) 59, 539 (1969); through *Chem. Abstr.* 71, 124707w (1969).

10. Monache, F. D., et al. *Ann. Chim.* (Rome), 60, 233 (1970); through *Chem. Abstr.* 73, 25690v (1970).

11. Mahajan, J. R. and G. A. Ferreira. *Ann. Acad. Brasil. Cienc.,* 43, 611 (1971) through *Chem. Abstr.* 77,140339g (1972).

12. Del Nunzio, M. J. *Aerosol Cosmet.* 7, 41, 7 (1985); through *Chem. Abstr.* 104, 56164q (1986).

DAMIANA

1. "Damiana." *Lawrence Review of Natural Products* (July 1996). St Louis, MO: Facts and Comparisons Inc.

2. Steinmetz, E. F. *Acta Phytother.* 7, 1 (1960).

3. Domínguez. X. A. and M. Hinojosa. "Mexican medicinal plants. XXVIII. Isolation of 5-hydroxy-7,3',4'-trimethoxy-flavone from *Turnera diffusa*." *Planta Med.* 30, 1 (August 1976): 68–71.

ERVA TOSTÃO

1. Jain, S. P., et al. "Ethnomedicinal plants of Jaunsar-Bawar Hills, Uttar Pradesh, India." *J. Ethnopharmacol.* 12, 2 (1984): 213–22.

2. Anis, M., et al. "Medicinal plantlore of Aligarh, India." *Int. J. Pharmacog.* 32, 1 (1994): 59–64.

3. Arseculeratne, S. N., et al. "Studies on medicinal plants of Sri Lanka. Part 14: Toxicity of some traditional medicinal herbs." *J. Ethnopharmacol.* 13, 3 (1985): 323-35.

4. Agarwal, R. R. "Chemical examination of punarnava or *Boerhaavia diffusa* Linn." *Proc. Acad. Sci.* 4 (1934): 73–76.

5. Mudgal, V. "Studies on medicinal properties of *Convolvulus pluricaulis* and *Boerhaavia diffusa*." *Planta Med.* 28 (1975): 62.

6. Gaitonde, B. B., et al. "Diuretic activity of punarnava (*Boerhaavia diffusa*)." *Bull Haffkine Inst* 2 (1974): 24.

7. Chowdhury, A., et al. "*Boerhaavia diffusa*--effect on diuresis and some renal enzymes." *Ann. Biochem. Exp. Med.* 15 (1955): 119–26.

8. Singh, R. P., et al. "Recent approach in clinical and experimental evaluation of diuretic action of punarnava (*B. diffusa*) with special reference to nephrotic syndrome." *J. Res. Edu. Ind. Med.* 7, 1 (1955): 29–35 (1992).

9. Devi, M. V., et al. "Effect of *Phyllanthus niruri* on the diuretic activity of punarnava tablets." *J. Res. Edu. Ind. Med.* 5, 1 (1986): 11–12.

10. Mishra, J. P., et al. "Studies on the effect of indigenous drug *Boerhaavia diffusa* Rom. on kidney regeneration." *Indian J. Pharmacy* 12 (1980): 59.

11. Chandan, B. K., et al. "*Boerhaavia diffusa*: a study of its hepatoprotective activity." *J. Ethnopharmacol.* 31, 3 (1991): 299–307.

12. Ramabhimaiah, S., et al. "Pharmacological investigations on the water soluble fraction of methanol extract of *Boerhaavia diffusa* root." *Indian Drugs* 21, 8 (1984): 343–44.

13. Hansen, K., et al. "In vitro screening of traditional medicines for anti-hypertensive effect based on inhibition of the angiotensin converting enzyme (Ace)." *J. Ethnopharmacol.* 48, 1 (1995): 43–51.

14. Dhar, M., et al. "Screening of Indian plants for biological activity: Part I." *Indian J. Exp. Biol.* 6 (1968): 232–47.

15. Sohni, Y., et al. "The antiamoebic effect of a crude drug formulation of herbal extracts against *Entamoeba histolytica* in vitro and in vivo." *J. Ethnopharmacol.* 45, 1 (1995): 43–52.

16. Anonymous. "Antifertility studies on plants." *Indian Counc. Med. Res.-Ann. Rept. Director General* (1978): 63–64.

17. Adesina, S. "Anticonvulsant properties of the roots of *Boerhaavia diffusa*." *Q. J. Crude Drug Res.* 17 (1979): 84–86.

18. Akah, P., et al. "Nigerian plants with anti-convulsant property." *Fitoterapia* 64, 1 (1993): 42–44.

19. Olukoya, D., et al. "Antibacterial activity of some medicinal plants from Nigeria." *J. Ethnopharmacol.* 39, 1 (1993): 69–72.

20. Aynehchi, Y. "Screening of Iranian plants for antimicrobial activity." *Acta Pharm. Suecica.* 19, 4 (1982): 303–8.

21. Vijayalakshimi, K., et al. "Nematicidal properties of some indigenous plant materials against second stage juveniles of *Meloidogyne incognita* (Koffoid and White) chitwood." *Indian J. Entomol.* 41, 4 (1979): 326–31.

22. Verma, H., et al. 1979. "Antiviral activity of *Boerhaavia diffusa* root extract and physical properties of the virus inhibitor." *Can. J. Bot.* 57 (1979): 926–32.

ESPINHEIRA SANTA

1. Flemming, K. "Increase of phagocytosis activity by *Maytenus laevis* leaves and Scholler-Tornesch lignine (Porlisan)." *Naturwissenschaften* (June 1965).

2. Hartwell, J. L. "Plants used against cancer: a survey." *Lloydia* 31 (1968): 114.

3. Lima, O. G. de, et al. "Substabcias antimicrobiano de plantas superiores. Comunicacao XXXI. Maitenina, novo antimicrobiano con acao antineoplastica, isolade de celastracea de pernambuco." *Revista do Instituto de Antibioticos (Recife)* 9 (1969): 17–25.

4. Lima, O. G. de, et al. "Antimicrobial substances from higher plants. XXXVI. On the presence of maytenin and pristimerine in the cortical part of the roots of *Maytenus ilicifolia* from the south of Brazil." *Revista do Instituto de Antibioticos (Recife)* (June 1971).

5. Monache, F. D., et al. "Maitenin: a new antitumoral substance from *Maytenus* sp." *Gazetta Chimica Italiana* 102 (1972): 317–20.

6. Wolpert-Defillipes, M. K., et al. "Initial studies on the cytotoxic action of maytansine, a novel ansa macrolide." *Biochemical Pharmacology* 24 (1975): 751–54.

7. Spjut, R. J. and R. E. Perdue, Jr. "Plant folklore: a tool for predicting sources of antitumor activity?" *Cancer Treatment Reports* 60 (1976): 979–85.

8. de Santana, C. F., et al. "Primeiras observacoes sobre o emprego da maitenina em pacientes cancerosos." *Revista do Instituto de Antibioticos (Recife)* 11 (1971): 37–49.

9. Melo, A. M., et al. "First observations on the topical use of primin, plumbagin and maytenin in patients with skin cancer." *Revista do Instituto de Antibioticos (Recife)* (December 1974).

10. F. Cabanillas, et al. "Phase I study of maytansine using a 3-day schedule." *Cancer Treatment Reports* 60 (1976): 1127–39.
11. Chabner, B. A., et al. "Initial clinical trials of mayansine, an antitumor plant alkaloid." *Cancer Treatment Reports* 62 (1978): 429–33.
12. O'Connell, M. J., et al. "Phase II trial of maytansine in patients with advanced colorectal carcinoma." *Cancer Treatment Reports* 62 (1978): 1237–38.
13. Suffnes, M. J., et al. "Current status of the NCI plant and animal product program." *Journal of Natural Products* 45 (1982): 1–14.
14. Crovetto, Paul Martinez. "Las plantas utilizadas en medicina popular en el noroeste de corrientes." *Miscelanea* 69. Tucuman, Argentina: Ministeris de Cultura y Educacion, Foundacion Miguel Lillo, 1981, 69.
15. Jones, Kenneth. *Pau d'Arco Immune Power from the Rainforest*. Rochester, VT: Healing Arts Press, 1995, 63.
16. Freise, F. W. "Plantas medicinais Brasileiras." *Boletim de Agricultura* 34 (1933): 410.
17. Souza-Formigoni, M. L., et al. "Antiulcerogenic effects of two *Maytenus* species in laboratory animals." *J. Ethnopharmacol.* (August 1991).
18. Oliveira, M. G., et al. "Pharmacologic and toxicologic effects of two *Maytenus* species in laboratory animals." *J. Ethnopharmacol.* (August 1991).
19. Shirota, O., et al. "Cytotoxic aromatic triterpenes from *Maytenus ilicifolia* and *Maytenus chuchuhuasca.*" *J. Nat. Prod.* (December 1994).

FEDEGOSO

1. Dennis, P. A. "Herbal medicine among the Miskito of eastern Nicaragua." *Econ. Bot.* 42, 1 (1988): 16–28.
2. Gupta, M. P., et al. "Ethnopharmacognostic observations on Panamanian medicinal plants. Part I." *Q. J. Crude Drug Res.* 17 3/4 (1979): 115–30.
3. Nagaraju, N., et al. "A survey of plant crude drugs of Rayalaseema, Andhra Pradesh, India." *J. Ethnopharmacol.* 29, 2 (1990): 137–58.
4. Bardhan, P., et al. "In vitro effect of an ayurvedic liver remedy on hepatic enzymes in carbon tetrachloride treated rats." *Indian J. Med.* Res. 82, 4 (1985): 359–64.
5. Elujoba, A., et.al, 1989. "Chemical and biological analyses of Nigerian *Cassia* species for laxative activity." *J. Pharm. Biomed. Anal.* 7, 12 (1989): 1453–57.
6. Gasquet, M., et al. "Evaluation in vitro and in vivo of a traditional antimalarial, 'Malarial 5.'" *Fitoterapia* 64, 5 (1993): 423.
7. Schmeda-Hirschmann, G., et al. "A screening method for natural products on triatomine bugs." *Phytother. Res.* 6, 2 (1989): 68–73.
8. Hussain, H., et al. "Plants in Kano ethomedicine: screening for antimicrobial activity and alkaloids." *Int. J. Pharmacog.* 29, 1 (1991): 51–6.
9. Caceres, A., et al. "Plants used in Guatemala for the treatment of dermatophytic infections. 1. Screening for antimycotic activity of 44 plant extracts." *J. Ethnopharmacol.* 31, 3 (1991): 263–76.
10. Saraf, S., et al. Antiheptatotoxic Activity of *Cassia occidentalis. Int. J. Pharmacog.* 32, 2 (1994): 178–83.
11. Sadique, J., et al. "Biochemical modes of action of *Cassia occidentalis* and *Cardiospermum halicacabum* in inflammation." *J. Ethnopharmacol.* 19, 2 (1987): 201–12.
12. Feng, P., et al. "Pharmacological screening of some West Indian medicinal plants." *J. Pharm. Pharmacol.* 14 (1962): 556–61.
13. Patney, N., et al. 1978. "A preliminary report on the role of liv-52, an indigenous drug, in serum B hepatitis (Australia antigen positive) cases." *Probe* 17, 2 (1978): 132–142.

14. Sama, S., et al. "Efficacy of an indigenous compound preparation (liv-52) in acute viral hepatitis—a double blind study." *Indian J. Med. Res.* 64 (1976): 738.
15. Sethi, J., et al. 1978. "Clinical management of severe acute hepatic failure with special reference to liv-52 in therapy." *Probe* 17, 2 (1978): 155–58.

GERVÃO

1. Robinson, R. D., et al. "Investigations of *Strongyloides stercoralis* filariform larvae in vitro by six commercial Jamaican plant extracts and tree anthelmintics." *West Indian Med. J.* 39, 4 (1990): 213–17.
2. Ayensu, E. S. *Medicinal Plants of the West Indies.* Unpublished manuscript, 110 pages. Washington, D.C.: Smithsonian Institution, Office of Biological Conservation, 1978.
3. Dragendorff, G. *Die Heilpflanzen der Verschiedenen Volker und Zeiten.* Stuttgart: F. Enke, 1898, 885 pages.
4. Asprey, G. F. and P. Thornton. "Medicinal plants of Jamaica. IV." *West Indian Med. J.* 4 (1955): 145–65.
5. Wong, W. "Some folk medicinal plants from Trinidad." *Econ. Bot.* 30 (1976): 103–42.
6. Simpson, G. E. "Folk medicine in Trinidad." *J Amer Folklore* 75 (1962): 326–40.
7. Subramanian, S. S., et al. "Chemical examination of the leaves of *Stachytarpheta indica*." *Indian J Pharm* 36 (1974): 15.
8. Feng, P. C., et al. "Pharmacological screening of some West Indian medicinal plants." *J. Pharm. Pharmacol.* 16 (1962): 115.
9. Robinson, R. D., et al. "Inactivation of *Strongyloides stercoralis* filariform larvae in vitro by six Jamaican plant extracts and three commercial anthelmintics." *West Indian Med. J.* 39, 4 (December 1990): 213–17.
10. Almeida, C. E., et al. "Analysis of antidiarrhoeic effect of plants used in popular medicine." *Rev. Saude Publica.* 29, 6 (December 1, 1995): 428–33.
11. Vela, S. M., et al. "Inhibition of gastric acid secretion by the aqueous extract and purified extracts of *Stachytarpheta cayennensis*." *Planta Med.* 63, 1 (February 1, 1997): 36–9.

GRAVIOLA

1. Feng, P.C., et al. "Pharmacological screening of some West Indian medicinal plants." *J. Pharm. Pharmacol.* 14 (1962): 556–61.
2. Meyer, T. M. "The alkaloids of *Annona muricata*." *Ing. Ned. Indie.* 8, 6 (1941): 64.
3. Carbajal, D., et al. "Pharmacological screening of plant decoctions commonly used in Cuban folk medicine." *J. Ethnopharmacol.* 33, 1/2 (1991): 21–4.
4. Misas, C. A. J., et al. "Contribution to the biological evaluation of Cuban plants. IV." *Rev. Cubana Med. Trop.* 31, 1 (1979): 29–35.
5. Sundarrao, K, et al. "Preliminary screening of antibacterial and antitumor activities of Papua New Guinean native medicinal plants." *Int. J. Pharmacog.* 31, 1 (1993): 3–6.
6. Heinrich, M., et al. "Parasitological and microbiological evaluation of Mixe Indian medicinal plants (Mexico)." *J. Ethnopharmacol.* 36, 1 (1992): 81–5.
7. Lopez, Abraham A. M. "Plant extracts with cytostatic properties growing in Cuba. I." *Rev. Cubana Med. Trop.* 31, 2 (1979): 97–104.
8. Bories, C. Et al. "Antiparasitic activity of *Annona muricata* and *Annona cherimolia* seeds." *Planta Med.* 57, 5 (1991): 434–36.
9. Antoun, M.D., et al. "Screening of the flora of Puerto Rico for potential antimalarial bioactives." *Int. J. Pharmacog.* 31, 4 (1993): 255–58.

10. Gbeassor, M., et al. "In vitro antimalarial activity of six medicinal plants." *Phytother. Res.* 4, 3 (1990): 115–17.

11. Tattersfield, F., et al. "The insecticidal properties of certain species of Annona and an Indian strain of *Mundulea sericea* (Supli)." *Ann. Appl. Biol.* 27 (1940): 262–73.

12. Hasrat, J. A., et al. "Isoquinoline derivatives isolated from the fruit of *Annona muricata* as 5-HTergic 5-HT1A receptor agonists in rats: unexploited antidepressive (lead) products." *J. Pharm. Pharmacol.* 49, 11 (November 1997): 1145–49.

13. Unpublished data, National Cancer Institute. Anon: Nat Cancer Inst Central Files (1976). From Napralert Files, University of Illinois, 1995.

14. Zeng, L., et al. "Five new monotetrahydrofuran ring acetogenins from the leaves of *Annona muricata*." *J. Nat. Prod.* 59, 11 (November 1996): 1035–42.

15. Rieser, M. J., et al. "Five novel mono-tetrahydrofuran ring acetogenins from the seeds of *Annona muricata*." *J. Nat. Prod.* 59, 2 (February 1996): 100–8.

16. Wu, F. E., et al. "Additional bioactive acetogenins, annomutacin and (2,4-trans and cis)-10R-annonacin-A-ones, from the leaves of *Annona muricata*." *J. Nat. Prod.* 58, 9 (September 1995): 1430–37.

17. Wu, F. E., et al. "New bioactive monotetrahydrofuran Annonaceous acetogenins, annomuricin C and muricatocin C, from the leaves of *Annona muricata*." *J. Nat. Prod.* 58, 6 (June 1995): 909–15.

18. Wu, F. E., et al. "Muricatocins A and B, two new bioactive monotetrahydrofuran Annonaceous acetogenins from the leaves of *Annona muricata*." *J. Nat. Prod.* 58, 6 (June 1995): 902–8.

19. Wu, F. E., et al. "Two new cytotoxic monotetrahydrofuran Annonaceous acetogenins, annomuricins A and B, from the leaves of *Annona muricata*." *J. Nat. Prod.* 58, 6 (June 1995): 830–36.

20. Rieser, M. J., et al. "Bioactive single-ring acetogenins from seed extracts of *Annona muricata*." *Planta Med.* 59, 1 (February 1993): 91–2.

21. Rieser, M. J., et al. "Muricatacin: a simple biologically active acetogenin derivative from the seeds of *Annona muricata* (Annonaceae)." *Tetrahedron Lett.* 32, 9 (1991): 1137–40.

GUARANA

1. Henman, A. R. "Guaraná (*Paullinia cupana* var. sorbilis): ecological and social perspectives on an economic plant of the central Amazon basin." *J. Ethnopharmacol.* (November 1982).

2. Belliardo, F., et al. "HPLC determination of caffeine and theophylline in *Paullinia cupana* Kunth (guarana) and *Cola* spp. samples." *Z. Lebensm. Unters. Forsch.* (May 1985).

3. Bydlowski, S. P., et al. "A novel property of an aqueous guaraná extract (*Paullinia cupana*): inhibition of platelet aggregation in vitro and in vivo." *Braz. J. Med. Biol Res.* (1988).

4. Bydlowski, S. P., et al. "An aqueous extract of guaraná (*Paullinia cupana*) decreases platelet thromboxane synthesis." *Braz. J. Med. Biol Res.* (1991).

5. Espinola, E. B., et al. "Pharmacological activity of guarana (*Paullinia cupana* Mart.) in laboratory animals." *J. Ethnopharmacol.* 55, 3 (February 1997): 223–29.

6. Galduróz, J. C., et al. "Acute effects of the *Paulinia cupana*, 'guaraná,' on the cognition of normal volunteers." *Rev. Paul. Med.* (July–September 1994).

7. Galduróz, J. C. , et al. "The effects of long-term administration of guarana on the cognition of normal, elderly volunteers." *Rev. Paul. Med.* (January–February 1996).

8. Benoni, H., et al. "Studies on the essential oil from guarana." *Z. Lebensm. Unters. Forsch.* (July 1996).

9. da Fonseca, C. A., et al. "Genotoxic and mutagenic effects of guarana (*Paullinia cupana*) in prokaryotic organisms." *Mutat. Res.* (May 1994).

GUAVA

1. Ponce-Macotela, M., et al. "In vitro effect against *Giardia* of 14 plant extracts." *Rev. Invest. Clin.* (September–October 1994).

2. Morales, M. A., et al. "Calcium-antagonist effect of quercetin and its relation with the spasmolytic properties of *Psidium guajava* L." *Arch. Med. Res.* (Spring 1994).

3. Lozoya, X., et al. "Quercetin glycosides in *Psidium guajava* L. leaves and determination of a spasmolytic principle." *Arch. Med. Res.* (Spring 1994).

4. Cáceres, A., et al. "Plants used in Guatemala for the treatment of gastrointestinal disorders. 3. Confirmation of activity against enterobacteria of 16 plants." *J. Ethnopharmacol.* (January 1993).

5. Lutterodt, G. D. "Inhibition of Microlax-induced experimental diarrhoea with narcotic-like extracts of *Psidium guajava* leaf in rats." *J. Ethnopharmacol.* (September 1992).

6. Lozoya, X., et al. "Model of intraluminal perfusion of the guinea pig ileum in vitro in the study of the antidiarrheal properties of the guava (*Psidium guajava*)." *Arch. Invest. Med.* (Mex) (April–June 1990).

7. Caceres, A., et al. "Plants used in Guatemala for the treatment of gastrointestinal disorders. 1. Screening of 84 plants against enterobacteria." *J. Ethnopharmacol.* (August 1990).

8. Lutterodt, G. D. "Inhibition of gastrointestinal release of acetylcholine by quercetin as a possible mode of action of *Psidium guajava* leaf extracts in the treatment of acute diarrhoeal disease." *J. Ethnopharmacol.* (May 1989).

9. Grover, I. S., et al. "Studies on antimutagenic effects of guava (*Psidium guajava*) in *Salmonella typhimurium*." *Mutat. Res.* (June 1993).

10. Lutterodt, G. D., et al. "Effects on mice locomotor activity of a narcotic-like principle from *Psidium guajava* leaves." *J. Ethnopharmacol.* (December 1988).

11. Roman-Ramos, R., et al. "Anti-hyperglycemic effect of some edible plants." *J. Ethnopharmacol.* (August 1995).

12. Cheng, J. T., et al. "Hypoglycemic effect of guava juice in mice and human subjects." *Am. J. Chin. Med.* (1983).

IPORURU

1. Anesini, C. and C. Perez. "Screening of plants used in Argentine folk medicine for antimicrobial activity." Catedra de Farmacologia, Facultad de Odontologia, Universidad de Buenos Aires, Argentina. *J. Ethnopharmacol.* 39 (1993): 119–28.

2. Ogungbamila, F. O., et al. "Smooth muscle–relaxing flavonoids from *Alchornea cordifolia*." *Acta Pharm. Nord.* 2, 6 (1990): 421–22.

JABORANDI

1. Mark Packer, M.D., et al. "Ophthalmology's botanical heritage." *HerbalGram* 35 (1995).

2. Coutinho, S. "Note sur un nouveau medicament diaphoretique et silagogue: le jaborandi du Bresil." *Therap.* 1 (1874): 165–67.

3. Ringold, S., et al. "On jaborandi." *Lancet* (January 30, 1875): 157–59.

4. Holmstedt, B., et al. "Jaborandi: an interdisciplinary approach." *J. Ethnopharmacology* 1 (1979): 3–21.
5. Yosipovitch, G, et al. "Sweat secretion, stratum corneum hydration, small nerve function and pruritus in patients with advanced chronic renal failure." *Br. J. Dermatol.* (October 1995).
6. Gangarosa, L. P. Sr., et al. "Iontophoresis for enhancing penetration of dermatologic and antiviral drugs." *J. Dermatol.* (November 1995).
7. Mishima, H. K., et al. "Ultrasound biomicroscopic study of ciliary body thickness after topical application of pharmacologic agents." *Am. J. Ophthalmol.* (March 1996).
8. Wollensak, J., et al. "One hundred years pilocarpine in ophthalmology." (Author's transl.) *Klin. Monatsbl. Augenheilkd.* (November 1976).
9. Holmstedt, B., et al. "Jaborandi: an interdisciplinary appraisal." *J. Ethnopharmacol.* (January 1979).
10. Gangarosa, L. P. Sr., et al. "Iontophoresis for enhancing penetration of dermatologic and antiviral drugs." *J. Dermatol.* (November 1995).
11. Tanzer, J. M., et al. "A pharmacokinetic and pharmacodynamic study of intravenous pilocarpine in humans." *J. Dent. Res.* (December 1995).
12. Shellard, E. J. "Jaborandi: a note on the contribution of E. M. Holmes to the identification of commercially available pilocarpus and species." *J. Ethnopharmacol.* (December 1979).
13. Holmstedt, B., et al. "Jaborandi: an interdisciplinary appraisal." *J. Ethnopharmacol.* (January 1979).
14. Link, H., et al. "Synthesis of the pilocarpus alkaloids isopilosin and pilocarpine as well as the absolute configuration of the (+)isopilosins.' *Helv. Chim. Acta.* (1972).
15. Vysotskaia, O. S., et al. "Quantitative determination of alkaloids of pilocarpus in plant raw materials and in semiproducts of pilocarpine production." *Farm. Zh.* (1966).
16. Croft, M. A., et al. "Aging effects on accommodation and outflow facility responses to pilocarpine in humans." *Arch. Ophthalmol.* (May 1996).
17. Levin, E. D. "Pergolide interactions with nicotine and pilocarpine in rats on the radial-arm maze." *Pharmacol. Biochem. Behav.* (December 1995).
18. Hung, L, et al. "Effect of pilocarpine on anterior chamber angles." *J. Ocul. Pharmacol. Ther.* (Fall 1995).
19. Kong, L., et al. "Clinical analysis of steroid glaucoma." *Yen Ko Hsueh Pao* (March 1995).
20. Lal, A., et al. "Pharmacodynamic effects of pilocarpine eye drop enhanced by decreasing its volume of instillation." *Indian J. Physiol. Pharmacol.* (July 1995).
21. Yosipovitch, G., et al. "Sweat secretion, stratum corneum hydration, small nerve function and pruritus in patients with advanced chronic renal failure." *Br. J. Dermatol.* (Ocotber 1995).

JATOBA

1. Silva, G. *Catalogo de Extractos Fluidos.* Rio de Janeiro: Araija e Cia.Ltd., 1930.
2. Gupta, M. P., et al. *Q.J. Drug Res.* 17 (1970): 115–30.
3. Arrhenius, S. P., et al. *Phytochemistry* 22 (1983): 471.
4. Arrhenius, S. P., et al. "Inhibitory effects of *Hymenaea* and *Copaifera* leaf resins on the leaf fungus, *Pestalotia subcuticulari.*" *Biochem. Syst. Ecol.* 11, 4 (1983): 361–66.

5. Marsaioli, A. J., et al. "Diterpenes in the bark of *Hymenaea courbaril*." *Phytochemisty* 14 (1975): 1882–83.

6. Giral, F., et al. "Ethnopharmacognostic observation on Panamanian medicinal plants." Part 1., *Q. J. Crude Drug Res.* 167, 3/4 (1979): 115–30.

7. Pinheiro de Sousa, M., et al. "Molluscicidal activity of plants from northeast Brazil." *Rev. Bras. Pesq. Med. Biol.* 7, 4 (1974): 389–94.

8. Rouquayrol, M. Z., et al. "Molluscicidal activity of essential oils from northeastern Brazilian plants." *Rev. Bras. Pesq. Med. Biol.* 13 (1980): 135–43.

9. Verpoorte, R., et al. "Medicinal plants of Surinam. IV. Antimicrobial activity of some medicinal plants." *J. Ethnopharmacol.* 21 3 (1987): 315–18.

10. Rahalison, L., et al. "Screening for antifungal activity of Panamanian plants." *Inst. J. Pharmacog.* 31 (1974): 68–76.

11. Caceres, A., et al. "Plants used in Guatemala for the treatment of dermatomucosal infections. 1: Screening of 38 plant extracts." *J. Ethnopharmacol.* 33, 3 (1991): 277–83.

12. Gupta, M. P. "Plants and traditional medicine in Panama." *Economic and Medicinal Plant Research,* vol 4. London: Academic Press Ltd., 1990.

13. Lopez, J. A. "Isolation of astilbin and sitosterol from *Hymenaea courbaril*." *Phytochemisty* 15 (1976): 2027F.

14. Closa, D., et al. "Prostanoids and free radicals in Cl4C-induced hepatotoxicity in rats: effect of astilbin." *Prostaglandins Leukot. Essent. Fatty Acids* 56, 4 (April 1997): 331–34.

JURUBEBA

1. Ripperger, H. "Structure of paniculonin A and B, two new spirostane glycosides from *Solanum paniculatum* L." *Chem. Ber.* 101, 7 (1968): 2450–58.

2. Ripperger, H. "Isolation of neochlorogenin and painculogenin from *Solanum paniculatum* L." Chem. Ber. 100, 5 (1967): 1741–52.

3. Ripperger, H. "Jurubin, a nitrogen containing steroidsaponin of a new structural type from *Solanum paniculatum* L; concerning the structure of paniculidin." *Chem. Ber.* 100, 5 (1967): 1725–40.

4. Meyer, K. F. Bernoulli. *Pharmac. Acta Helvetiae* 36 (1961): 80–96.

5. Leekning, M. E. and M. A. Rocca. *Rev. Fac. Farm. Adont. Araraquara* 2, 2 (1968): 299–300.

6. Siqueira, N. S. and A. Macan. *Trib. Farm. Curitiba.* 44, 1–2 (1976): 101–4.

7. Cambiachi, S., et al. *Ann. Chim.* (Rome) 61, 1 (1971): 99–111.

8. Costa, Aloisio F. *Farmacognosia,* vol. 2, 3d ed. Fundacaoe Calouste-Gulbenkian, 1975. 712–3.

9. Costa, A. O. *Rev. Bras. Farm.* 21 (1940): 404–16.

10. Penna, Meira. *Dicionario Brasileiro de Plantas Medininais,* 3d ed. Rio de Janeiro: Livraria Kosmos Editora, 1946.

11. Barros, G. S. G., et al. *Rev. Bra. Farm.* 4 (1970): 195–204.

12. Barros, G. S. G., et al. *J. Pharm. Pharmac.* 22 (1970): 116–22.

MACA

1. Rea, J. "Raices andinas: maca." In H. Bermejo and J. E. Leon, eds., *Cultivos Marginados, Otra Perspectiva de 1492.* (1992).

2. King, Steven. "Ancient Buried Treasure of the Andes." *Garden* (November/December 1986).

3. Report of an ad hoc panel of the Advisory Committee on Technical Innovation, Board on Science and Technology for International Development, National Research Council, 1989. *Lost Crops of the Incas: Little-Known Plants of the Andes with Promise for Worldwide Cultivation.*

4. Johns, T. "The anu and the maca." *Journal of Ethnobiology* 1 (1981):208–212.

5. Quiros, C., et al. "Physiological studies and determination of chromosome number in maca, *Lepidium meyenii.*" *Economic Botany* 50, 2 (1996): 216–23.

6. Leon, J. 1964. "The 'maca' (*Lepidium meyenii*), a little-known food plant of Peru." *Economic Botany* 18 (1986): 122–27.

7. Chacon, R. C. 1961. *Estudio Fitoquimico de* Lepidium meyenii. Dissertation, Univ., Nac. Mayo de San Marcos, Peru, 1986.

8. Dini, A., et al. "Chemical composition of *Lepidium meyenii.*" *Food Chemistry* 49 (1994): 347–49.

9. "Plant medicine's importance stressed by CSU professor." *HerbalGram* (Spring 1989): 12.

10. Steinberg, P. *Phil Steinberg's Cat's Claw News* 1, 2 (July/August1995).

11. Gomez, A. "Maca, es alternativa nutricional para el ano 2000." *Informe Ojo con su Salud* (Lima, Peru) 58 (August 15, 1997).

12. Chacon, G. "La maca (*Lepidium peruvianum Chacon* sp. Nov.) y su habitat." *Revista Peruana de Biologia* 3 (1990): 171–272.

MACELA

1. Vargas, V., et al. "Genotoxicity of plant extracts." *Mem. Inst. Oswaldo Cruz Rio De Janeiro* 86, 11 (1991): 67–70.

2. Rocha, M., et al. "Effects of hydroalcoholic extracts of *Portulaca pilosa* and *Achyrocline satureoides* on urinary sodium and potassium excretion." *J. Ethnopharmacol.* 43, 3 (1994): 179–83.

3. Saggese, D. *Medicinal Herbs of Argentina,* 10th ed. Rosario: Antognazzi & Co., 1959, 1–189.

4. Gonzalez, A., et al. "Biological screening of Uruguayan medicinal plants." *J. Ethnopharmacol.* 39, 3 (1993): 217–20.

5. Hirschmann, G. S. "The constituents of *Achyrocline satureoides* Dc." *Rev. Latinoamer. Quim.* 15, 3 (1984): 134–35.

6. Mesquita, A., et al. "Flavonoids from four compositae species." *Phytochemistry* 25, 5 (1986): 1255–56.

7. Simoes, C. M., 1988. "Antiinflammatory action of *Achyrocline satureoides* extracts applied topically." *Fitoterapia* 59, 5 (1988): 419–21.

8. Simoes, C. M., et al. 1988. "Pharmacological investigations on *Achyrocline satureoides* (Lam). Dc., compositae." *J. Ethnopharmacol.* 22, 3 (1988): 281–93.

9. de Souza, C. P., et al. "Chemoprophylaxis of schistosomiasis: molluscicidal activity of natural products." *An. Acad. Brasil. Cienc.* 56, 3 (1984): 333–38.

10. Vargas, V. M. F., et al. "Mutagenic and genotoxic effects of aqueous extracts of Achyrocline satureoides in prokaryotic organisms." *Mutat. Res.* 240, 1 (1990): 13–18.

11. Wagner, H., et al. "Immunostimulating polysaccharides (heteroglycans) of higher plants." *Arzneim-Forsch.* 35, 7 (1985): 1069–75.

12. Wagner, H., et al. "Immunostimulating polysaccharides (heteroglycanes) of higher plants/preliminary communication." *Arzneim-Forsch.* 34 6 (1984): 659–61.

13. Arisawa, M. "Cell growth inhibition of KB cells by plant extracts." *Nat Med* 48, 4 (1994): 338–47.

14. Abdel-Malek, S., et al. "Drug leads from the Kallawaya herbalists of Bolivia. 1. Background, rationale, protocol and anti-HIV activity." *J. Ethnopharmacol.* 50 (1996): 157–66.

MANACÁ

1. Ruppelt, B. M., et al. "Pharmacological screening of plants recommended by folk medicine as anti-snake venom—I. Analgesic and anti-inflammatory activities." *Mem. Inst. Oswaldo Cruz* (1991).
2. Iyer, R. P., et al. "*Brunfelsia hopeana* I: Hippocratic screening and antiinflammatory evaluation." *Lloydia* (July–August 1977).

MARACUJA (Passionflower)

1. Lutomski, J., 1960. "Alkaloidy *Pasiflora incarnata* L." Dissertation, Institute for Medicinal Plant Research, Pozan, 1960.
2. *HerbClip: Passion Flower.* "An herbalist's view of passionflower." American Botanical Council, Austin, Texas April 10, 1996.

MARACUJA (Passion fruit)

1. *HerbalGram* 27 (1992): "Passion–Passion Pop."
2. Zúñiga, Rojas J. "Oil seeds from the American tropics." *Arch. Latinoam Nutr.* 31, 2 (June 1981): 350–70.
3. Spencer, K. C., et al. "Cyanogenesis of *Passiflora edulis.*" J. Agric. Food Chem. 31, 4 (July–August 1983): 794–96.
4. Lutomski, J., et al. "Pharmacochemical investigations of the raw materials from genus Passiflora. Phytochemical investigations on raw materials of *Passiflora edulis* from a flavicarpa." (Author's transl.) *Planta Med.*, 27, 3 (May 1975): 222–25.
5. Lutomski, J., et al. "Pharmacochemical investigations of the raw materials from *Passiflora* genus. 2. The pharmacochemical estimation of juices from the fruits of *Passiflora edulis* from a flavicarpa." *Planta Med.*, 27, 2 (March 1975): 112–21.

MUIRA PUAMA

1. Dias Da Silva, Rodolpho. "Medicinal plants of Brazil. Botanical and pharmacognostic studies. Muira puama." *Rev. Bras. Med. Pharm.* 1, 1 (1925): 37–41.
2. Penna, M. 1930. *Notas Sobre Plantas Brasileriras.* Rio de Janeiro: Araujo Penn & Cia., 1930, 258.
3. Anselmino, Elisabeth. "Ancestral sources of muira-puama." *Ach. Pharm.* 271 (1933): 296–314.
4. *British Herbal Pharmacopoeia.* West York, England: British Herbal Medicine Association, 1983, 132–33.
5. "Muira puama, *Ptychopetalum olacoides.*" Brazilian Pharmacopeia. Rio de Janeiro, Brazil, 1956.
6. Youngken, H. W. "Observations on muira puama." *J. Am. Pharm. Assoc.* 10 (1921): 690–2.
7. Olofsson, Erif. "Action of extract of *Liriosma ovata* on the blood pressure, vessels and respiration of the rabbit." *Compt. Rend. Soc. Biol.* 97 (1927): 1639–40.
8. Gaebler, H. "Revival of the drug muira puama." *Deut. Apoth.* 22, 3 (1979): 94–6.
9. Iwasa, J., et al. "Constituents of muira puama." *Yakungaka Zasshi* (Japan) 89, 8 (1969): 1172–74.
10. Auterhoff, H., et al. "Components of muira puama." *Arch. Pharm. Ber. Dtsch. Pharm. Ges.* 301, 7 (1968): 481–89.

11. Auterhoff, H., et al. "Components of muira puama II." *Arch. Pharm. Ber. Dtsch. Pharm. Ges.* 302, 3 (March 1969): 209–12.
12. Auterhoff, H., et al. 1971. "Lipophilic constituents of muira puama." *Arch. Pharm. Ber. Dtsch. Pharm. Ges.* 304, 3 (March 1971): 223–28.
13. Steinmetz, E. "Muira puama." *Quart. J. Crude Drug Res.* 11, 3 (1971): 1787–89.
14. Ninomiya, Ruriko, et al. "Studies of Brazilian crude drugs." *Shoyakugaku Zasshi* (Japan) 33, 2 (1979): 57–64.
15. Bucek, E., et al. "Volatile constituents of *Ptychopetalum olacoides* root oil." *Planta Med.* 53, 2 (1989): 231.
16. Waynberg, J. "Contributions to the Clinical Validation of the Traditional Use of *Ptychopetalum guyanna*." Presented at the First International Congress on Ethnopharmacology, Strasbourg, France, June 5–9, 1990.
17. Werbach, Melvyn R., M.D., and Michael Murray, N.D. *Botanical Influences on Illness: A Sourcebook of Clinical Research.* Tarzana, CA: Third Line Press, 1994, 200.
18. Waynberg, J. "Male sexual asthenia--interest in a traditional plant-derived medication." *Ethnopharmacology* (March 1995).

MULATEIRO

1. Lorenzi, H. *Arvores Brasilieras.* Editora Plantarum LTDA, 1992.
2. Luna, L. E. "The healing practices of a Peruvian shaman." *Journal of Ethnopharmacology* 112 (1984): 123–33.

MULLACA

1. Vasina, O. E., et al. "Withasteroids of *Physalis.* VII. 14-alpha-hydroxyixocarpanolide and 24,25-epoxywithanolide D." Chem. Nat. Comp. 22, 5 (1987): 560–65.
2. Chen, C. M., et al. "Withangulatin A, a new withanolide from *Physalis angulata.*" *Heterocycles* 31, 7 (1990): 1371–75.
3. Shingu, K., et al. "Physagulin C, a new withanolide from *Physalis angulata* L." *Chem. Pharm. Bull.* 39, 6(1991): 1591–93.
4. Shingu, K., et al. "Three new withanolides, physagulins A, B and D, from *Physalis angulata* L." *Chem. Pharm. Bull.* 40, 8 (1992): 2088–91.
5. Shingu, K., et al. "Three new withanolides, physagulins E, F and G, from *Physalis angulata* L." *Chem. Pharm. Bull.* 40, 9 (1992): 2448–51.
6. Basey, K., et al. "Phygrine, an alkaloid from *Physalis* species." *Phytochemistry* 31, 12 (1992): 4173–76.
7. Lin, Y. S., et al. "Immunomodulatory activity of various fractions derived from Physalis angulata L. extract." *Amer. J. Chinese Med.* 20, 3/4 (1992): 233–43.
8. Chiang, H., et al. "Antitumor agent, physalin F, from *Physalis angulata* L." *AntiCancer Res.* 12, 3 (1992): 837–43.
9. Chiang, H., et al. "Inhibitory effects of physalin B and physalin F on various human leukemia cells in vitro." *AntiCancer Res.* 12, 4 (1992): 1155–62.
10. Anonymous. "Biological Assay of Antitumor Agents from Natural Products." Sabstr Seminar on the Development of Drugs from Medicinal Plants, Organized by the Department of Medical Science Department at Thai Farmer Bank, Bangkok Thailand, 1982, 129.
11. Otake, T., et al. "Screening of Indonesian plant extracts for anti-human immunodeficiency virus-type 1 (HIV-1) activity." *Phytother. Res.* 9, 1(1995): 6–10.
12. Kusumoto, I. T., et al. "Screening of some Indonesian medicinal plants for inhibitory effects on HIV-1 protease." *Shoyakugaku Zasshi* 46, 2 (1992): 190–93.

13. Kusumoto, I., et al. "Inhibitory effect of Indonesian plant extracts on reverse tran-scriptase of an RNA tumour vVirus (I)." *Phytother. Res.* 6, 5 (1992): 241–44.
14. Kurokawa, M., et al. "Antiviral traditional medicines against herpes simplex virus (HSV-1), poliovirus, and measles virus in vitro and their therapeutic efficacies for HSV-1 infection in mice." *Antiviral Res.* 22, 2/3 (1993): 175–88.
15. Hussain, H., et al. "Plants in Kano ethomedicine: screening for antimicrobial activ-ity and alkaloids." *Int. J. Pharmacog.* 29, 1 (1991): 51–56.
16. Ogunlana, E. O., et al. "Investigations into the antibacterial activities of local plants." *Planta Med.* 27 (1975): 354.
17. Cox, P. A. "Pharmacological activity of the Samoan ethnopharmacopoeia." *Econ. Bot.* 43, 4 (1989): 487–97.
18. Cesario De Mello, A., et al. "Presence of acetylcholine in the fruit of *Physalis angu-lata* (Solanaceae)." *Cienc. Cult.* (Sao Paulo) 37, 5 (1985): 799–805.
19. Kone-Bamba, D., et al. "Hemostatic activity of 216 plants used in traditional medi-cine in the Ivory Coast." *Plant. Med. Phytother.* 21, 2 (1987): 122–30.

MULUNGU

1. Santos, W. O., et al. "Pesquisas de Substancias Cadioativas em Plantas Xerofilas Medicinais." IX Simposio de Plantas Medicinais do Brasil, Rio de Janeiro-RL, Brasil, September 1–3, 1986, 45.
2. Pohill, R. M., P. H. Raven. *Advances in Legume Systematics,* Part 2. Kew, England: Royal Botanic Gardens, 1981.
3. Sanzen. T., et al. "Expression of glycoconjugates during intrahepatic bile duct de-velopment in the rat: an immunohistochemical and lectin-histochemical study." *Hepatology* 3 (September 22, 1995): 944–51.
4. Lee, R. F., et al. "The metabolism of glyceryl (35 S)sulfoquinovoside by the coral tree, *Erythrina crista-galli*, and alfalfa, *Medicago sativa*." *Biochim. Biophys. Acta* 261, 1 (January 28, 1972): 35–37.
5. Inamura, H., M. Ho, and H. Ohashi. *Gifu Daigaku Nogakubu Kenyu Hokoku* 77 (1981) (C. A. 96:196524y).

MUTAMBA

1. Dominguez, X. A., et al. "Screening of medicinal plants used by Huastec Mayans of northeastern Mexico." *J. Ethnopharmacol.* 13, 2 (1985): 139–56.
2. Caceres, A., et al. "Diuretic activity of plants used for the treatment of urinary ail-ments in Guatemala." *J. Ethnopharmacol.* 19, 3 (1987): 233–45.
3. Caceres, A, et al. "Screening of antimicrobial activity of plants popularly used in Guatemala for the treatment of dermatomucosal diseases." *J. Ethnopharmacol.* 20, 3 (1987): 223–37.
4. Vieira, J. E. V., et al. "Pharmacologic screening of plants from northeast Brazil. II." *Rev. Brasil. Farm.* 49 (1968): 67–75.
5. Caceres, A. et al. "Plants used in Guatemala for the treatment of gastrointestinal disorders. 1. Screening of 84 plants against enterobacteria." *J. Ethnopharmacol.* 30, 1 (1990): 55–73.
6. Heinrich, M., et al. 1992. "Parasitological and microbiological evaluation of Mixe Indian medicinal plants." (Mexico) *J. Ethnopharmacol.* 36, 1 (1992): 81–85.
7. Caceres, A., et al. "Plants used in Guatemala for the treatment of respiratory diseases. 2: Evaluation of activity of 16 plants against gram-positive bacteria." *J. Ethnopharmacol.* 39, 1 (1993): 77–82.

8. Caceres, A., et al. "Plants used in Guatemala for the treatment of gastrointestinal disorders. 3. Confirmation of activity against enterobacteria of 16 plants." *J. Ethnopharmacol.* 38, 1 (1993): 31–38.

9. Caceres, A., et al. "Anti-gonorrhoeal activity of plants used in Guatemala for the treatment of sexually transmitted diseases." *J. Ethnopharmacol.* 48, 2 (1995): 85–88.

10. Pinheiro De Sousa, M., et al. "Molluscicidal activity of plants from northeast Brazil." *Rev. Brasil. Pesq. Med. Biol.* 7, 4 (1974): 389–94.

11. Nascimento, S. C., et al. "Antimicrobial and cytotoxic activities in plants from Pernambuco, Brazil." *Fitoterapia* 61, 4 (1990): 353–55.

12. Tseng, C. F. "Inhibition of in vitro prostaglandin and leukotriene biosyntheses by cinnamoyl-beta-phenethylamine and N-acyldopamine derivatives." *Chem. Pharm. Bull.* 40 (1992) 2: 396–400.

13. Hor, M., et al. "Inhibition of intestinal chloride secretion by proanthocyanidins from Guazuma ulmifolia." *Planta Med.* 61, 3 (1995): 208–12.

14. Hor, M., et al. "proanthocyanidin polymers with antisecretory activity and proanthocyanidin oligomers from *Guazuma ulmifolia* bark." *Phytochemistry* 42, 1 (1996): 109–19.

NETTLE

1. "Nettles." *Lawrence's Review of Natural Products.* St. Louis, MO. Facts and Comparison, Inc., February 1989.

2. Herb of the Month. *Urtica dioica* Monograph, Bastyr University, Department of Botanical Medicine, May 1996.

3. Tyler, Varro E. *Herbs of Choice.* Pharmaceutical Press, 1994.

4. Tyler, Varro E. "Secondary products: physiologically active compounds, a congress review." *HerbalGram* 36, 60–61.

5. Koch E. and A. Biber. "Pharmacological effects of saw palmetto and urtica extracts for benign prostatic hyperplasia." *Urologe* 34, 2 (1994): 90–95.

6. Hryb, D., et al. "The effect of extracts of the roots of the stinging nettle (Urtica dioica) on the interaction of SHBG with its receptor on human prostatic membranes." *Planta Med.* 61 (1995): 31–32.

7. Gansser, D. "Plant constituents interfering with human sex hormone–binding globulin. Evaluation of a test method and its application to Urtica dioica root extracts." *Z. Natur.Forsch.* [C] 50, 1–2 (1995): 98–104.

8. Hirano, T. "Effects of stinging nettle root extracts and their steroidal components on the Na+,K(+)-ATPase of the benign prostatic hyperplasia." *Planta Med.* 60, 1 (1994): 30–33.

9. Vahlensieck, W. Jr. "Drug therapy of benign prostatic hyperplasia." *Fortschr. Med.* 114, 31 (1996): 407–11.

PATA DE VACA

1. Juliane, C. "Acao hipoglicemiante da unha-de-vaca." *Rev. Med. Pharm. Chim. Phys.* 2, 1 (1929): 165–69.

2. Juliane, C. "Acao hipoglicemiante de 'bauhinia forficata' link, novos estudos experimentails." *Rev. Sudam Endocrin. Immol. Quimiot.* 14 (1931): 326–34.

3. Costa, O. A. "Estudo farmacoquimico da unha-de-vaca." Rev. Flora Medicinal 9, 4 (1945): 175–89.

4. Almeida, R. and Agra, M. F. 1984. "Levantamento da Flora Medicinal de Uso no Tratamento da Diabete e Alguns Resultados Experimentais." VIII Simposio de Plantas Medicinais do Brasil, September 4–6, 1984, Manaus-AM, Brazil, 23.

5. Miyake, E. T., et al. "Caracterizacao farmacognostica de pata-de-vaca (*Bauhinia fortificata*)." Rev. Bras. Farmacogn. 1, 1 (1986): 56–68.

PAU D'ARCO

1. Jones, Kenneth. *Pau D'Arco: Immune Power from the Rain Forest*. Rochester, VT: Healing Arts Press, 1995, 54–8.
2. Gentry, Alwyn. "A synopsis of bignoniaceae ethnobotany and economic botany." *Annals of the Missouri Botanical Garden* 79 (1992): 53–64.
3. Rao, K. V., et al. "Recognition and evaluation of lapachol as an antitumor agent." *Canc. Res.* 28 (1968): 1952–4.
4. Block, J. B., et al. "Early clinical studies with lapachol (NSC-11905)." *Cancer Chemother. Rep.* 4 (1974): 27–8.
5. Linardi, M. D. C., et al. "A lapachol derivative active against mouse lympocyte leukemia P-388." *J. Med. Chem* 18, 11 (1975): 1159–62.
6. Santana, C. F., et al. "Preliminary observation with the use of lapachol in human patients bearing malignant neoplasms." *Revista do Instituto de Antibioticos* 20 (1971): 61–8.
7. Beckstrom-Sternberg, Stephen M., and James A Duke. "The Phytochemical Database." ACEDB version 4.3: July 1994. National Germplasm Resources Laboratory (NGRL), Agricultural Research Service (ARS), U.S. Department of Agriculture.
8. de Lima, O. G., et al. "Primeiras observacoes sobre a acao antimicrobiana do lapachol." *Anais da Sociedade de Biologica de Pernambuco* 14 (1956): 129–35.
9. de Lima, O. G., et al. "Una nova substancia antibiotica isolada do 'Pau d'Arco,' *Tabebuia* sp." *Anais da Sociedade de Biologica de Pernambuco* 14 (1956): 136–40.
10. Burnett, A. R., et al. "Naturally occuring quinones. The quinonoid constituents of *Tabebuia avellanedae.*" *J. Chem. Soc.* (C) (1967): 2100–4.
11. Gershon, H., et al. "Fungitoxicity of 1,4-naphthoquinonoes to *Candida albicans* and *Trichophyton menta* grophytes." *Can. J. Microbiol.* 21 (1975): 1317–21.
12. Binutu, O. A., et al. "Antimicrobial potentials of some plant species of the *Bignoniaceae* family." *Afr. J. Med.* Sci. 23, 3 (1994): 269–73.
13. Linhares, M. S., et al. "Estudo sobre of efeito de substancias antibioticas obitdas de *Streptomyces* e vegatais superiores sobre o herpesvirus hominis." *Revista Instituto Antibioticos, Recife* 15 (1975): 25–32.
14. Lagrota, M., et al. "Antiviral activity of lapachol." *Rev. Microbiol.* 14 (1983): 21–26.
15. Schuerch, A. R., et al. "B-Lapachone, an inhibitor of oncornavirus reverse transcriptase and eukarotic DBA polymerase-a. Inhibitory effect, thiol dependency and specificity." *Eur. J. Biochem.* 84 (1978): 197–205.
16. Austin, F. R. "Schistosoma mansoni chemoprophylaxis with dietary lapachol." *Am. J. Trop. Med. Hyg.* 23 (1979): 412–19.
17. Gilbert, B., et al. "Schistosomiasis. Protection against infection by terpenoids." *An. Acad. Brasil. Cienc.* 42 (Suppl) (1970): 397–400.
18. Oga, S., et al. "Toxicidade e atividade anti-inflamatoria de *Tabebuia avellanedae* Lorentz ('Ipe Roxo')." *Rev. Fac. Farm. Bioquim.* 7 (1969): 47–53.
19. Taylor, Leslie. Personal observations in Manaus, Belem, and Sau Paulo, Brazil.
20. Awang, D. V. C. "Commerical taheebo lacks active ingredient." *Information Letter* 726 (August 13, 1987); *Can. Pharm. J.* 121 (1991): 323–26.

PEDRA HUME CAA

1. Martins de Toledo, O. *Tese de Doutoramento*. Faculdade de Medicina de Sao Paulo. Sao Paulo, Brazil, 1929.
2. Coutinho, A. B. *Tese de Catedra*. Faculdade de Medicina de Recife. Recife, Brazil, 1938.

3. Mendes dos Reis Arruda, L., et al. "Efeito Hipoglicemiante Induzido pelo Extracto das Raizes de *Myrcia citrifolia* (Pedra-Hume-Caa), Esudo Famacologico Preliminar." V Simposio de Plantas Medicinais do Brasil, Sao Paulo-SP, Brazil, September 4–6, 1978, 74.

4. Brune, U., et al. "*Myrcia spaerocarpa*, D.C., Planta Diabetica." V Simposio de Plantas Medicinais do Brasil, Sao Paulo-SP, Brazil, September 4–6, 1978, 74.

5. Russo, E. M., et al. "Clinical trial of *Myrcia uniflora* and *Bauhinia forficata* leaf extracts in normal and diabetic patients." *Braz. J. Med. Biol. Res.* (1990).

6. Pepato, M. T., et al. "Assessment of the antidiabetic activity of *Myrcia uniflora* extracts in streptozotocin diabetic rats." *Diabetes Res.* (1993).

PICAO PRETO

1. Neves, J. L., et al. "Contribuicao ao Estudo de *Bidens pilosa*." VII Simposio de Plantas Medicinais do Brasil, Belo Horizonte-MG, Brazil, September 1–3, 1982, 90.

2. Rabe, T. "Antibacterial activity of South African plants used for medicinal purposes." *J. Ethnopharmacol.* 56, 1 (1997): 81–87.

3. Alvarez, L., et al. "Bioactive polyacetylenes from *Bidens pilosa*." *Planta Med.* 62, 4 (1996): 355–57.

4. Jager, A. K., et al. "Screening of Zulu medicinal plants for prostaglandin-synthesis inhibitors" *J. Ethnopharmacol.* 52, 2 (1996): 95–100.

5. Chin, H. W., et al. "The hepatoprotective effects of Taiwan folk medicine 'ham-hong-chho' in rats." *Am. J. Chin. Med.* 24, 3–4 (1996): 231–40.

6. Chih, H. W., et al. "Anti-inflammatory activity of Taiwan folk medicine 'ham-hong-chho' in rats." *Am. J. Chin. Med.* 23, 3–4 (1995): 273–78.

7. Geissberger, P., et al. "Constituents of *Bidens pilosa* L.: do the components found so far explain the use of this plant in traditional medicine?" *Acta Trop.* 48, 4 (1991): 251–61.

8. Sarg, T. M., et al. "Constituents and biological activity of *Bidens pilosa* L. grown in Egypt." *Acta Pharm. Hung.* 61, 6 (1991): 317–23.

9. Wat, C. K., et al. "Ultraviolet-mediated cytotoxic activity of phenylheptatriyne from *Bidens pilosa* L." *J. Nat. Prod.* 42, 1 (1979): 103–11.

10. Arnason, T., et al. "Photosensitization of *Escherichia coli* and *Saccharomyces cerevisiae* by phenylheptatriyne from *Bidens pilosa*." *Can. J. Microbiol.* 26, 6 (1980): 698–705.

SAMAMBAIA

1. Rayward, J. "An extract of the fern *Polypodium leucotomos* inhibits human peripheral blood mononuclear cells proliferation in vitro." *Int. J. Immunopharmacol.* 19, 1 (1997): 9–14.

2. Sempere J. M. "Effect of anapsos (*Polypodium leucotomos* extract) on in vitro production of cytokines." *Br. J. Clin. Pharmacol.* 43, 1 (1997): 85–89.

3. Hostettmann, K., et al. *Phytochemistry of Plants Used in Traditional Medicine.* Proceedings of the Phytochemical Society of Europe. Oxford, NY: Oxford University Press, 1995.

4. Piñeiro, Alvarez B. "Two years personal experience in anapsos treatment of psoriasis in various clinical forms." *Med. Cutan. Ibero. Lat. Am.* (1983).

5. Padilla, H. C. "A new agent (hydrophilic fraction of *Polypodium leucotomos*) for management of psoriasis." *Int. J. Dermatol.* 13, 5 (1974): 276–82.

6. Tuominen, M., et al. "Effects of calaguala and an active principle, adenosine, on platelet activating factor." *Planta Med.* 58, 4 (1992): 306–10.

7. Vasange, M., et al. "A sulphonoglycolipid from the fern *Polypodium decumanum* and its effect on the platelet activating-factor receptor in human neutrophils." *J. Pharm. Pharmacol.* 49, 5 (1997): 562–66.

8. Vasange-Tuominen, M., et al. "The fern *Polypodium decumanum,* used in the treatment of psoriasis, and its fatty acid constituents as inhibitors of leukotriene B4 formation." *Prostaglandins Leukot. Essent. Fatty Acids* 50, 5 (1994): 279–84.

SANGRE DE GRADO

1. Perdue, G. P., et al. "South American plants II: taspine isolation and anti-inflammatory activity." *J. Pharm. Sci.* (January 1979).
2. Vlietinck, A. J. and R. A. Dommisse, eds. Advances in Medicinal Plant Research. Stuttgart: Wiss. Verlag, 1985.
3. Vaisberg, A. J., et al. "Taspine is the cicatrizant principle in sangre de grado extracted from *Croton lechleri.*" *Planta Med.* (April 1989).
4. Porras-Reyes, B. H., et al. "Enhancement of wound healing by the alkaloid taspine defining mechanism of action." *Proc. Soc. Exp. Biol. Med.* 203, 1 (1993): 18–25.
5. Itokawa, H., et al. "A cytotoxic substance from sangre de grado." *Chem. Pharm. Bull.* (Tokyo) 39, 4 (1991): 1041–42.
6. Pieters, L., et al. "Isolation of a dihydrobenzofuran lignan from South American dragon's blood (*Croton* spp.) as an inhibitor of cell proliferation." *J. Nat. Prod.* (June 1993).
7. Chen, Z.P., et al. "Studies on the anti-tumour, anti-bacterial, and wound-healing properties of dragon's blood." *Planta Med.* (December 1994).

SARSAPARILLA

1. Hobbs, Christopher. "Sarsaparilla, a literature review." HerbalGram 17 (1988).
2. Lung, Albert and Steven Foster. *Encyclopedia of Common Natural Ingredients.* New York: John Wiley & Sons, Inc., 1996.
3. Thurman, F. M. "The treatment of psoriasis with sarsaparilla compound." *New England Journal of Medicine* 337 (1942): 128–33.
4. D'Amico, M. L. "Ricerche sulla presenza di sostanze ad azione antibiotica nelle piante superiori." *Fitoterapia* 21, 1 (1950): 77–79.
5. Fitzpatrick, F. K. "Plant substances active against mycobacterium tuberculosis." *Antibiotics and Chemotherapy* 4, 5 (1954): 528–36.
6. Rollier, R. "Treatment of lepromatous leprosy by a combination of DDS and sarsaparilla (*Smilax ornata*)." *Int. J. Leprosy* 27 (1959): 328–40.
7. Ageel, A. M., et al. "Experimental studies on antirheumatic crude drugs used in Saudi traditional medicine." *Drugs Exp. Clin. Res.* 15 (1989): 369–72.
8. Rafatullah, S., et al. "Hepatoprotective and safety evaluation studies on sarsaparilla." *Int. J. Pharmacognosy* 29 (1991): 296–301.
9. Harnischfeger, G., et al. "*Smilax* Species--Sarsaparille." In *Bewahrte Pflanzendrogen in Wissenschaft* und Medizin. Bad Homburg/Melsungen: Notamed Verlag, 1983, 216–25.
10. Tschesche, R. "Advances in the chemistry of antibiotic substances from higher plants." In H. Wagner and L. Horhammer, *Pharmacognosy and Phytochemisty.* New York: Springer Verlag, 1971, 274–76.
11. Willard, Terry. *The Wild Rose Scientific Herbal.* Alberta: Wild Rose College of Natural Healing, 1991, 307.
12. Botanical Monograph, "Sarsaparilla (*Smilax sarsaparilla*)." *American Journal of Natural Medicine* 3, 9 (1996).
13. Newal, Carol, Linda Anderson, and J. David. Phillipson. *Herbal Medicine: A Guide for Health-care Professionals.* Cambridge, England: The Pharmaceutical Press, 1996.

SIMARUBA

1. Brendler, Thomas. *Heilpflanzen—Herbal Remedies.* CD ROM. Berlin, Germany: Institut für Phytopharmaka Gmbh, 1996.
2. Shepheard, S., et al. "Persistent carriers of *Entameba histolytica.*" Lancet (1918): 501.
3. Spencer, C. F. et al. "Survey of plants for antimalarial activity." *Lloydia* 10 (1947): 145–74.
4. Duriez, R. et al. "Glaucarubin in the treatment of amebiasis." *Presse Med.* 70 (1962): 1291.
5. Unpublished data, National Cancer Institute. Anon: Nat. Cancer Inst. Central Files (1976), from the NAPRA report on simaruba, University of Illinois.
6. Polonsky, J. "The isolation and structure of 13,18-dehydroglaucarubinone, a new antineoplastic quassinoid from *Simarouba amara.*" *Experientia* 34, 9 (1978): 1122–23.
7. Ghosh, P. C., et al. 1977. "Antitumor plants. IV. Constituents of *Simarouba versicolor.*" *Lloydia* 40, 4 (July 1977): 364–69.
8. Wright C. W. "Use of microdilution to assess in vitro antiamoebic activities of *Brucea javanica* fruits, *Simarouba amara* stem, and a number of quassinoids." *Antimicrob. Agents Chemother.* 32, 11 (1988): 1725–29.
9. O'Neill, M. J. "Plants as sources of antimalarial drugs, Part 6. Activities of *Simarouba amara* fruits." *J. Ethnopharmacol.* 22, 2 (1988): 183–90.
10. Caceres, A. "Plants used in Guatemala for the treatment of gastrointestinal disorders. 1. Screening of 84 plants against enterobacteria." *J. Ethnopharmacol.* 30, 1 (1990): 55–73.
11. Franssen, F. F. "In vivo and in vitro antiplasmodial activities of some plants traditionally used in Guatemala against malaria." *Antimicrob. Agents Chemother.* 41, 7 (1997): 1500–3.

STEVIA

1. Bridel, M., et al. *J. Pharm. Chem.* 14 (1931): 99.
2. Samuelsson, Gunnar. *Drugs of Natural Origin.* Stockholm: Swedish Pharmaceutical Press, 1992.
3. Lung, A. and S. Foster. *Encyclopedia of Common Natural Ingredients.* New York: Wiley & Sons, 1996.
4. FDA Import Alert No. 45-06 (May 17, 1991).
5. Blumenthal, Mark. "Perspectives on FDA's new stevia policy, after four years, the agency lifts its ban—but only partially." *Whole Foods Magazine* (February 1996).
6. Melis, M. S. "A crude extract of *Stevia rebaudiana* increase the renal plasma flow of normal and hypertensive rats." *Braz. J. Med. Biol. Res.* 5 (May 29, 1996): 669–75.
7. Melis, M. S. "Chronic administration of aqueous extract of *Stevia rebaudiana* in rats: renal effects." *J. Ethnopharmacol.* (July 28, 1995).
8. Melis, M. S. "Stevioside effect on renal function of normal and hypertensive rats." *J. Ethnopharmacol.* (June 1992).
9. Melis, M.S., et al. "Effect of calcium and verapamil on renal function of rats during treatment with stevioside." *J. Ethnopharmacol.* (July 1991).
10. Curi, R., et al. "Effect of *Stevia rebaudiana* on glucose tolerance in normal adult humans." Braz. J. Med. Biol Res (1986).
11. Yamamoto, N. S., et al. "Effect of steviol and its structural analogues on glucose production and oxygen uptake in rat renal tubules." *Experientia* (January 15, 1985).
12. Boeckh, E. M. A., et al. "Avaliacao Clinica do Efeito Cronico do Edulcorante Natural *Stevia rebaudiana* Bertoni Sobre o Teste de Tolerancia a Glicose,

Parametros Clinicos e Eletrocardiograficos em Individuos Normais." V
Simposio de Plantas Medicinais do Brasil, Sao Paulo-SP, Brazil, September 4–6,
1978, 208.

13. Humbolt, G., et al. "Steviosideo: Efeitos Cardio-circulatorios em Ratos." V
Simposio de Plantas Medicinais do Brasil, Sao Paulo-SP, Brazil, September 4–6,
1978, 208.

SUMA

1. Record number 0079-00504 Nova Genera et Species Plantarum 542 43. Pl. 140, 142
(1826).

2. De Oliveira, Fernando. "*Pfaffia paniculata* (Martius) Kuntze--Brazilian ginseng."
Rev. Bras. Farmacog. 1, 1 (1986) 86–92.

3. Hobbs, Christopher. "Adaptogens—herbal gems to help us adapt." *Let's Live*
(1996).

4. Anuario Naturista. *Los Productos Naturales,* 5th ed. Quito: Mundo Naturista, 1992.

5. Nishimoto, N., et al. "Constituents of 'Brazil ginseng' and some *Pfaffia* species."
Tennen Yuki Kagobutsu Toronkai Keon Yoshishu (Japan) 10 (1988):17–24.

6. Nishimoto, N., et al. "Three ecdysteroid glycosides from *Pfaffia*." *Phytochemistry*
27, 6 (1988): 1665–68.

7. Beta-Ecdysone from *Pfaffia paniculata*. Japanese patent number (84 10,600).
January 20, 1984, by Wakunaga Pharmaceutical Co., Ltd.

8. De Oliveira, F. G., et al. "Contribution to the pharmacognostic study of Brazilian
ginseng *Pfaffia paniculata*." An. Farm. Chim. 20, 1–2 (1980): 277–361.

9. Nakai, Shiro, et al. "Pfaffosides. Part 2. Pfaffosides, nortriterpenoid saponins from
Pfaffia paniculata." *Phytochemisty* 23, 8 (1984): 17–35.

10. Nishimoto, N., et al. "Pfaffosides and nortriterpenoid saponins from *Pfaffia paniculata*." *Phytochemistry* 1984 23, 1 (1984): 139–42.

11. Takemoto, T., et al. "Pfaffic acid, a novel nortriterpene from Pfaffia paniculata
Kuntze." *Tetrahedron Lett*. 24, 10 (1983): 1057–60.

12. Antitumor pfaffosides from Brazilian carrots. Japanese patent number (84
184,198). October 19, 1984, by Rohto Pharmaceutical Co., Ltd.

13. Pfaffic acid and its derivatives. Japanese patent number (84 10,548). January 20,
1984, by Rohto Pharmaceutical Co., Ltd.

TAYUYA

1. Ruppelt, B. M., et al. "Pharmacological screening of plants recommended by folk
medicine as anti-snake venom--I. Analgesic and anti-inflammatory activities."
Mem. Inst. Oswaldo Cruz 86, Suppl. 2 (1991): 203–5.

2. Balbach, A. *As Plantas Curam*. Rio de Janeiro, Brazil: Bertram Publishers, 1982.

3. Bauer, R. and H. Wagner. *Dtsch. Apoth. Ztg*. 123 (1983): 1313.

4. Bauer, R., et al. "Cucurbitacins and flavone C-glycosides from *Cayaponia tayuya*."
Phytochemisty (1984): 1587–91.

5. Himeno, E., et al. "Structures of cayaponosides A, B, C and D, glucosides of new
nor-cucurbitacins in the roots of *Cayaponia tayuya*." *Chem. Pharm. Bull*. (Tokyo)
(October 1992).

6. Huguet, A. I., et al. "Superoxide scavenging properties of flavonoids in a non-
enzymic system." *Z. Natur. Forsch*. [C] (January–February 1990).

7. Konoshima, T., et al. "Inhibitory effects of cucurbitane triterpenoids on Epstein-
Barr virus activation and two-stage cacinogenesis of skin tumor." *Biol. Pharm.
Bull*. (February 1995).

VASSOURINHA

1. Laurens, A., et al. "Antimicrobial activity of some medicinal species of Dakar markets." *Pharmazie* 40, 7 (1985): 482–85.

2. Singh, J., et al. "Antifungal activity of *Mentha spicata*." *Int. J. Pharmacog.* 32, 4 (1994): 314–19.

3. Ramesh, P., et al. "Flavonoids of *Scoparia dulcis* and *Stemodia viscosa*." Curr. Sci. 48 (1979): 67.

4. Mahato, S., et al. "Triterpenoids of *Scoparia dulcis*." *Phytochemistry* 20 (1981): 171–73.

5. Hayashi, T., et al. "Scopadulcic acid-A and -B, new diterpenoids with a novel skeleton, from a Paraguayan crude drug 'typycha kuratu' (*Scoparia dulcis* L.)." *Tetrahedron Lett.* 28, 32 (1987): 3693–96.

6. Kawasaki, M. "Structure of scoparic acid A, a new labdane-type diterpenoid from a Paraguayan crude drug 'typycha kurata' (*Scoparia dulcis* L.)." *Chem. Pharm. Bull.* 35, 9 (1987): 3963–66.

7. Hayashi, T. "Structures of new diterpenoids from a Paraguayan crude drug 'typycha kuratu' (Scoparia dulcis L.)." *Tennen Yuki Kagobutsu Toronkai Koen Yoshishu* 29 (1987): 544–51.

8. Hayashi, T. "Antiviral agents of plant origin. III. Scopadulin, a novel tetracyclic diterpene from *Scoparia dulcis* L." *Chem. Pharm. Bull.* 38, 4 (1990): 945–47.

9. Ahmed, M. "Diterpenoids from *Scoparia dulcis*." *Phytochemistry* 29, 9 (1990): 3035–37.

10. Hayashi, T. "Scopadulciol, an inhibitor of gastric H+, K+-atpase from *Scoparia dulcis,* and its structure-activity relationships." *J. Nat. Prod.* 54 3 (1991): 802–9.

11. Hayashi, T. "Scoparic acid A, a beta-glucuronidase inhibitor from *Scoparia dulcis.*" *J. Nat. Prod.* 55, 12 (1992): 1748–55.

12. Hayashi, T. "A new vhemotype of *Scoparia dulcis*." *Phytochemistry* 32, 2 (1993): 349–52.

13. Jain, H. C. "Indian plants with oral hypoglycaemic activity." *Abstr. Internat. Res. Cong Nat Prod Coll Pharm, Chapel Hill, NC, University of North Carolina (July 7–12, 1985): Abstr-152.

14. Freire, S., et al. "Sympathomimetic effects of *Scoparia dulcis* L. and catecholamines isolated from plant extracts." *J. Pharm. Pharmacol.* 48, 6 (1996): 624–28.

15. Freire, S., et al. "Analgesic and antiinflammatory properties of *Scoparia dulcis* L. extracts and glutinol in rodents." *Phytother. Res.* 7, 6 (1993): 408–14.

16. Nishino, H, 1993. "Antitumor-promoting activity of scopadulcic acid B, isolated from the medicinal plant *Scoparia dulcis* L." *Oncology* 50, 2 (1993): 100–3.

17. Hayashi, T, 1990. "Antiviral agents of plant origin. III. Scopadulin, a novel tetracyclic diterpene from *Scoparia dulcis* L." *Chem. Pharm. Bull.* (Tokyo) 38, 4 (1990): 945–47.

18. Hayashi, K. "In vitro and in vivo antiviral activity of scopadulcic acid B from Scoparia dulcis, Scrophulariaceae, against herpes simplex virus type 1." *Antiviral Res.* 9, 6 (1988): 345–54.

19. Hasrat, J., et al. "Medicinal plants in Surianame: screening of plant extracts for receptor binding activity." *Phytomedicine* 4, 1 (1997): 59–65.

YERBA MATE

1. "Mate." *The Review of Natural Products* (February 1997). Facts and Comparisons Group.
2. Wichtl, Max. *Herbal Drugs and Phytopharmaceuticals.* Boca Raton, FL: CRC Press, 1994.
3. Alikaridis F. "Natural constituents of *Ilex* species." *J. Ethnopharmacol.* 20, 2 (1987): 121–44.
4. Fossati, C. "On the virtue and therapeutic properties of 'yerba-mate' (*Ilex paraguayensis* or *paraguariensis* St. Hilaire 1838)." *Clin. Ter.* 78, 3 (1976): 265–72.
5. Tenorio Sanz, M.D. "Mineral elements in mate herb (*Ilex paraguariensis* St. H.)." *Arch. Latinoam Nutr.* 41, 3 (1991): 441–54.
6. Swanston-Flatt, S. K. "Glycaemic effects of traditional European plant treatments for diabetes. Studies in normal and streptozotocin diabetic mice." *Diabetes Res.* 10, 2 (1989): 69–73.
7. Gugliucci, A. "Antioxidant effects of *Ilex paraguariensis:* induction of decreased oxidability of human LDL in vivo." *Biochem. Biophys. Res. Commun.* 224, 2 (1996): 338–44.
8. Gugliucci, A. "Low-density lipoprotein oxidation is inhibited by extracts of *Ilex paraguariensis.*" *Biochem. Mol. Biol. Int.* 35, 1 (1995): 47–56.
9. Kraemer, K. H. "Matesaponin 5, a highly polar saponin from *Ilex paraguariensis.*" *Phytochemistry* 42, 4 (1996): 1119–22.
10. Schenkel, E.P. "Triterpene saponins from mate, *Ilex paraguariensis.*" *Adv. Exp. Med. Biol.* 405 (1996): 47–56.
11. Gosmann, G. "Triterpenoid saponins from *Ilex paraguariensis.*" *J. Nat. Prod.* 58, 3 (1995): 438.

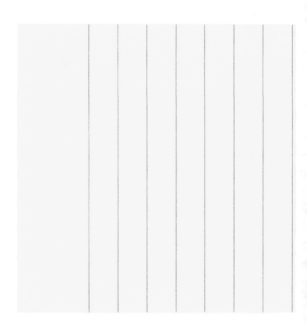

References

BOTANY/ETHNOBOTANY/TRIBAL USES

Acero, D. *Prinipales Plantas Utiles de la Amazonia Columbiana.* Bogata: Proyecto Radargrametrico del Amazonas, 1979.

Arvigo, Rosita and Michael Balick. *Rainforest Remedies, One Hundred Healing Herbs of Belize.* Twin Lakes, WI: Lotus Press, 1993.

Asprey, G. F. and P. Thornton, P. "Medicinal plants of Jamaica. III." *West Indian Med. J.* 4 (1955): 69–92.

Ayensu, E. S. *Medicinal Plants of the West Indies.* Unpublished manuscript: 110 pages. Washington, D.C.: Office of Biological Conservation, Smithsonian Institution, 1978.

Balee, William. *Footprints of the Forest Ka'apor Ethnobotany—The Historical Ecology of Plant Utilization by an Amazonian People.* New York: Columbia University Press, 1994.

Beckstrom-Sternberg, Stephen M., James A. Duke, and K. K. Wain. "The Ethnobotany Database." (ACEDB version 4.3-data version July 1994). National Germplasm Resources Laboratory (NGRL), Agricultural Research Service (ARS), U.S. Department of Agriculture.

Berry, Paul E., Bruce Holst, and Kay Yatskievych. *Flora of the Venezuelan Guayana.* Missouri Botanical Garden, 1995.

Branch, L. C. and I. M. F. da Silva, 1983. "Folk medicine of Alter do Chao, Para, Brazil." *Acta Amazonica* 13 (5/6): 737–97.

Coee, F., et al. "Ethnobotany of the Garifuna of eastern Nicaragua." *Econ. Bot.* 50, 1 (1996): 71–107.

Correa, Pio. *Dicionario de Plantas Uteis do Brasil e Exoticas Cultivadas,* vols. 1–6, Brasilia: IBDF, 1984.

de Feo, V. "Medicinal and magical plants in the northern Peruvian Andes." *Fitoterapia* 63 (1992): 417–40.

Dennis, P. "Herbal medicine among the Miskito of eastern Nicaragua." *Econ. Bot.* 42, 1 (1988): 16–28.

Duke, James and Rudolfo Vasquez. *Amazonian Ethnobotanical Dictionary.* Boca Raton, FL: CRC Press Inc., 1994.

Duke, J. A. *Handbook of Northeastern Indian Medicinal Plants.* Boston, MA: Quarterman Publications, 1986.

Duke, J. A. *Isthmian Ethnobotanical Dictionary,* 2d ed., 1978.

Forero, P. L. "Ethnobotany of the Cuna and Waunana indigenous communities." *Cespedesia* 9, 33 (1980): 115–02.

Garcia-Barriga, H. *Flora Medicinal de Columbia, Botanica-Medica.* Ins. Cein. Nat. Bogota. 3 vols. (1974–5).

Gentry, Alwyn H. *A Field Guide to the Families and Genera of Woody Plants of Northwest South America.* Chicago, IL: University of Chicago Press, 1993.

Gentry, Alwyn H. *Woody Plants of Northwest South America (Colombia, Ecuador, Peru).*Chicago, IL: The University of Chicago Press, 1993.

Girago, IL: The University of Chicago Press, 1993.

cuador, Peru).est South America. azil." ch Servic *J. Ethnopharmacol.* (September 1991).

Grenand, P., Moretti, C., Jacquemin, H. *Pharmacopées Traditionelles en Guyane: Créoles, Palikur, Waypi.* Editorial l-ORSTROM, Coll. Mem No. 108. Paris, France, 1987.

Hirschmann, G., et al. "A survey of medicinal plants of Minas Gerais." *Brazil. J. Ethnopharmacol.* 29, 2 (1990): 159–72.

Joyce, Christopher. *Earthly Goods: Medicine-Hunting in the Rainforest.* New York: Little, Brown, & Company, 1994.

Lewis, Walter H., and Memory Lewis. *Medical Botany.* New York: John Wiley & Sons, Inc., 1977.

Maxwell, Nicole. *Witch Doctor's Apprentice: Hunting for Medicinal Plants in the Amazon,* 3d ed. New York: Citadel Press, 1990.

Morton, J. F. *Major Medicinal Plants: Botany, Culture and Uses.* Springfield, IL: Charles C. Thomas Publishing, 1977.

Plotkin, Mark, J. *Tales of a Shaman's Apprentice.* Middlesex, England: Penguin Books, 1993.

Ramirez, V., et al. *Vegetales Empleados en Medicina Tradicional Norperuana.* Trujillo, Peru: Banco Agrario Del Peru and Nacional Universidad Trujillo, June, 1988.

Rutter, R. A. *Catalogo de Plantas Utiles de la Amazonia Peruana.* Yarinacocha, Peru: Instituto Linguistico de Verano, 1990.

Schultes, R. E. "Gifts of the Amazon flora to the world." *Arnoldia* 50, 2 (1990): 21–34.

Schultes, R. E. and Raffauf. *The Healing Forest: Medicinal and Toxic Plants of the Northwest Amazonia.* Portland: R. F. Dioscorides Press, 1990.

Soukup, J. *Vocabulary of the Common Names of the Peruvian Flora and Catalog of the Genera.* Lima: Editorial Salesiano, 1970.

Van den Berg, E. *Plantas Medicinais na Amazonia.* Belem: Museu Goeldi, 1983.

Vasquez, M. R. *Useful Plants of Amazonian Peru.* Second Draft. Filed with USDA's National Agricultural Library, 1990.

USES IN HERBAL MEDICINE IN EUROPE AND THE UNITED STATES

Balch, James F. and Phyllis A. Balch. *Prescription for Nutritional Healing.* Garden City Park, NY: Avery Publishing Group, 1990.

Bartram, Thomas. *Encyclopedia of Herbal Medicine.* Dorset, England: Ed Grace Publishers, 1995.

Beckstrom-Sternberg, Stephen M., and James A. Duke. "The Phytochemical Database." (ACEDB version 4.3—data version July 1994). National Germplasm Resources Laboratory (NGRL), Agricultural Research Service (ARS), U.S. Department of Agriculture.

Bruneton, J. *Pharmacognosy, Phytochemistry, Medicinal Plants*. Hampshire, England: Intercept, Ltd., 1995.

Duke, J. A. *CRC Handbook of Medicinal Herbs*. Boca Raton, FL: CRC Press, 1985.

Duke, J. A. and K K. Wain. *Medicinal Plants of the World*. Computer index with more than 85,000 entries. 3 vols., 1981, p. 1654.

Easterling, J. *Traditional Uses of Rainforest Botanicals*. 1993.

Flynn, Rebecca and Mark Roest. *Your Guide to Standardized Herbal Products*. Prescott, AZ: One World Press, 1995.

Grieve, Mrs. M. M. *A Modern Herbal*. New York: Dover Publications, 1971.

Heinerman, John. *Heinerman's Encyclopedia of Healing Herbs & Spices*. New York: Parker Publishing Co., 1996.

Hobbs, Christopher. "Herbal Prescriber." 1995. (Software).

Hoffman, David. *The Herbal Handbook*. Rochester, VT: Healing Arts Press, 1987.

Hoffman, David. *The New Holistic Herbal*. Rockport, MA: Element Books, Inc., 1991.

Lawrence Review of Natural Products. St. Louis, MO: Facts and Comparisons Inc.

List, P. H. and L. Horhammer. *Hager's Handbuch der Pharmazeutischen Praxis*, vols. 2–6. Berlin: Springer-Verlag, 1969–79.

Lucas, Richard, M. *Miracle Medicine Herbs*. West Nyak, NY: Parker Publishing, 1991.

Lung. A. and S. Foster. *Encyclopedia of Common Natural Ingredients*. New York: John Wiley & Sons, 1996.

Mindell, Earl. *Earl Mindell's Herb Bible*. New York: Simon & Shuster, 1992.

Mowrey, Daniel B., Ph.D. *Herbal Tonic Therapies*. New Canaan, CT: Keats Publishing, Inc., 1993.

Mowrey, Daniel., *The Scientific Validation of Herbal Medicine*. New Canaan, CT: Keats Publishing, Inc., 1986.

Murray, Michael T., N.D. *The Healing Power of Herbs*. Rocklin, CA: Prima Publishing, 1995.

Samuelsson, Gunnar. *Drugs of Natural Origin*. Stockholm: Swedish Pharmaceutical Press, 1992.

Schauenberb, Paul, and Ferdinand Paris. *Guide to Medicinal Plants*. Cambridge, England: Keats Publishing, 1977.

Schwontkowski, Donna. "Herbal treasures from the Amazon," parts 1, 2, and 3. *Healthy & Natural Journal* (1996).

Schwontkowski, Donna. *Herbs of the Amazon: Traditional and Common Uses*. Utah: Science Student Braintrust Publishing, 1993.

Werbach, Melvyn R., M.D., and Murray, Michael T., N.D. *Botanical Influences on Illness—A Sourcebook of Clinical Research*. Tarzana, CA: Third Line Press, 1994.

Wichtl, M. *Herbal Drugs and Phytopharmaceuticals*. Boca Roton, FL: CRC Press, 1994.

World Perservation Society. *Powerful and Unusual Herbs from the Amazon and China*. Gainesville, FL: The World Preservation Society, Inc., 1993.

USES IN HERBAL MEDICINE IN SOUTH AMERICA AND CENTRAL AMERICA

de Almeida, E. R. *Plantas Medicinais Brasileiras, Conhecimentos Populares E Cientificos*. São Paulo: Hemus Editora Ltda., 1993.

Arvigo, Rosita and Michael Balick. *Rainforest Remedies: One Hundred Healing Herbs of Belize*. Twin Lakes, WI: Lotus Press, 1993.

Bernardes, Antonio. *A Pocketbook of Brazilian Herbs*. Rio de Janeiro: A Shogun Editora e Arta Ltda, 1984.

Branch, L. C. and I. M. F. da Silva. "Folk medicine of Alter do Chao, Para, Brazil." *Acta Amazonica* 13, 5/6 (1983): 737–97. Manaus.

Coimbra, Raul. *Manual de Fitoterapia*, 2d ed. Sao Paulo, Brasil: Dados Internacionais de Catalogacao na Pulicacao, 1994.

Correa, Pio. *Dicionario das Plantas Uteis do Brasil e das Exoticas Cultivadas*, vol. 2. Rio de Janeiro: Ministerio da Agricultura, 1931.

Correa, Pio. *Dicionario de Plantas Uteis do Brasil e Exoticas Cultivadas,* vols. 1–6. Brasilia: IBDF, 1984.

Cruz, G. L. *Dicionario das Plantas Uteis do Brasil,* 5th ed. Rio de Janeiro: Bertrand, 1995.

Cruz, G. L. *Livro Verde das Plantas Medicinais e Industriais do Brasil*, vol. 2, 1st ed. Brazil: Belo Horizonte, 1965.

Girón, L M., et al. "Ethnobotanical survey of the medicinal flora used by the Caribs of Guatemala." *J. Ethnopharmacol.* (September 1991).

Kember, Mejia and Elsa Reng. *Plantas Medicinales de Uso Popular en la Amazonia Peruana.* Lima: AECI and IIAP, 1995.

Matos, F. J. Abreu. *Farmacias Vivas: Sistema de Utilizaco de Plantas Medicinais Projetado Para Pequenas Comunidades.* Fortaleza, Brazil: Edicoes UFC, 1994.

Mors, W. B. and C.T. Rissine. *Useful Plants of Brazil.* San Francisco: Holden-Day, Inc., 1966.

de Rios, Marlene Dubkin. *Amazon Healer: The Life and Times of an Urban Shaman.* Garden City Park, NY: Avery Publishing Group, 1992.

Robineau, L., ed. *Towards a Caribbean Pharmacopoeia.* Enda Caribe, Santo Domingo: TRAMIL-4 Workshop, UNAH, 1991.

Roig, J. T. *Plantas Medicinales, Aromaticas o Venenosas de Cuba.* La Habana: Cientifico-Tecnica, 1988, 1125.

Rutter, R. A. *Catalogo de Plantas Utiles de la Amazonia Peruana.* Yarinacocha, Peru: Instituto Linguistico de Verano, 1990.

Silva, M. *Catalogo de Extractos Fluidos.* Rio de Janeiro: Araija e Cia, Ltd., 1930.

Smith, Nigel, J. Williams, Donald Plucknett, and Jennifer Talbot. *Tropical Forests and Their Crops.* New York: Comstock Publishing, 1992.

de Sousa, M. P, M. E. And F. J. Matos, et al. *Constituintes Quimicos Ativos de Planta Med.icinais Brasileiras.* Fortaleza, Brasil: Laboratorio de Produtos Naturais, 1991.

Taylor, Leslie. Personal field notes from interviews of *curanderos,* shamans, and herbalists in Peru, Brazil, and Ecuador, 1994 to 1998.

Valdizan, H. and A. Maldonado. *La Medicina Popular Peruana.* Lima: Imp. Torres Aquirre, 1982.

Index

D

M

Maca, 143-146
  ethnic uses of, 253
  nutritional value of, 145
  properties of, 243
McCaleb, Rob, 212
Macela, 147-150
  ethnic uses of, 253
  properties of, 243
Maceration, 237
Madagascar periwinkle, 17-18
Magnesium, 216
Malaria, xxxiv
  carqueja for, 77
  deforestation and, 4
  fedegoso for, 111
  mullaca for, 167, 168
  mutamba for, 175
  pau d'arco for, 183
  simaruba for, 206-207, 208
  vassourinha for, 222
Malaysia, 10
Manacá, 151-153
  ethnic uses of, 253
  properties of, 243
Manaceine, 152
Manacine, 152
Maracua grande, 159
Maracuja (passionflower), 154-157
  ethnic uses of, 253
  properties of, 243
Maracuja (passion fruit), 158-160
  ethnic uses of, 253
  properties of, 243
Marajo Island, 8
Marcela, 147
Maytansine, 107-108
Mayteine, 107-108
Maytenus krukovit, 94
Maytenus species, 107
Medical Botany (Lewis & Lewis)
Medicinal properties, xviii
Melanoma. *See* Skin cancer

Memory disorders
  catuaba and, 87
  guarana and, 126
Mendelsohn, Robert, 22-23
Menopause, xxxiv
  maca and, 145
  suma for, 215
Menorrhagia. *See also* Dysmenorrhea/ dysmenorrhagia
Menstrual disorders, xxxiv. *See also* Dysmenorrhea/dysmenor- rhagia; Premenstrual syndrome (PMS)
  abuta for, 33
  Brazilian peppertree for, 61
  chuchuhuasi for, 95
  fedegoso for, 111
  guava and, 128
  maca and, 145
  maracuja (passionflower) for, 155
  muira puama for, 163
  rainforest menstrual pain relief remedy, 236
  suma for, 215
  vassourinha for, 221, 222
Merck Pharmaceutical Company, 19
Methionine, 67-68
Midwives' herb, 31
Migraines, xxxv
  guarana for, 123
  vassourinha for, 222
Milton, John P., 160
Minerals
  in suma, 216
  in yerba mate, 228
Mitraphylline, 83
Mmroxylon balsamum. See Balsam of Tolu
A Modern Herbal (Grieve), 134
Molluscicides
  jatoba, 138
  macela, 148
  mutamba, 175

Monardes, 154
Mononucleosis, xxxv
  suma for, 215
Monoterpenes, 148
Monsanto, 19
Monteiro da Silva, J., 218-219
Moonshine Trading Co., 261
Morphinism, 155
Mouth sores, xiv
  picao preto for, 191
  sangre de grado for, 199
Mouthwash, 71
Mowrey, Daniel B., 159, 227
Muira puama, 161-164
  ethnic uses of, 253
  properties of, 243
Muirapuamine, 162, 163
Mulateiro, 165-166
  ethnic uses of, 253
  properties of, 243
Mullaca, 167-170
  ethnic uses of, 254
  properties of, 244
Mulungu, 171-173
  ethnic uses of, 254
  properties of, 244
Muscle pain, xxli, xxxv
  amor seco for, 42
  andiroba, 47
  iporuru for, 130
  muira puama for, 161
Mutamba, 174-176
  ethnic uses of, 254
  properties of, 244
Mycosis, 191
Myrcia species, 188

N

National Cancer Institute, 18, 19
  graviola, use of, 121
Nations, James D., 187
Nausea, xxxv

Vertigo, xxxix
Veterinary practice, 84
Vianna, Gilney, 4
Vinho de jatoba, 137
Virend, 199
Visions of the Rainforest
    (Heinzman), 63, 120
Vitamin C
    in acerola, 35-36
    in cajueiro, 71
    in camu-camu, 74
    in guava, 128
Vomiting, 98
Von Martius, Theodore, 124
Vulneraries, xxxix
Brazilian peppertree, 61

W

Walnut Access, 263
Ward's Pond Farm, 263
Warts, xxxix
    cajueiro for, 70
Water pollution, 4
Waynberg, J., 163
Weber, A., 134

Weight loss
    picao preto for, 191
    yerba mate for, 227
Whitaker, Julian, 83-84
Whitworth, Eugene, 81
Whooping cough, 194
Wild-harvesting medicinal
    plants, 26
Wilson, Edward O.,
    7, 17
Wood chipboard industry, 10
Worker's Party, Mato
    Grosso, 4
World Bank, 15
World Health Organization
    (WHO), 82
World Wide Fund for Nature, 4
Worldwide Uses table, xix-xx
Wounds, xxxix
    amor seco for, 41
    andiroba, 47
    balsam of Tolu for, 54
    Brazilian peppertree
        for, 61
    cat's claw for, 81
    fedegoso for, 111

mulateiro and, 165
mutamba for, 175
sangre de grado
    for, 199
sarsaparilla for, 203
simaruba for, 207
tayuya for, 219
vassourinha
    for, 221

Y

Yeast infections. *See also*
    Candidiasis
    pau d'arco for, 183
    rainforest fungal/yeast
        remedy, 234
Yellow fever, xxxix
    manacá for, 152
Yerba mate, 226-229
    ethnic uses of, 256-257
    properties of, 245

Z

Zinc, 216